Rapid Review
Neuroscience

Rapid Review Series

Series Editor
Edward F. Goljan, MD

Behavioral Science, Second Edition
Vivian M. Stevens, PhD; Susan K. Redwood, PhD; Jackie L. Neel, DO;
Richard H. Bost, PhD; Nancy W. Van Winkle, PhD; Michael H. Pollak, PhD

Biochemistry, Second Edition
John W. Pelley, PhD; Edward F. Goljan, MD

Gross and Developmental Anatomy, Second Edition
N. Anthony Moore, PhD; William A. Roy, PhD, PT

Histology and Cell Biology, Second Edition
E. Robert Burns, PhD; M. Donald Cave, PhD

Microbiology and Immunology, Second Edition
Ken S. Rosenthal, PhD; James S. Tan, MD

Neuroscience
James A. Weyhenmeyer, PhD; Eve A. Gallman, PhD

Pathology, Second Edition
Edward F. Goljan, MD

Pharmacology, Second Edition
Thomas L. Pazdernik, PhD; Laszlo Kerecsen, MD

Physiology
Thomas A. Brown, MD

USMLE Step 2
Michael W. Lawlor, MD, PhD

USMLE Step 3
David Rolston, MD; Craig Nielsen, MD

Rapid Review
Neuroscience

James A. Weyhenmeyer, PhD

Professor, Cell and Developmental Biology, Neuroscience, and Pathology
College of Medicine and School of Molecular and Cell Biology
Associate Vice President
University of Illinois
Urbana, Illinois

Eve A. Gallman, PhD

Adjunct Assistant Professor, Cell and Developmental Biology and Neuroscience
College of Medicine and School of Molecular and Cell Biology
University of Illinois
Urbana, Illinois

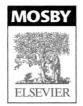

1600 John F. Kennedy Blvd.
Suite 1800
Philadelphia, PA 19103-2899

RAPID REVIEW NEUROSCIENCE
Copyright © 2007 by Mosby, Inc., an affiliate of Elsevier Inc.

ISBN-10: 0-323-02261-8
ISBN-13: 978-0-323-02261-3

NOTICE

Knowledge and best practice in this field are constantly changing. As new research and experience broaden our knowledge, changes in practice, treatment and drug therapy may become necessary or appropriate. Readers are advised to check the most current information provided (i) on procedures featured or (ii) by the manufacturer of each product to be administered, to verify the recommended dose or formula, the method and duration of administration, and contraindications. It is the responsibility of the practitioner, relying on their own experience and knowledge of the patient, to make diagnoses, to determine dosages and the best treatment for each individual patient, and to take all appropriate safety precautions. To the fullest extent of the law, neither the Publisher nor the Authors assume any liability for any injury and/or damage to persons or property arising out or related to any use of the material contained in this book.

Library of Congress Cataloging-in-Publication Data

Weyhenmeyer, James A.
   Neuroscience / James A. Weyhenmeyer, Eve A. Gallman.—1st ed.
      p. ; cm.—(Rapid review series)
   ISBN 0-323-02261-8
      1. Neurosciences—Outlines, syllabi, etc. 2. Neurosciences—Examinations, questions, etc.
   I. Gallman, Eve A. II. Title. III. Series.
      [DNLM: 1. Nervous System—Examination Questions. WL 18.2 W547n 2007]
   RC343.6.W49 2007
   612.80076—dc22

                                            2006041965

Publishing Director: Linda Belfus
Acquisitions Editor: James Merritt
Developmental Editor: Katie DeFrancesco
Design Direction: Steven Stave

Printed in the United States of America.

Last digit is the print number: 9 8 7 6 5 4 3 2 1

To my wife, Jan, and my children, James and Jonathan, for their continued support and patience

JAW

To my husband, Kurt, who keeps life interesting

EAG

To our students. After all, they are the point of this endeavor.

Figure Credits

Brodmann K: Vergleichende Lokalisation lehre der Grosshirnrinde in ihren Prinzipien dargestelt auf Grund des Zellenbaues. Leipzig, Germany: JA Barth, 1909.
Figure 16-1

Burns ER, Cave MD: Rapid Review Histology and Cell Biology, 1st ed. Philadelphia: Mosby, 2002.
Figures 4-1 and 4-3

Fitzgerald MJT, Folan-Curran J: Clinical Neuroanatomy and Related Neuroscience, 4th ed. Philadelphia: Saunders, 2001.
Figures 7-4 and 7-8

Gilman AG, Goodman LS, Rall TW, Murad F: Goodman and Gilman's The Pharmacological Basis of Therapeutics, 7th ed. New York: Macmillan, 1985.
Figure accompanying Table 6-1

Gilroy J: Basic Neurology, 3rd ed. New York: McGraw-Hill, 2000.
Figure 16-4

Goetz C: Textbook of Clinical Neurology, 2nd ed. Philadelphia: Saunders, 2003.
Figures accompanying Test 2, Questions 3 and 41

Haines DE: Fundamental Neuroscience, 2nd ed. New York: Churchill Livingstone, 2002.
Figures 1-4 to 1-7A, 2-3, 2-4, 3-4, 3-7, 7-1, and 12-3

Hardman JG, Limbird LE: Goodman and Gilman's The Pharmacologic Basis of Therapeutics, 10th ed. New York: McGraw-Hill, 2001.
Figures 6-1 and 6-2

Jarvis C: Physical Examination and Health Assessment, 4th ed. Philadelphia: Saunders, 2003.
Figure 7-9

Kandel ER, Schwartz JH, Jessel TM: Principles of Neural Science, 4th ed. New York: McGraw-Hill, 2000.
Figures 5-2, 8-4, and 8-5

Nadeau SE, Ferguson TS, Valenstein E, et al: Medical Neuroscience. Philadelphia: Saunders, 2004.
Figure 15-3 and figures accompanying Test 2, Questions 28–31

Nolte J: The Human Brain, 5th ed. Philadelphia: Mosby, 2002.
Figures 1-3, 1-7 to 1-10, 2-5, 3-2, 5-4, 5-6 to 5-8, 10-1, and the figure accompanying Test 1, Question 30.
Tables 11-3 to 11-9, 12-1, 13-5, and 13-6

Nolte J, Angevine JB: The Human Brain in Photographs and Diagrams, 2nd ed. Philadelphia: Mosby, 2000.
Figures 3-6, 7-6, 7-7, and the figures accompanying Test 1, Questions 3–5, 9, 38, 49, and Test 2, Questions 12 and 18
Tables 3-1 to 3-6, and 3-8

Orrison WW, Jr: Neuroimaging, vol 2. Philadelphia: Saunders, 2000.
Figure accompanying Test 2, Question 40

Penfield W, Rasmussen T: The Cerebral Cortex of Man. New York: Macmillan, 1950.
Figures 1-13 and 8-2

Waxman SG: Clinical Neuroanatomy, 25th ed. New York: McGraw-Hill, 2002.
Figure 10-3

Woolsey TA, Hanaway J, Gado MJ: The Brain Atlas, 2nd ed. New York: Wiley, 2003.
Figure 16-2

Series Preface

The *Rapid Review Series* has received high critical acclaim from students studying for the United States Medical Licensing Examination (USMLE) Step 1 and high ratings in *First Aid for the USMLE Step 1*. We have created a learning system, including a print and electronic package, that is easier to use and more concise than other review products on the market.

SPECIAL FEATURES

Book

- **Outline format:** Concise, high-yield subject matter is presented in a study-friendly format. In addition, key words and phrases appear in bold throughout.
- **High-yield margin notes:** Key content that is most likely to appear on the exam is reinforced in the margin notes.
- **High-quality visual elements:** Abundant two-color schematics, black and white images, and summary tables enhance your study experience.
- **Two-color design:** The two-color design helps highlight important elements, making studying more efficient and pleasing.
- **Two practice examinations:** Two sets of 50 USMLE Step 1–type clinically oriented, multiple-choice questions (including images where necessary) and complete discussions (rationales) for all options are included.

New! Online Study and Testing Tool

- **350 USMLE Step 1–type MCQs:** Clinically oriented, multiple-choice questions that mimic the current board format are presented. These include images where necessary, and complete rationales for all answer options. All the questions from the book are included so you can study them in the most effective mode for you!

- **Test mode:** Select from randomized 50-question sets or by subject topics for an exam-like review session. This mode features a 60-minute timer to simulate the actual exam, a detailed assessment report that can be printed or saved to your hard drive, and direct links to all or only incorrect questions. The links include your answer, the correct answer, and full rationales for all answer options, so you can fully analyze your test session and learn from your mistakes.
- **Study mode:** Like the test mode, in the study mode you can select from randomized 50-question sets or by subject topics to create a dynamic study session. This mode features unlimited attempts at each question, instant feedback (either on selection of the correct answer or when using the "Show Answer" feature), complete rationales for all answer options, and a detailed progress report that can be printed or saved to your hard drive.
- **Online access:** Online access allows you to study from an internet-enabled computer wherever and whenever it is convenient. This access is activated through registration on www.studentconsult.com with the pincode printed inside the front cover.

Student Consult

- **Full online access:** You can access the complete text and illustrations of this book on www.studentconsult.com.
- **Save content to your PDA:** Through our unique Pocket Consult platform, you can clip selected text and illustrations and save them to your PDA for study on the fly!
- **Free content:** An interactive community center with a wealth of additional valuable resources is available.

Acknowledgments

The authors would like to thank Jason Malley for his enthusiasm and encouragement as we began this process, and for introducing us to Susan Kelly. We thank Susan for her tireless and always good-humored efforts to organize and drive us forward. It is a tribute to her dedication to this project that she continued to hound us even after she had moved on to other projects and passed us on to the very capable hands of James Merritt and Katie DeFrancesco. We are pleased to acknowledge Therese Grundl, who helped us see our words through the readers' eyes, Matt Chansky, for transforming our illegible scribbles into the illustrations that grace this text, and our administrative assistant, Heidi Rockwood, who has been invaluable to keeping this project on target. Finally, we thank our students and friends who began so many conversations with, "So, is that book done yet?" and then offered the advice, support, and encouragement that allow us to answer, "Yes, it is!"

James A. Weyhenmeyer, PhD
Eve A. Gallman, PhD

Contents

CHAPTER 1

Development and Anatomy of the Nervous System

I. **Development of Central Nervous System**
  A. **Neural tube**
    1. **Formation** (Fig. 1-1 and Table 1-1)
      a. Neural plate arises from ectodermal tissue and invaginates to form neural groove.
      b. Three primary vesicles (prosencephalon, mesencephalon, and rhombencephalon) form by week 3.
        • Flexures appear; mesencephalic flexure will be retained into adult brain, causing the relationship between the neuraxis and the body to change within the head (Fig. 1-2).
      c. Five secondary vesicles (telencephalon, diencephalon, mesencephalon, metencephalon, and myelencephalon) are apparent by week 6.
    2. **Neurulation** (fusion of neural tube) occurs between days 20 and 28, beginning at the cervical region and progressing both rostrally and caudally.
      a. **Alar plate** (posterior) gives rise to cranial nerve sensory nuclei and spinal cord posterior horn (Fig. 1-3).
      b. **Basal plate** (anterior) gives rise to cranial nerve motor nuclei and spinal cord anterior horn.
      c. **Neural crest** cells remain external to tube and give rise to neurons and glia of peripheral nervous system.
    3. **Cranial closure** is complete by days 24 to 26.
    4. **Caudal closure** is complete by days 26 to 28.
      a. Any disruption of neurulation can prevent cranial closure of the neural tube, which causes **anencephaly,** or can prevent closure of the spinal region of the tube, which causes varying degrees of **spina bifida.**
      b. **Holoprosencephaly** occurs after neural tube closure and is generally fatal.
  B. **Neural tube defects** (Table 1-2)
    1. Give rise to up to 1% of all congenital malformations
    2. Risk factors include maternal **diabetes,** maternal **folic acid insufficiency,** and hypothermia.
    3. Frequently cause **hydrocephalus** because cerebrospinal fluid (CSF) flow is obstructed (see Chapter 2)

A developmental defect that prevents cranial closure causes **anencephaly.**

A developmental defect that prevents spinal closure causes varying degrees of **spina bifida.**

Folic acid supplementation before and during pregnancy reduces risk for neural tube defects.

Hydrocephalus frequently accompanies neural tube defects.

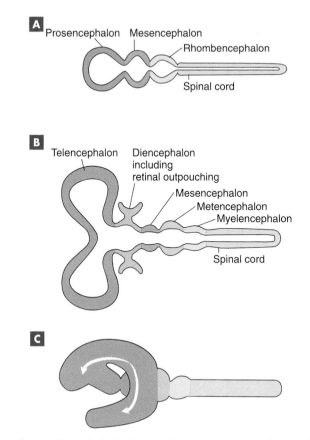

1-1: A, *Three-vesicle stage of neural tube development, dorsal view.* **B,** *Five-vesicle stage, dorsal view.* **C,** *Five-vesicle stage, sagittal view. Telencephalon will expand (arrows) to give rise to hemispheres.*

TABLE 1-1:
Developmental
Origins of Adult
Brain

Primary Vesicles	Secondary Vesicles	Divisions of Adult Brain
Prosencephalon	Telencephalon	Cerebral cortex (two hemispheres), portions of basal ganglia
	Diencephalon	Thalamus, hypothalamus, subthalamus, and epithalamus
Mesencephalon	Mesencephalon	Mesencephalon (midbrain)
Rhombencephalon	Metencephalon	Pons and cerebellum
	Myelencephalon	Medulla oblongata

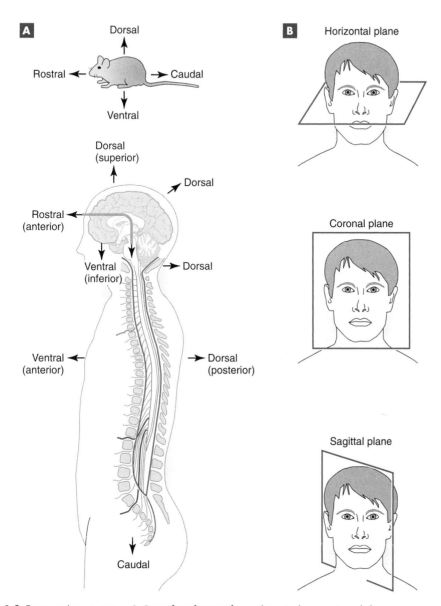

1-2: Terms used in orientation. **A, Dorsal and ventral** are relative to the neuraxis and change relationship to the body at the head; **anterior and posterior** are relative to the body and change relationship to the neuraxis in the head; **rostral and caudal** are relative to the neuraxis; **superior and inferior** are relative to the body. **B,** Planes of section are referenced to the body.

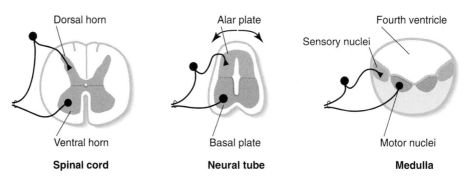

1-3: *Formation of motor and sensory regions. Green, basal plate leads to motor nuclei. Gray, alar plate leads to sensory nuclei.*

TABLE 1-2:
Developmental Origin of Neural Defects

Developmental Stage	Potential Defect
First trimester Week 3: neural groove, primary vesicle Week 4: neural tube closure Day 22: cervical tube closure Days 24–26: anterior tube closure Days 26–28: posterior tube closure Week 5: five-vesicle stage, optic vesicle apparent	Neural tube defects that are incompatible with life Anencephaly: failure of anterior tube to close Spina bifida: extent depends on timing Arnold-Chiari malformation and encephalocele are related to skull formation. Holoprosencephaly: range of rare and usually fatal defects resulting from failure of full development and separation of telencephalic structures; can occur as a result of failure of ventral induction within first 2 months of development
Weeks 6–7: basal ganglia expand; hemispheres expand, insular cortex apparent Weeks 8–16: major neuronal proliferation and migration; cerebral cortex, major sulci, lobes, corpus callosum	 Lissencephaly: abnormal or absent gyri
Second trimester	Porencephaly: major circulatory defect, frequently near longitudinal fissure and/or central sulcus
Third trimester	Multicystic encephalopathy: rare, fatal occurrence of multiple cysts within both white and gray matter

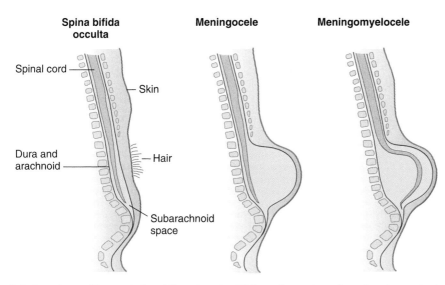

1-4: *Sagittal view of lower spinal cord illustrating spina bifida occulta, meningocele, and meningomyelocele.*

- Shunts are used to treat hydrocephalus in children who have neural tube defects.
4. Cause **elevated maternal serum alpha-fetoprotein** (AFP) during weeks 16 to 18:
   a. Elevated amniotic fluid AFP with accompanying elevated acetylcholinesterase confirms elevated serum AFP finding.
   b. Decreased AFP indicates chromosomal abnormalities, including Down syndrome.
5. Fetal ultrasonography assists in accurate determination of gestational age and can detect many neural tube defects as early as week 14.
6. **Specific anomalies**
   a. **Spina bifida occulta:** incomplete closure of vertebrae (Fig. 1-4; see Chapter 2)
      (1) Skin dimples over the affected vertebrae, and/or a tuft of hair grows.
      (2) Latex allergy is common with spina bifida owing to excessive neonatal exposure to latex rubber.
   b. **Meningocele:** protruding CSF-filled sac covered by pia and arachnoid; no direct neural involvement
   c. **Meningomyelocele:** neural tissue protrudes into CSF-filled sac covered by pia and arachnoid.

II. **Anatomy of Spinal Cord**
   A. **External anatomy** (Fig. 1-5A)
      1. Extends caudally from medulla, exits cranial cavity through foramen magnum, and tapers into conus medullaris.

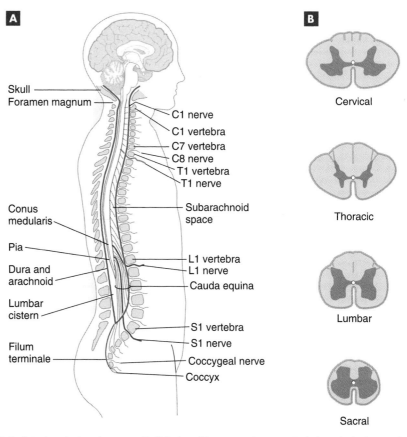

<table>
<tr><td>**A**</td></tr>
</table>

Skull
Foramen magnum
C1 nerve
C1 vertebra
C7 vertebra
C8 nerve
T1 vertebra
T1 nerve
Subarachnoid space
Conus medularis
Pia
L1 vertebra
L1 nerve
Dura and arachnoid
Cauda equina
Lumbar cistern
S1 vertebra
S1 nerve
Filum terminale
Coccygeal nerve
Coccyx

B

Cervical

Thoracic

Lumbar

Sacral

1-5: A, Spinal cord external anatomy. **B,** Spinal cord in cross-section at cervical, thoracic, lumbar, and sacral levels. Dark green, gray matter; light green, white matter.

Newborn spinal cord extends farther within vertebral column than adult spinal cord.

2. **Filum terminale,** formed as an extension of the meningeal coverings, extends from the tip of the conus medullaris to anchor the spinal cord to the vertebral column at the dorsal surface of the coccyx.
3. Thirty-one pairs of spinal nerves: 8 cervical, 12 thoracic, 5 lumbar, 5 sacral, and 1 coccygeal
   • Each spinal root is deflected caudally to exit the vertebral column below the corresponding numbered vertebra.
4. Enlarged at levels that innervate extremities
   a. **Cervical enlargement** (C5–T1) innervates arm.
   b. **Lumbosacral (lumbar) enlargement** (L2–S3) innervates leg.
5. Covered by three meningeal layers separated by two spaces
   a. **Spinal dura mater** extends from meningeal dura surrounding brain.
      (1) Continuous with the epineurium that surrounds the spinal nerves.
      (2) **Epidural space** lies above spinal dura and beneath inner vertebral surface.

(a) Unlike the cranial epidural space, a potential space that opens when blood forces the periosteal dura away from the skull, the spinal epidural space is a true space that exists normally.

(b) The lumbar epidural space is discontinuous because the spinal dura contacts the periosteum of the laminae.

> **Epidural anesthesia** is delivered by a needle that passes through the ligamentum flavum between two adjacent vertebrae but does not penetrate the underlying dura.

b. **Arachnoid** membrane adheres to spinal dura.
   (1) **Subarachnoid space** containing CSF lies between arachnoid and pia mater.
   (2) **Lumbar puncture** penetrates arachnoid to enter the subarachnoid space.
c. **Pia mater** adheres to spinal cord surface.
   (1) The pia and arachnoid are continuous with the perineurium that surrounds individual nerve fascicles in a spinal nerve.
   (2) Denticulate ligaments connect arachnoid and pia, suspending the spinal cord, much as arachnoid trabeculae suspend the brain.

6. Spinal cord ends at lumbar vertebra while dural sheath extends to S2 vertebra, leaving an enlargement of the subarachnoid space, the **lumbar cistern,** that is the source of CSF in lumbar puncture (see Fig. 1-5A).

> At birth, the cord extends to the L3 vertebra, and puncture must be done no higher than L4-L5 intervertebral space. In the adult, the cord extends to the L1 vertebra, and puncture may be done at the L2-L3 or L3-L4 space (Fig. 1-6).

7. **Surface grooves**
   a. **Posterior median sulcus:** runs shallowly down middle of dorsal surface
   b. **Posterior intermediate sulcus:** divides each dorsal column into fasciculus gracilis and fasciculus cuneatus
   c. **Posterolateral sulcus:** line of attachment of dorsal roots
   d. **Anterolateral sulcus:** line of attachment of ventral roots
   e. **Anterior median fissure:** runs deep on ventral midline; contains anterior spinal artery

B. Cross-sectional features (see Figs. 1-5B and 1-6)
   1. **Gray matter** appears as a central butterfly or H shape.
      a. **Posterior horn** receives sensory inputs, integrates nociceptive input, and contains cell bodies that project pain input centrally as spinothalamic tract.
      b. **Central region** contains intermediolateral gray matter (autonomic preganglionic cell bodies) and dorsal nucleus (spinocerebellar projecting neurons).
      c. **Anterior horn** contains cell bodies of alpha and gamma motor neurons and is, therefore, enlarged in cervical and lumbosacral regions (see Fig. 1-5)

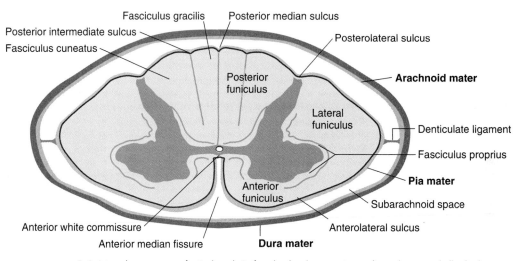

1-6: *Internal components of spinal cord. Surface landmarks: posterior median sulcus runs shallowly down middle of posterior surface; posterior intermediate sulcus divides each dorsal column into fasciculus gracilis and fasciculus cuneatus; posterolateral sulcus is the line of attachment of dorsal roots; anterolateral sulcus is the line of attachment of ventral roots; anterior median fissure runs deep on ventral midline and contains anterior spinal artery.*

2. **White matter** surrounds gray matter
   a. **Posterior funiculus** contains dorsal columns (fine touch, vibration, and proprioception).
      (1) **Fasciculus gracilis,** carrying input from lower body, is seen at all levels.
      (2) **Fasciculus cuneatus,** carrying input from **upper body,** appears from T6 rostrally to C1.
   b. **Lateral funiculus** contains corticospinal tracts (voluntary motor control), major spinocerebellar tracts (proprioception for muscle coordination,) and anterolateral system (spinothalamic and other pain-related pathways).
   c. **Anterior funiculus** contains reticulospinal, vestibulospinal, and tectospinal tracts (motor control).
C. **Spinal defects**
   1. **Syringomyelia:** enlarging cyst within central spinal cord, most frequently cervical

Syringomyelia: motor loss + loss of pain

   a. **Segmental loss of pain and temperature** (hands and arms) because crossing spinothalamic fibers damaged.
   b. **Weakness, fasciculations, and paralysis** (hands and arms) if cyst expands to anterior horn
   c. **Hyperreflexia in lower limb** if cyst expands into lateral funiculus to involve descending corticospinal tracts

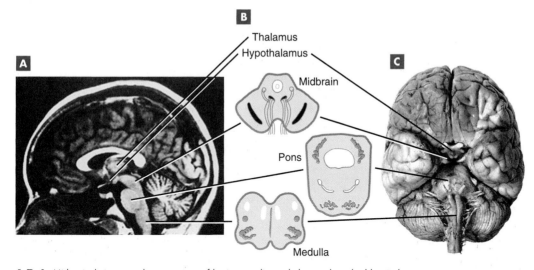

1-7: A, Midsagittal view reveals components of brainstem, diencephalon, and cerebral hemisphere. **B,** Brainstem cross-sectional anatomy is distinctive at midbrain, pons, and medulla. **C,** Brainstem and hypothalamus are visible on ventral brain.

2. Spina bifida (see section I, B and Chapter 2)

D. **Localizing signs**
1. Upper motor neuron axons descend ipsilaterally to target lower motor neurons.
   - **Spinal lesions yield ipsilateral motor deficits,** which may include lower motor neuron signs at the level of the lesion with upper motor neuron signs below the lesion.
2. Fine touch, vibration, and proprioception ascend in ipsilateral posterior columns, while pain and temperature ascend in the contralateral anterolateral system.
   - **Spinal hemisections (e.g., Brown-Séquard) yield crossed sensory deficits** (e.g., loss of vibration sensation in ipsilateral leg and loss of pain sensation in contralateral leg).

III. **Anatomy of Brainstem**
A. **Overview** (Fig. 1-7)
1. Extends from posterior commissure, rostrally, through midbrain, pons, and medulla, to pyramidal decussation caudally.
2. Contained within the infratentorial space (posterior fossa), bounded by tentorial notch superiorly and foramen magnum inferiorly
3. Cerebellum is within this space and is generally considered with brainstem.
4. Contains all cranial nuclei, except olfactory, optic, and spinal accessory
B. **Medulla** (Fig. 1-8)
1. **Motor nuclei and associated cranial nerves**
   a. **Control of ipsilateral tongue:** hypoglossal nucleus and nerve (CN XII)

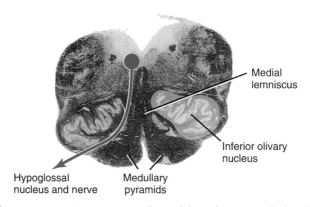

Medial
lemniscus

Inferior olivary
nucleus

Hypoglossal
nucleus and nerve

Medullary
pyramids

1-8: *Medulla in cross-section. Note major ascending and descending tracts and selected motor nuclei.*

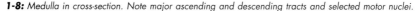

     b. **Speech and swallowing:** nucleus ambiguus and glossopharyngeal and vagus nerves (CN IX, X)

     c. **Salivation:** inferior salivatory nucleus and glossopharyngeal nerve (CN IX)

2. **Sensory nuclei and associated cranial nerves**

     a. **Pain, temperature, and crude touch** from ipsilateral face and anterior dura: spinal trigeminal nucleus; trigeminal, facial, glossopharyngeal, and vagus nerves (CN V, VII, IX, X)

     b. **Vestibular and auditory inputs:** vestibular and cochlear nuclei and vestibulocochlear nerve (CN VIII)

     c. **Taste:** nucleus of solitary tract (rostral portion); facial, glossopharyngeal, and vagus nerves (CN VII, IX, X)

     d. **Visceral sensory input,** including blood oxygen and arterial pressure: nucleus of solitary tract (caudal portion) and glossopharyngeal and vagus nerves (CN IX)

3. **Descending motor tracts**

     a. **Corticospinal tracts** controlling contralateral body run in medullary pyramids.

        • Corticospinal axons leave medulla and enter contralateral spinal cord through **pyramidal decussation** in caudal medulla.

     b. **Sympathetic** tracts descend from hypothalamus toward preganglionic cell bodies within ipsilateral spinal cord.

4. **Ascending sensory tracts**

     a. **Medial lemniscus,** located medially, carries fine touch, vibration, and proprioception from contralateral body.

     b. **Nucleus cuneatus and nucleus gracilis,** located dorsally in caudal medulla, receive fine touch, vibration, and proprioception from ipsilateral body.

     c. **Spinothalamic tract,** located laterally, carries pain and temperature from contralateral body.

5. **Raphe nuclei:** source of serotonin

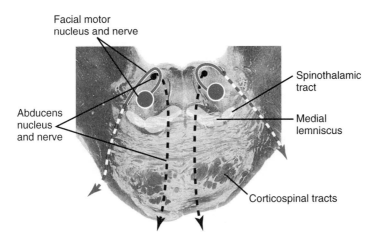

1-9: *Pons in cross-section. Note major ascending and descending tracts and selected motor nuclei.*

C. **Pons** (Fig. 1-9)
  1. **Motor nuclei and associated cranial nerves**
     a. **Mastication:** trigeminal motor nucleus, trigeminal nerve (CN V)
     b. **Eye abduction:** abducens nucleus, abducens nerve (CN VI)
     c. **Facial expression, including eye blink:** facial motor nucleus, facial nerve (CN VII)
     d. **Tearing and salivation:** superior salivatory nucleus, facial nerve
  2. **Sensory nuclei and associated cranial nerves**
     a. **Fine touch, vibration, and proprioception from face and anterior dura:** main trigeminal nucleus, trigeminal nerve (CN V)
     b. **Vestibular input:** vestibular nucleus and vestibulocochlear nerve (CN VIII)
  3. **Descending motor tracts: corticospinal tracts** controlling contralateral body run in pontine base
  4. **Ascending sensory tracts**
     a. **Medial lemniscus** (dorsomedial) carries find touch, vibration, and proprioception from contralateral body.
     b. **Spinothalamic tract** (dorsolateral) carries pain and temperature from contralateral body.
  5. **Pontocerebellar tracts:** relay cortical inputs to contralateral cerebellum through pontine nuclei
  6. **Locus coeruleus:** component of arousal system and source of norepinephrine
  7. **Raphe nuclei:** source of serotonin
D. **Midbrain** (Fig. 1-10)
  1. **Motor nuclei and associated cranial nerves**
     a. **Eye movement:** oculomotor nucleus and nerve and trochlear nucleus and nerve (CN III, IV)

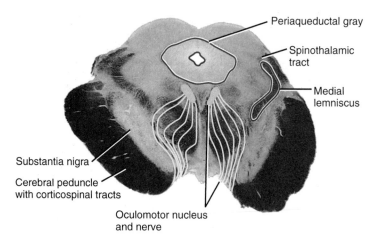

Periaqueductal gray

Spinothalamic tract

Medial lemniscus

Substantia nigra

Cerebral peduncle with corticospinal tracts

Oculomotor nucleus and nerve

1-10: *Midbrain in cross-section. Note major ascending and descending tracts and selected motor nuclei.*

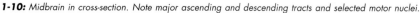

  b. **Eyelid retraction:** oculomotor nucleus and nerve (CN III)

  c. **Pupil constriction and lens thickening:** Edinger-Westphal nucleus and oculomotor nerve, parasympathetic fibers (CN III)

 2. **Ascending sensory tracts**

  a. **Medial lemniscus** (dorsolateral) carries fine touch, vibration, and proprioceptive from contralateral body.

  b. **Spinothalamic tract** (dorsolateral), contiguous with medial lemniscus dorsolaterally, carries pain and temperature from contralateral body.

 3. **Descending motor tracts: corticospinal tracts** controlling contralateral body run in cerebral peduncles

 4. **Periaqueductal gray:** component of intrinsic analgesia system

 5. **Substantia nigra:** component of basal ganglia and source of dopamine

 6. **Raphe nuclei:** source of serotonin

 7. **Red nucleus:** source of rubrospinal tract

 8. **Tectum** (includes superior and inferior colliculi): contributes to saccadic eye movements, pupillary light reflex, and reflex orientation to auditory stimuli

E. **Cerebellum** (see Chapter 10)

 1. Connected to brainstem by three pairs of peduncles

 2. Consists of anterior, posterior, and flocculonodular lobes

 3. Controls movement of **ipsilateral** body

F. **Anatomic defects**

 1. **Arnold-Chiari type II malformation**

  a. Results from abnormally small posterior fossa

  b. Possible displacement of cerebellar tonsils and brainstem downward through foramen magnum

 2. **Encephalocele:** herniation of underlying meninges and brain tissue resulting from congenital, traumatic, or postoperative gap in skull

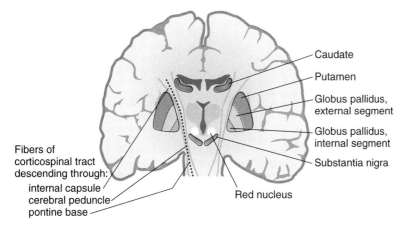

1-11: *Cerebral hemispheres and brainstem, coronal section. Broken line,* fibers of corticospinal tract.

G. **Localizing signs**
1. **Alternating hemiplegia** (upper motor neuron signs on one side of body and lower motor neuron signs on opposite side of head) localizes damage to brainstem.
   a. **Damage to ventromedial medulla** causes paralysis of ipsilateral tongue (CN XII) and contralateral body (pyramids).
   b. **Damage to ventral midbrain** causes paralysis of ipsilateral eye (CN III) and contralateral lower face, tongue, and body (cerebral peduncles).
2. **Damage to dorsolateral medulla,** due to infarct of posterior inferior cerebellar artery (PICA) or vertebral artery, causes multiple signs known as **lateral medullary syndrome** (see Table 3-4)
3. **Cerebellar** signs, including **ataxia,** localize damage to ipsilateral cerebellum.

IV. **Anatomy of Cerebral Hemispheres**
A. **Hypothalamus** (see Fig. 1-7)
1. Bounded medially by the third ventricle, laterally by the internal capsule, rostrally by lamina terminalis, caudally by the midbrain, and superiorly by hypothalamic sulcus
2. Visible on ventral brain surface, extending from optic chiasm through infundibular stalk to mammillary bodies
B. **Thalamus** (see Figs. 1-7, 8-1, and 9-2)
1. Bounded medially by the third ventricle, laterally by the internal capsule, superiorly by fornix and lateral ventricle, and inferiorly by hypothalamic sulcus
2. Consists, functionally, of multiple subnuclei
C. **Basal ganglia** (Fig. 1-11; see also Figs. 8-1 and 9-2 and Chapter 9)
1. Consists, functionally, of several related nuclear groups: caudate, putamen, globus pallidus (external and internal), subthalamic nucleus, and substantia nigra

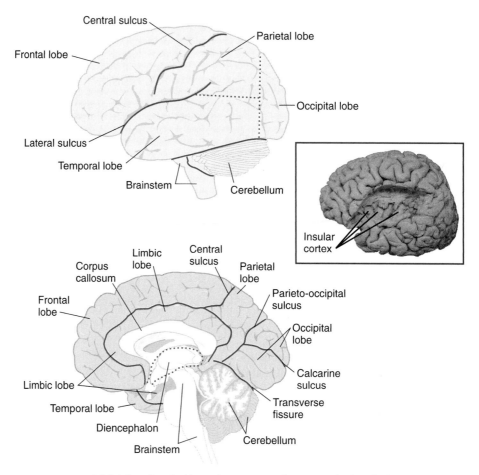

1-12: *Lobes of cerebral hemispheres. Inset, Insular cortex within lateral sulcus.*

Caudate and putamen atrophy in Huntington disease

Substantia nigra appears pale in histologic specimens in Parkinson disease.

2. **Caudate:** forms lateral wall of lateral ventricle
3. **Putamen and globus pallidus** (collectively, the lentiform nucleus) lie medial to the insular cortex and are separated from the caudate by the anterior limb of the internal capsule and from the thalamus by the posterior limb of the internal capsule.
4. **Substantia nigra,** within midbrain, is separated from globus pallidus by internal capsule.

D. **Cerebral cortex** (Fig. 1-12)
   1. **Frontal lobe**
      a. Bounded posteriorly by central sulcus and inferiorly by lateral sulcus
      b. Primary **motor** strip resides within **precentral gyrus.**
      c. Frontal eye fields control voluntary saccades to contralateral side (see Chapter 12).
      d. Language production requires posterior inferior frontal lobe (Broca area), **usually in left hemisphere.**

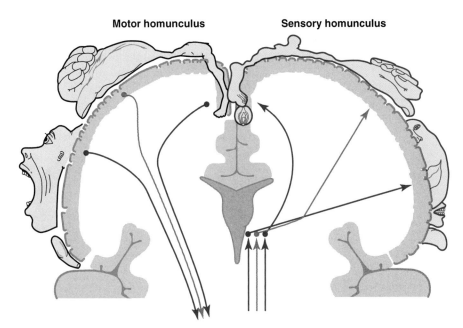

1-13: *Motor homunculus and sensory homunculus.*

2. **Parietal lobe**
   a. Bounded anteriorly by central sulcus and posteriorly by parieto-occipital sulcus (medially) and imaginary line from parieto-occipital sulcus, superiorly, to preoccipital notch, inferiorly
   b. Primary **sensory** strip resides within **postcentral gyrus.**
3. **Occipital lobe**
   a. Bounded anteriorly by parietal lobe.
   b. **Primary visual cortex** located medially within **occipital lobes.**
4. **Temporal lobe**
   a. Bounded superiorly by lateral sulcus
   b. Spoken language interpretation requires **superior temporal lobe** (Wernicke area), usually within left hemisphere.
5. **Insular cortex** lies within lateral sulcus (see Fig. 1-12, inset).
6. **Limbic cortex** (see Fig. 1-7)
   a. Includes cingulate gyrus, visible on medial cortex
   b. Processes **memories,** emotions, and aspects of chronic pain
E. **Localizing signs**
   1. **Sensory deficit** with no motor paralysis may arise from contralateral thalamic damage.
   2. **Basal ganglia damage** causes contralateral signs (e.g., hemiballismus).
   3. **Aphasias** result from damage to dominant (generally left) hemisphere.
   4. **Gerstmann syndrome** (acalculia, finger agnosia, left–right confusion, agraphia) results from damage to **dominant parietal lobe.**
   5. **Hemi-neglect** syndromes result from damage to **nondominant parietal lobe.**

6. **Complex partial seizures** commonly begin within hippocampal region of medial temporal lobe.
7. **Herniation of the medial temporal lobe** (uncus) through the tentorial notch is caused by large supratentorial masses or cerebral edema.
8. **Scotomas in contralateral visual field** may result from occipital lobe damage.
   • By using a homunculus as a reference, clinicians can predict that damage to medial locations within the primary sensory and primary motor cortices will cause paralysis and loss of sensation in the contralateral leg (Fig. 1-13).

Ventricles, Cerebrospinal Fluid, and Meninges

I. **Ventricles**
   A. **Development**
      1. Walls of neural tube develop into central nervous system (CNS), while fluid-filled core becomes ventricular system.
      2. **Cavities in vesicles** become ventricles (Fig. 2-1).
         a. **Lateral ventricles:** cavities within telencephalon, one in each hemisphere, that extend from anterior horn (frontal lobe) through the body (parietal lobe), back into posterior horn (occipital lobe), and finally down and forward into inferior horn (temporal lobe).
         b. **Third ventricle:** cavity separating right and left diencephalon
         c. **Fourth ventricle:** cavity of rhombencephalon between pons and cerebellum extending as far caudal as medulla
         d. **Central canal:** continuation of neural tube cavity into the spinal cord; although functional during early fetal development, it closes during the late stages of development.
   B. **Anatomy**
      1. Ventricles are continuous compartments within the brain that are **filled with cerebrospinal fluid** (CSF).
      2. **Interventricular foramen** (foramina of Monro) connects each lateral ventricle directly to third ventricle.
      3. **Cerebral aqueduct** connects third and fourth ventricles.
      4. Two **lateral apertures** (foramina of Luschka) and **median aperture** (foramen of Magendie) connect fourth ventricle to subarachnoid space.
      5. **Central canal** is a continuation of neural tube cavity into the spinal cord; although functional during early fetal development, it later closes.

II. **Cerebrospinal Fluid**
   A. **Composition**
      1. **Produced** by **choroid plexus** (Fig. 2-2A)
      2. **Clear,** odorless, and **acellular;** *not* an ultrafiltrate of plasma
      3. Glucose concentration normally about **two thirds that of serum concentration**
      4. **Protein** is *not* transported into ventricles across choroid plexus and is minimal.
      5. **Changes in composition may indicate disease.**
         a. **Increased protein** frequently occurs in **meningitis, tumor,** or **demyelinating disorder.**

↓ CSF glucose: bacterial, tuberculous, and fungal meningitis

↑ CSF protein: demyelination, CNS tumors, infection

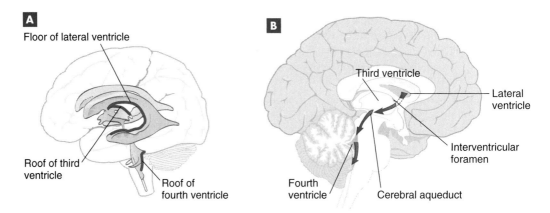

2-1: *Major cavities of ventricular system and points of communication between ventricles. Each lateral ventricle, consisting of anterior horn, body, posterior horn, and inferior horn, extends through frontal, parietal, occipital, and temporal lobes of one hemisphere. Extension of the posterior horn varies.*

2-2: *Choroid plexus and cerebrospinal fluid (CSF) flow.* **A,** *Choroid plexus (green) within lateral ventricles is continuous with choroid plexus in the roof of the third ventricle. Choroid plexus is also in the roof of the fourth ventricle.* **B,** *Direction of CSF flow through ventricular system (arrows). CSF flows from lateral ventricle through* **interventricular foramen** *into third ventricle, third ventricle through* **cerebral aqueduct** *into fourth ventricle, and fourth ventricle through* **median and lateral apertures** *into subarachnoid space. Left hemisphere, midsagittal section.*

  b. **Bacterial meningitis: CSF cloudy; decreased glucose levels in CSF**
  (Table 2-1)

> Xanthochromia results when red blood cells lyse within the CSF, suggesting subarachnoid hemorrhage. If blood in the CSF is caused by traumatic lumbar puncture, the CSF will be clear after centrifugation.

B. **Course**
  1. Flows through ventricular system and escapes into subarachnoid space
  (Fig. 2-2B)

	White Blood Cells	Protein	Glucose
Normal	0–5 (all lymphocytes)	<50 mg/dL	50–75 mg/dL
Bacterial meningitis	50–10,000 (neutrophils)	Highly increased	Decreased
Viral meningitis	20–500 (lymphocytes)	Slightly increased	Normal
Fungal meningitis	50–10,000 (mixed or lymphocytes)	Increased	Slightly decreased
Tubercular meningitis	50–10,000 (mixed)	Increased	Decreased

2. Absorbed into venous system through **arachnoid villi**
   a. Arachnoid villi form as outpouchings of arachnoid membrane and subarachnoid space that extend through the overlying dura into venous sinuses, especially the superior sagittal sinus (Fig. 2-3).
   b. Arachnoid villi are one-way valves, allowing CSF flow from subarachnoid space to venous blood due to hydrostatic and colloidal osmotic pressure gradients.

> Arachnoid villi: compromised by congenital defects, infection, trauma, and aging, producing hydrocephalus

C. **Function**
   1. Transports hormones and removes metabolic waste products
   2. **Cushions and floats brain**

> Coup–countercoup brain injury occurs due to blow to head (e.g., motor vehicle crash). Brain collides with skull (coup) and rebounds against opposite side of skull (countercoup). Countercoup injury is frequently worse than initial coup injury.

   3. **Sensitive to changes in intracranial pressure** (ICP)
      a. **Normal pressure** (lateral decubitus): 6 to 13 mmHg (90–180 mm H_2O)
      b. Minimal changes in ICP accompany every arterial pulse and are accommodated by minor shifts of CSF from skull into subarachnoid space.
      c. Major changes in intracranial fluid volume are usually accommodated by the brain shrinking, if the changes occur slowly.
   4. **Responses to increased ICP**
      a. **Bradycardia and hypertension** as cerebral blood flow becomes compromised (ICP > 40–50 mmHg)
      b. **Respiration slows and becomes irregular** as brainstem respiratory centers are compressed.
      c. **Papilledema** results from compression of retinal vein as it courses through subarachnoid space with optic nerve.
      d. **Brain herniations**
         (1) **Subfalcial herniation:** medial portion of one hemisphere may be forced under falx cerebri.
         (2) **Temporal lobe herniation:** inferior and medial portion of the temporal lobe (uncus) forced through tentorial notch.
            (a) **Ipsilateral pupillary dilation (mydriasis)** after compression of parasympathetic fibers within oculomotor nerve

> ↑ Intracranial pressure: papilledema, hypertension, bradycardia, morning headache, projectile vomiting

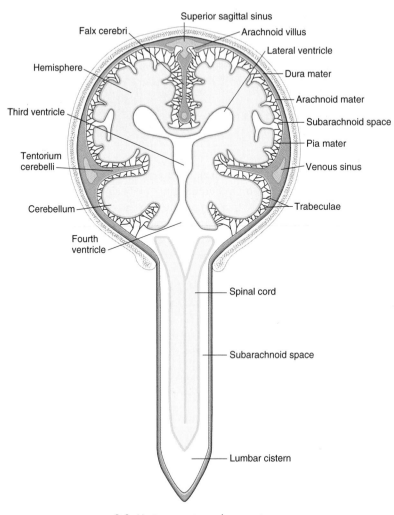

Falx cerebri
Superior sagittal sinus
Arachnoid villus
Hemisphere
Lateral ventricle
Dura mater
Arachnoid mater
Third ventricle
Subarachnoid space
Pia mater
Tentorium cerebelli
Venous sinus
Cerebellum
Trabeculae
Fourth ventricle
Spinal cord
Subarachnoid space
Lumbar cistern

2-3: Meninges, septa, and venous sinuses.

(b) **Ipsilateral paresis** as contralateral cerebral peduncle is forced against a free edge of the tentorium

(c) **Homonymous hemianopia** caused by compression of posterior cerebral artery (occipital lobe infarction)

(3) **Tonsillar herniation:** tonsils of cerebellum push into foramen magnum, compressing brainstem.

Lumbar puncture: contraindicated in presence of papilledema; risk for tonsillar herniation

III. **Meninges**

    A. **Dura mater** (see Fig. 2-3)

        1. **Two fused layers**

            a. **Outer periosteal layer:** tightly adherent to skull; around spinal cord periosteal layer is replaced by vertebral periosteum

      b. **Inner meningeal layer:** surrounds brain and spinal cord; fused to periosteal layer around brain

      c. **Venous sinuses** lie between layers.

      d. **Spinal epidural space:** lies between meningeal dura and vertebral periosteum

  2. **Four septa**

      a. **Falx cerebri** inserts into longitudinal fissure, between the cerebral hemispheres.

      b. **Falx cerebelli** inserts between cerebellar hemispheres.

      c. **Diaphragma sellae** forms roof of hypophysis fossa (sella turcica) and is perforated by the infundibular stalk that extends from the hypothalamus to the pituitary gland.

      d. **Tentorium cerebelli:** transverse septum that separates cerebral hemispheres (superior) from brainstem and cerebellum (inferior)

  3. **Blood supply to dura and skull**

      a. Ophthalmic arteries that branch from internal carotids supply anterior cranial fossa.

      b. Occipital branch of external carotid supplies posterior cranial fossa.

      c. **Middle meningeal artery,** fed by the external carotid artery, supplies middle cranial fossa.

      d. **Epidural hematoma**

          (1) Probable cause: **rupture of middle meningeal artery** following **temporal skull fracture**

          (2) Blood is forced, under arterial pressure, between skull and dura.

          (3) **May be rapidly life-threatening**

      e. **Subdural hematoma**

          (1) Probable cause: **rupture of bridging veins** that drain blood from brain to venous sinuses; almost always secondary to head trauma

          (2) Blood may force a space between the dura and arachnoid or split the dura.

          (3) Ranges from a **mild, slowly evolving chronic hematoma** to a **rapidly progressing medical emergency** characterized by fluctuating levels of consciousness

          (4) Occurs as a **complication of delivery and postnatal trauma** in newborns and in **shaken-baby syndrome.**

> Perimacular retinal folds are strongly suggestive of shaken-baby syndrome.

  4. **Sensory innervation of cranial dura mater**

      a. Anterior: **trigeminal nerve**

      b. Posterior: **second and third cervical roots**

B. **Arachnoid mater**

  1. Tightly fused to overlying dura with no intervening space

  2. Avascular, although bridging veins pass through

Epidural hematoma: rupture of middle meningeal artery; subdural hematoma: trauma may tear bridging veins

Some headache pain is mediated by trigeminal innervation of the dura.

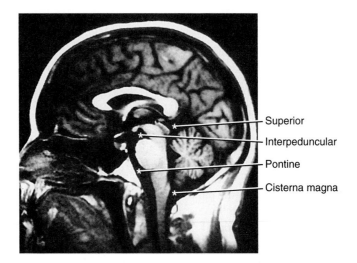

2-4: *Major subarachnoid cisterns. Magnetic resonance image, midsagittal view.*

C. **Pia mater**
1. Tightly adheres to brain and spinal cord, following all contours
2. Surrounds cerebral arteries and initial portions of penetrating branches (Virchow-Robin space)

D. **Subarachnoid space**
1. CSF-filled space **between arachnoid and pia**
2. **Subarachnoid cisterns:** enlargements of subarachnoid space (Fig. 2-4)
   a. **Cisterna magna,** posterior to medulla, receives CSF as it escapes from fourth ventricle.
   b. Spinal cord ends at **L1–L2 in adults** and **below L2 in children;** spinal dural and arachnoid sheath extends to S2, leaving **large lumbar cistern.**
3. **Subarachnoid hemorrhage**
   a. Probable cause: **rupture of a congenital arterial berry aneurysm** at the junction of communicating branches with main cerebral artery
   b. Symptom: **sudden severe headache ("worst headache of my life")**
   c. **May be life-threatening**

E. **Meningitis**
1. Mild and self-limiting (e.g., some viral infections) to life-threatening (e.g., bacterial infection)
2. Signs and symptoms: **nuchal rigidity,** Kernig sign, Brudzinski sign, fever, headache (see Figs. 17-2 and 17-3)

F. **Meningioma**
1. Typically benign, encapsulated tumor
2. Accounts for more than 20% of intracranial tumors in adults
3. More common in **women**

Virchow-Robin space: access of leukemic cells to brain parenchyma

Lumbar puncture in adults: performed at L3-L4 or L4-L5 intervertebral space

Subarachnoid hemorrhage: "Worst headache of my life!"

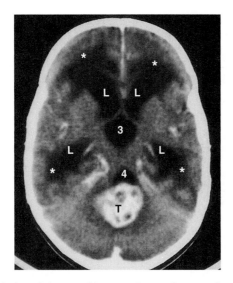

2-5: *Noncommunicating hydrocephalus caused by tumor. Computed tomography scan, horizontal view. Because the tumor blocks the fourth ventricle, all four ventricles expand. Asterisks, areas of edema. L, Lateral ventricle; T, tumor; 3, third ventricle; 4, fourth ventricle.*

IV. **Hydrocephalus**
   A. Excessive accumulation of CSF; can be genetic, congenital, or acquired
   B. **Signs of hydrocephalus**
      1. Vary with cause and age
      2. **Infants:** enlarged head, vomiting, seizures, upward gaze palsy with downwardly deviated eyes ("sunsetting")
      3. **Adults:** vomiting, papilledema, blurred or double vision, urinary incontinence, imbalance or gait ataxia, dementia
   C. **Causes**
      1. **Excess production of CSF (rare):** caused by choroid plexus papilloma; occurs in children
      2. **Noncommunicating hydrocephalus:** obstruction within the ventricular system, preventing communication with subarachnoid space (Fig. 2-5)
         • Most common form
      3. **Communicating hydrocephalus:** CSF exits to subarachnoid space but is not reabsorbed into the venous system.
         a. Obstruction of CSF flow within subarachnoid space
         b. **Reduced CSF reabsorption**
            (1) Decreased arteriovenous pressure difference
            (2) Blockage of arachnoid villi (e.g., after infection or subarachnoid hemorrhage)
      4. **Normal-pressure hydrocephalus:** ICP increases, causing chronic enlargement of ventricles, and then re-equilibrates in a high-normal range; occurs in adults

CSF obstruction leading to hydrocephalus: congenital defects, infection, trauma

Triad for normal-pressure hydrocephalus: dementia, gait ataxia, urinary incontinence

Normal-pressure hydrocephalus: causes reversible dementia

5. **Compensatory hydrocephalus** (hydrocephalus ex vacuo)
   a. When **brain atrophies,** CSF fills the space.
   b. Occurs in **neurodegenerative disorders** (e.g., Alzheimer disease, Huntington disease)

V. **Developmental Anomalies in Ventricular System**
   A. **Spina bifida**
      1. Developmental defect that **prevents vertebral column from closing**
      2. Associated with **herniation of meninges** and **occasionally of spinal cord**
      3. **Signs and symptoms:** weakness, atrophy, loss of sensation and tendon reflexes in legs, bladder and bowel dysfunction
   B. **Meningocele**
      1. **Herniating meningeal sac** filled with CSF
      2. **Signs and symptoms:** usually related to other developmental malformations or hydrocephalus
   C. **Meningomyelocele**
      1. **Herniated spinal cord** in association with **meningocele**
      2. **Signs and symptoms:** weakness, atrophy, loss of sensation and tendon reflexes in legs, bladder and bowel dysfunction
   D. **Encephalocele**
      1. **Protrusion of brain and/or meninges** through anomalous midline clefts in cranium
      2. **Signs and symptoms:** variable
   E. **Arnold-Chiari malformation**
      1. Displacement of intracranial tissue toward spinal cord
      2. Frequently associated with **syringomyelia** (cavitation of central canal)
      3. **Signs and symptoms**
         a. Weakness, atrophy and ataxia in legs, visual disturbances (e.g., perception that stationary objects are moving or blurring of fixed objects)
         b. May occur in first few months of life; usually associated with other developmental malformations or hydrocephalus
   F. **Dandy-Walker syndrome**
      1. **Diagnostic triad**
         a. Cerebellar vermis small (hypoplasia) or absent (agenesis)
         b. Fourth ventricle enlarged (cyst)
         c. Posterior fossa enlarged
      2. **Causes**
         a. First-trimester exposure to rubella, alcohol
         b. Genetic defect in some cases

3

Vasculature

I. **Internal Carotid System (Anterior Circulation)**
  A. **Internal carotid arteries** (Figs. 3-1 and 3-2)
    1. **Anatomy**
      a. Arise from **common carotid arteries**
        (1) Left common carotid arises from aortic arch
        (2) Right common carotid arises from brachiocephalic branch off aorta.
      b. Run through carotid canal in base of skull to enter middle cranial fossa, continue through cavernous sinus, carotid siphon, along medial side of anterior clinoid process, and then immediately lateral to optic chiasm

> **Aneurysm of the internal carotid artery** near its bifurcation compresses the lateral edge of the optic chiasm, producing **unilateral nasal field hemianopsia.**

    2. **Function:** carry **about 80% of total cerebral blood flow** and supply anterior and middle cerebral hemispheres and diencephalon
  B. **Hypophysial arteries**
    1. **Anatomy:** arise from internal carotid arteries in cavernous sinus
    2. **Function:** supply infundibulum and give rise to pituitary portal system
  C. **Ophthalmic arteries**
    1. **Anatomy:** arise from internal carotids and pass through optic foramen
    2. **Function:** supply eye, frontal area of scalp, frontal and ethmoidal paranasal sinuses, and parts of nose
  D. **Posterior communicating arteries**
    1. **Anatomy:** arise from internal carotid or proximal middle cerebral arteries
    2. **Function:** form part of arterial circle by connecting to posterior cerebral arteries
  E. **Anterior choroidal arteries**
    1. **Anatomy:** arise from internal carotid or proximal middle cerebral arteries
    2. **Function:** supply choroid plexus in lateral ventricle, optic tract, amygdala, hippocampus, globus pallidus, lateral geniculate nucleus, ventral thalamus, subthalamus, and internal capsule

> Anterior choroidal arteries are prone to **thrombosis** because of their small diameter and lengthy course through the subarachnoid space.

Unilateral nasal field hemianopsia: aneurysm of internal carotid artery

Ophthalmic artery disruption: partial or complete blindness in ipsilateral eye

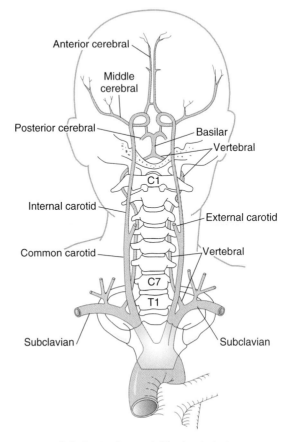

3-1: *Arteries that supply blood to the brain.*

F. **Middle cerebral artery**
   1. **Anatomy:** larger of the two terminal branches of the internal carotid (Fig. 3-3 and Table 3-1)
   2. **Function**
      a. Branches that enter lateral sulcus and emerge supply the superior (frontal and parietal) and inferior (temporal) aspects of the lateral convexity of the cerebral cortex (Fig. 3-4).
      b. Penetrating lateral striate (lenticulostriate) branches supply deep structures, including portions of caudate, putamen, globus pallidus, and internal capsule (Fig. 3-5)

   > **Stress:** In hypertension, stress on the lenticulostriate vessels produces aneurysms. Rupture of an aneurysm produces an intracerebral hematoma.

Middle cerebral artery disruption: sensory-motor deficits in contralateral upper body and head

G. **Anterior cerebral arteries**
   1. **Anatomy:** smaller of the two terminal branches of the internal carotids; run superior to optic chiasm and enter the longitudinal fissure (Table 3-2)

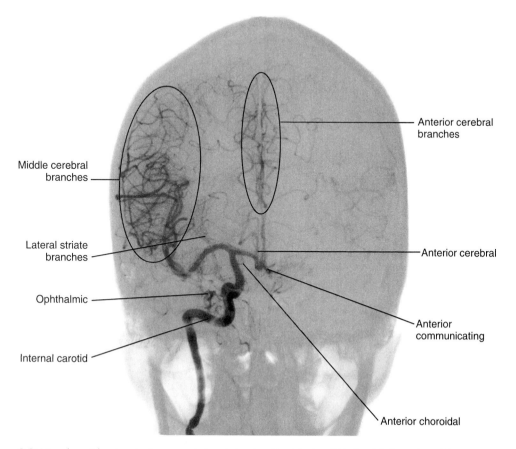

Anterior cerebral
branches

Middle cerebral
branches

Lateral striate
branches

Ophthalmic

Internal carotid

Anterior cerebral

Anterior
communicating

Anterior choroidal

3-2: *Internal carotid system. Angiogram, anteriaposterior view. Dye introduced into the right internal carotid artery has filled all branches.*

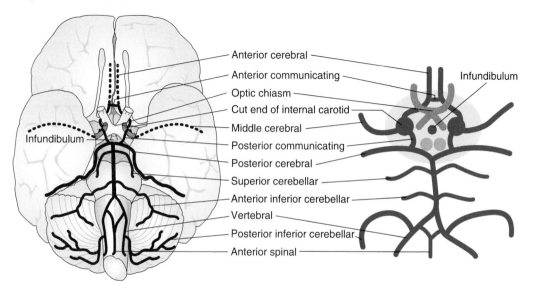

Anterior cerebral

Anterior communicating

Optic chiasm

Cut end of internal carotid

Middle cerebral

Posterior communicating

Posterior cerebral

Superior cerebellar

Anterior inferior cerebellar

Vertebral

Posterior inferior cerebellar

Anterior spinal

Infundibulum

Infundibulum

3-3: *Vertebrobasilar system and arterial circle. Left, Brain, ventral view; right, major arteries.*

TABLE 3-1:
Middle Cerebral Artery Occlusion

Site of Occlusion	Regions Affected	Signs and Symptoms
	Motor area for upper body Somatosensory cortex for upper body	Paresis or paralysis of contralateral face, hand, and arm Sensory deficits involving contralateral face, hand, and arm
	Axons of coronal radiata projecting from somatic motor area for lower limb (*left arrow*) Axons from thalamic ventroposterolateral nucleus to somatosensory cortex for lower limb (*right arrow*)	Paresis of contralateral leg Sensory deficit involving contralateral leg
	Frontal lobe of **dominant** hemisphere (usually left hemisphere) related to speech production (Broca area)	Expressive aphasia (nonfluent or motor aphasia)
	Superior temporal lobe areas of **dominant** hemisphere related to interpretation of speech	Receptive aphasia, fluent aphasia
	Angular gyrus and parieto-occipital cortex of **dominant** hemisphere Supramarginal or angular gyrus	Acalculia, agraphia, finger agnosia, right-left disorientation (collectively referred to as Gerstmann syndrome) Loss or impairment of optokinetic reflex
	Parietal lobe of **nondominant** hemisphere	Contralateral neglect (hemi-neglect), anosognosia
	Frontal eye fields in frontal lobe	Transient loss of voluntary saccadic eye movement to contralateral side
	Optic radiation within temporal lobes (Meyer loop)	Superior quadrantanopsia
	Optic radiation within parietal and temporal lobes	Homonymous hemianopia
	Upper portion of posterior limb of internal capsule and adjacent corona radiata	Capsular (pure motor) hemiplegia

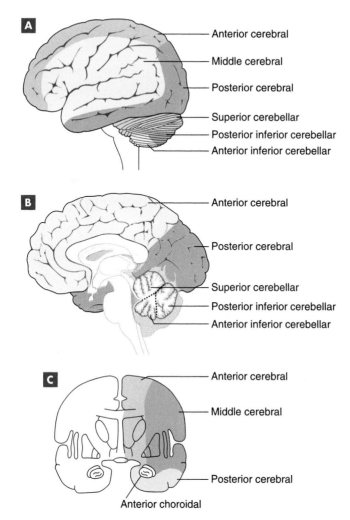

3-4: *Areas of the brain supplied by the cerebral and cerebellar arteries. **A,** Lateral view; **B,** medial view; **C,** coronal view.*

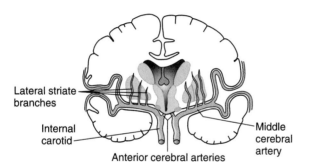

3-5: *Middle cerebral artery and branches. Penetrating lateral striate branches supply subcortical regions, including much of the basal ganglia and internal capsule. M₁ to M₄, segments of cerebral artery.*

TABLE 3-2:
Anterior Cerebral Artery Occlusion

	Regions Affected	Signs and Symptoms
	Motor area for lower body	Paresis or paralysis of contralateral leg and foot
	Somatosensory cortex for lower body	Sensory impairment (paresthesia or anesthesia) involving contralateral foot and leg
	Fibers coursing from arm and hand area of motor cortex through corona radiata (*left arrow*)	Mild paresis of contralateral arm
	Fibers coursing to arm and hand area of somatosensory cortex through corona radiata (*right arrow*)	Mild sensory impairment of contralateral arm
	Superior frontal gyrus (*upper*) and anterior cingulate gyrus (*lower*), bilaterally	Urinary incontinence

2. **Function**
   a. Pericallosal branch supplies cingulate gyrus and corpus callosum
   b. Callosomarginal branch supplies cortical regions that include primary sensory and motor cortex for lower extremity.
   H. **Anterior communicating artery**
      1. **Anatomy:** arise from proximal anterior cerebral arteries
      2. **Function:** form part of arterial circle by connecting anterior cerebral arteries

II. **Vertebrobasilar System (Posterior Circulation)**
   A. **Vertebral arteries** (Fig. 3-6; see also Figs. 3-1 and 3-3)
      1. **Anatomy:** arise from right and left subclavian arteries and merge to form **basilar artery**
      2. **Function:** carry about 20% of total cerebral blood flow and supply brainstem and posterior cerebral hemispheres
   B. **Anterior spinal artery** (Fig. 3-7; see also Fig. 3-3)

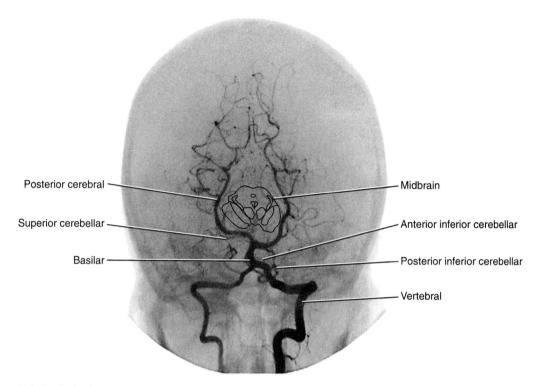

Posterior cerebral — Midbrain

Superior cerebellar — Anterior inferior cerebellar

Basilar — Posterior inferior cerebellar

— Vertebral

3-6: *Vertebrobasilar system. Angiogram, anteroposterior view. Dye introduced into the left vertebral artery has filled the vertebrobasilar system.*

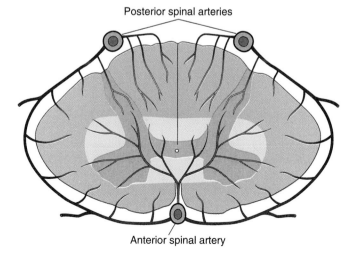

Posterior spinal arteries

Anterior spinal artery

3-7: *Arteries that supply of the spinal cord. Light green area, spinal territory supplied by branches of anterior spinal artery; dark green area, spinal territory supplied by branches of posterior spinal arteries.*

TABLE 3-3:
Medial Medullary Syndrome

Likely cause: occlusion of branches of anterior spinal artery (illustrated)
or paramedian branches of basilar artery

Regions and Structures Affected	Signs and Symptoms
Hypoglossal nucleus or nerve (CN XII)	Paralysis and eventual atrophy of tongue ipsilateral to lesion
Corticospinal tracts within medullary pyramids	Paralysis of contralateral arm and leg
Medial lemniscus	Loss of touch, vibration, and proprioception from contralateral arm and leg

1. **Anatomy:** merging branches from both vertebral arteries arise at level of medulla and run caudally down anterior medulla and spinal cord
   a. Receives collateral supply from radicular arteries
   b. Great segmental medullary artery, a direct branch of the aorta and the largest radicular artery, joins about T10-L2.
2. **Function:** supplies medial medulla and anterior horn and ventral and lateral spinal cord
   a. Disruptions to flow within anterior spinal artery are most frequently caused by **aortic disease,** with infarct most likely in thoracic and lumbar region.
   b. Infarct at medullary level causes **medial medullary syndrome** (Table 3-3)

Anterior spinal artery infarct at cervical level: incompatible with life

C. **Posterior spinal arteries**
   1. **Anatomy:** arise from vertebral or posterior inferior cerebellar arteries at level of medulla and run caudally down posterolateral medulla and spinal cord
   2. **Function:** supply posterior columns, posterolateral spinal tracts, and posterior horn

   The posterior spinal arteries receive collateral circulation from numerous paired radicular arteries, forming a resilient supply that **rarely occludes.**

D. **Posterior inferior cerebellar arteries**
   1. **Anatomy:** arise from vertebral arteries, occasionally, basilar artery, at level of medulla

TABLE 3-4:
Posterior Inferior Cerebellar Artery Syndrome

Likely cause: infarct of posterior inferior cerebellar artery or vertebral artery

Regions and Structures Affected	Signs and Symptoms
Spinal trigeminal nucleus and spinal trigeminal tract (CN V)	Loss of pain and temperature from ipsilateral face
Fibers from contralateral spinal trigeminal nucleus	Possible loss of pain and temperature from contralateral face
Spinothalamic tract	Loss of pain and temperature from contralateral body
Descending autonomic (sympathetic) fibers	Horner syndrome (miosis, ptosis, anhydrosis) on ipsilateral face
Glossopharyngeal (CN IX) and vagus (CN X) and nucleus ambiguus (motor nucleus for CN IX and CN X)	Dysphagia, dysarthria, loss of gag reflex ipsilateral to lesion
Vestibular nucleus and connections to cerebellum	Vertigo, nausea, nystagmus
Cerebellum and/or inferior cerebellar peduncle	Limb ataxia ipsilateral to lesion

2. **Function:** supply lateral medulla, posterior cerebellar hemisphere, inferior vermis, deep cerebellar nuclei, and choroid plexus of fourth ventricle
   - Disruption to flow causes posterior inferior cerebellar artery syndrome, also called lateral medullary (Wallenberg) syndrome (Table 3-4).
E. **Basilar artery**
   1. **Anatomy:** formed from merging of vertebral arteries at pontomedullary junction, runs along midline of anterior pons, and bifurcates at rostral border of pons to form posterior cerebral arteries
   2. **Function:** supplies majority of pons and, occasionally, medial rostral medulla.
      - Infarction involving a penetrating branch of basilar artery causes one of several pontine syndromes (Tables 3-5 and 3-6)
F. **Anterior inferior cerebellar arteries**
   1. **Anatomy:** arise from caudal basilar artery
   2. **Function:** supply inferior cerebellum, deep cerebellar nuclei, and cochlear nuclei at dorsal pontomedullary junction

TABLE 3-5:
Medial Pontine Syndromes

Cause: infarct affecting paramedian branches from basilar artery

Regions and Structures Affected	Signs and Symptoms
Descending corticospinal tracts and corticobulbar tract to hypoglossal nucleus (CN XII)	Paralysis of arm, leg, tongue, contralateral to lesion
Ascending medial lemniscus	Loss of tactile sense, proprioception, vibratory sense from body contralateral to lesion (limited to face and upper body with rostral lesions)
Middle cerebellar peduncle	Limb and gait ataxia, ipsilateral to lesion
Medial longitudinal fasciculus	Internuclear ophthalmoplegia (eye ipsilateral to lesion does not adduct on lateral gaze)
Descending corticobulbar tract to facial motor nucleus (CN VII)	Paralysis of lower contralateral face
Abducens nerve (CN VI)	Diplopia on ipsilateral lateral gaze, convergent strabismus
Lateral gaze center (paramedian pontine reticular formation)	Paralysis of conjugate gaze ipsilateral to lesion

G. **Labyrinthine arteries**
   1. **Anatomy:** arise from basilar artery, pass through internal acoustic meatus, and ramify throughout labyrinth of inner ear
   2. **Function:** supply inner ear labyrinth
H. **Pontine arteries**
   1. **Anatomy:** arise as paramedian and circumferential penetrating branches from basilar artery
   2. **Function:** supply pontine base and tegmentum
I. **Superior cerebellar arteries**
   1. **Anatomy:** arise from rostral basilar artery
   2. **Function:** supply superior cerebellum, pons, superior cerebellar peduncle, and tectum of midbrain (see Table 3-6)
J. **Posterior cerebral arteries** (Tables 3-7 and 3-8)
   1. **Anatomy:** arise as terminal bifurcation of basilar artery
   2. **Function:** major blood supply to midbrain and inferior temporal and occipital lobes

TABLE 3-6:
Dorsal and Lateral Pontine Syndromes

Cause: infarct affecting anterior cerebellar artery (caudal), circumferential arteries (middle), or superior cerebellar artery (rostral)

Regions and Structures Affected	Signs and Symptoms
Middle or superior cerebellar peduncle	Limb and gait ataxia, ipsilateral to lesion
Spinothalamic tract	Loss of pain and temperature from contralateral body Loss of pain and temperature from contralateral face with more rostral lesions
Medial lemniscus (lateral aspect)	Loss of touch, proprioception, vibratory sense from lower body, contralateral to lesion
Descending autonomic (sympathetic) fibers	Horner syndrome (miosis, ptosis, anhydrosis) ipsilateral to lesion
Facial motor nucleus and/or nerve (CN VII) (caudal pons)	Paralysis of ipsilateral face (upper and lower)
Cochlear nerve or nucleus (CN VIII) (caudal pons)	Tinnitus or deafness, ipsilateral to lesion
Vestibular nerve or nucleus (CN VIII) (caudal pons)	Nystagmus, vertigo
Descending fibers of spinal trigeminal tract (caudal pons)	Loss of pain and temperature from ipsilateral face
Trigeminal motor nucleus and/or nerve (CN V) (rostral pons)	Paralysis of ipsilateral muscles of mastication
Trigeminal nerve or nucleus (CN V) (rostral pons)	Loss of sensation (touch and pain) from ipsilateral face

Occlusion of a posterior cerebral artery produces a contralateral hemianopia with macular sparing

III. **Arterial Circle (of Willis)** (see Fig. 3-3)
   A. **Connects anterior and posterior circulations**
      1. Proximal portions of **posterior cerebral arteries** form caudal portion of circle.

TABLE 3-7:
Posterior Cerebral Artery (Peripheral Branches) Occlusion

Regions and Structures Affected	Signs and Symptoms
Primary visual cortex or optic radiation	Homonymous hemianopia (with possible macular sparing) contralateral to damage
Bilateral occipital lobe with possible involvement of parieto-occipital region	Bilateral homonymous hemianopia, cortical blindness with denial of blindness
Dominant primary visual cortex and posterior part of corpus callosum	Dyslexia without agraphia, color anomia
Inferomedial portions of temporal lobe bilaterally or on the dominant side only (i.e., hippocampal region) Note: anterior choroidal artery is also a major supply for the hippocampal region.	Memory loss
Inferomedial temporal lobe	Prosopagnosia
Dominant visual cortex	Difficulty integrating complex visual scenes

Aneurysm on posterior communicating artery: causes compression lesion of CN III.

2. **Posterior communicating arteries** connect posterior cerebral arteries to **internal carotid arteries** close to origin of middle and anterior cerebral arteries.
3. Proximal portions of **anterior cerebral arteries** form part of rostral circle.
4. **Anterior communicating artery** connects the anterior cerebral arteries to complete the circle.

> Bifurcations within the circle of Willis are the most common site for congenital berry aneurysms. Ruptures of these aneurysms account for up to 80% of all subarachnoid hemorrhages.

Large aneurysm within arterial circle can cause bitemporal hemianopsia.

B. **Provides variable protection**
1. **Protects against vascular compromise** because anastomosing vessels allow for alternate sources of blood if one source is damaged
2. Protects during **slow occlusion** of one participating vessel but **will not protect against acute** (e.g., embolic) **occlusions**

TABLE 3-8:
Posterior Cerebral Artery (Central Branches) Occlusion

Regions and Structures Affected	Signs and Symptoms
Ventral posterior nucleus of thalamus (medial and lateral) in territory of thalamogeniculate artery	Thalamic syndrome: sensory loss (all modalities), spontaneous pain, dysesthesias
Subthalamic nucleus or its connections to globus pallidus	Choreoathetosis, hemiballismus, contralateral to damage
Oculomotor nucleus or nerve (CN III) in midbrain	Third nerve palsy (eye down and out, ptosis, mydriasis)
Cerebral peduncle	Contralateral hemiplegia
Tectum of midbrain	Paralysis or paresis of vertical eye movement; slowed, diminished pupillary responses to light
Upper motor neuron tracts in cerebral peduncle caudal to red nucleus of midbrain	Decerebrate posturing

An incomplete arterial circle occurs in up to half of the population because one posterior communicating artery or one anterior cerebral artery segment is of small diameter or is completely missing.

IV. **Venous Drainage of Cerebral Hemispheres** (Fig. 3-8)
   A. **Superficial veins**
      1. Drain surface of cerebral cortex
      2. Superior anastomotic vein drains parietal lobe to superior sagittal sinus.
      3. Inferior anastomotic vein drains posterior inferior temporal lobe into the transverse sinus.
      4. Superficial middle cerebral vein drains temporal lobe into the cavernous sinus
   B. **Deep veins**
      1. Drain subcortical regions of cerebral cortex
      2. Internal cerebral vein drains caudate nucleus, thalamus, choroid plexus of lateral ventricle into great cerebral vein.

Insidious severe headache without neurologic signs: intracranial sinus or venous thrombosis

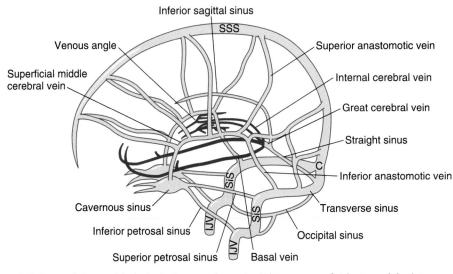

3-8: *Venous drainage of the brain.* Dark green, *deep veins;* light green, *superficial veins and dural sinuses.* C, confluence; IJV, internal jugular vein; SiS, sigmoid sinus; SSS, superior sagittal sinus.

> On imaging studies, use the **venous angle** to locate the interventricular foramen.

3. Basal vein drains insula, inferior basal ganglia, and inferior frontal lobe into great cerebral vein.
4. Great cerebral vein receives basal veins and tributaries from the cerebellum and brainstem before emptying into straight sinus.

C. **Venous sinuses**
   1. Carry blood from superficial and deep systems to internal jugular veins
   2. **Superior sagittal sinus,** at intersection of falx cerebri and overlying periosteal dura, collects superficial venous drainage

> Severe trauma with **tearing of the superior sagittal sinus** can force venous blood into the epidural space.

   3. **Inferior sagittal sinus,** formed along the free border of falx cerebri overlying corpus callosum, receives tributaries from medial aspects of cerebral hemispheres and drains into straight sinus
   4. **Straight sinus,** at junction of posterior falx cerebri and tentorium, collects deep venous drainage
   5. **Transverse sinuses,** formed at intersection of tentorium cerebelli and overlying periosteal dura, receive venous blood from superior sagittal sinus
      • Transverse sinuses fit within a groove on occipital bone and are continuous with sigmoid sinus that runs through posterior fossa on mastoid portion of petrous bone and empties into internal jugular vein at jugular foramen.

6. **Cavernous sinuses,** on either side of sphenoid bone, receive blood from ophthalmic veins, superficial middle cerebral veins, and diaphragma sellae and drain into transverse sinuses and internal jugular veins through superior and inferior petrosal sinuses, respectively.

> Lesions within the cavernous sinuses may cause ocular palsies affecting the oculomotor (CN III), trochlear (CN IV), and abducens (CN VI) nerves. Involvement of the trigeminal nerve (CN V) may lead to facial numbness.

7. **Occipital sinus,** at the falx cerebelli, drains into the confluence of sinuses.

V. **Blood Barriers**
   A. **Blood–brain barrier**
      1. **Brain capillaries** limit diffusion between blood and brain parenchyma.
         a. Endothelial cells are induced to form **tight junctions** by astrocytic end-feet.
         b. **Glucose** is actively transported from capillaries by astrocytes
         c. **Plasma proteins** and macromolecules are excluded from brain parenchyma.

> The ability of the blood–brain barrier to exclude most molecules is critical to preventing brain edema

      2. **Disruptions**
         a. **Access by infectious agents** (viruses, bacteria, fungi)
         b. **Osmotic challenges** can circumvent the barrier.

> During treatment with some forms of chemotherapy, hyperosmolar mannitol solution shrinks capillary endothelial cells, which disrupts the barrier and allows more of the drug to reach the tumor.
>   **Dye introduced during angiography** leaks into the brain at areas of rapid vascularization (e.g., tumors) because the capillaries there do not have a patent barrier.
>   **Kernicterus** in Rh-hemolytic disease is a danger because the barrier is not well developed in **newborns.** Free unconjugated bilirubin is lipid soluble.

   B. **Blood–CSF barrier:** specialized ependymal cells with tight junctions line the choroid plexus, actively transporting some substances into the ventricles while forming a barrier to general diffusion from the capillaries into the ventricles.
   C. **Arachnoid barrier:** arachnoid membrane forms an impermeable barrier around the brain and spinal cord that prevents blood from the body or the meningeal arteries from directly contacting central nervous system.

VI. **Vascular Compromise after Cerebrovascular Disease**
   A. **Cerebrovascular disease**

Hypotonia and hyporeflexia become hyperreflexia days to weeks after a stroke

> Cerebrovascular disease, or stroke, is an abrupt or rapid onset of neurologic deficit of vascular origin. Patients frequently present with focal neurologic signs that may remain fixed, rapidly improve, or progressively worsen.
>
> A patient may be asymptomatic after a stroke in which collateral flow compensates for partial or total arterial occlusion or when infarct or hemorrhage is in a silent region.

     1. **Stages of ischemic injury**
       a. **Acute** (within seconds of arterial occlusion): minimal changes in neurons, neuropil, and microvasculature (reversible)
       b. **Delayed** (6 hours after arterial occlusion): presence of red (eosinophilic) neurons (sign of apoptosis) indicates irreversible neuronal injury.
     2. **Transient ischemic attack** (TIA): transient focal neurologic deficit attributed to a specific vascular supply
       a. Frequent cause: **emboli from atherosclerotic plaques** in common or internal carotid arteries

Immediate treatment of TIA can prevent permanent brain damage

       b. **Symptoms usually last for 2 to 15 minutes** but no longer than 24 hours; permanent damage begins within minutes, although immediate administration of drugs, such as tissue plasminogen activators ("clot busters"), can prevent permanent damage

> **Transient blindness** is one of a wide range of problems caused by TIA. Patients may report that they feel a curtain is falling on their vision (amaurosis fugax).

     3. **Factors influencing outcome of ischemic crisis**
       a. **Age:** because of plasticity of the brain, a child typically recovers more rapidly and more completely than an adult.
       b. **Temperature:** reducing brain temperature by 1 degree can protect brain tissue.

> During neurosurgery, brain temperature is reduced by 7°F to 10°F to protect the brain during periods of incomplete or deficient cerebral blood flow.

Arterial vasospasm: subarachnoid hemorrhage, migraines, and cocaine use

       c. **Treatment initiated within 4 to 6 hours** of onset has the greatest likelihood of reversible stroke-related damage.
     4. **Ischemic strokes:** caused by cerebral infarction or vasospasm.
     5. **Hemorrhagic strokes:** caused by intracranial hemorrhage
   B. **Cerebral infarction**

> Cerebral infarct results from ischemia caused by occlusion or severe hypoperfusion of the contributing artery. It produces a clearly defined area of necrosis in the distribution of a cerebral artery and is the most frequent cause of stroke.

1. **Overview**
   a. **Anoxia**
      (1) Anoxic anoxia: low inspired P_{O_2}
      (2) Anemic anoxia: hemoglobin reduced
      (3) Histotoxic anoxia: cyanide poisoning
      (4) Ischemic anoxia: no blood flow
         (a) Hemodynamic failure results from cardiac disease (e.g., myocardial infarction).
         (b) Major artery stenosis
         (c) Last common path for all forms of hypoxia; severe hypoxia is rapidly followed by severe hypotension and cardiac arrest.

   > **Hypoxemia** (low arterial blood oxygen) results in tissue hypoxia or anoxia. **Ischemic anoxia** (caused by loss of blood flow) leads to tissue anoxia and local accumulation of metabolic products (e.g., lactic acid) and pH changes.

   b. **Selective vulnerability of neurons**
      (1) Neurons can tolerate ischemia for only **3 to 4 minutes** before damage is permanent
      (2) Some neurons (e.g., pyramidal cells of the CA1 region of the **hippocampus**) are particularly vulnerable to anoxia damage.
      (3) **Glutamate toxicity:** glutamate promotes ischemic cell necrosis by **persistent opening of calcium channels** (*N*-methyl-D-asparate receptors) which activates calcium-dependent proteases and lipoxygenases and caspases, causing **apoptosis.**

2. **Thrombotic infarct**
   a. **Atherothrombotic occlusion** occurs most frequently in the **internal carotid** (carotid siphon) and rostral basilar arteries.
   b. **Carotid occlusion** may be asymptomatic if the arterial circle is patent and occlusion is gradual.

   > In a patient with an incomplete arterial circle (e.g., from congenital defect or stenosis), an infarct from carotid occlusion may range from small distal lesion to the entire hemisphere. **Atherosclerosis of the basilar artery is often fatal** because the posterior circulation does not have same anastomotic protection as the anterior. **Thrombotic occlusion** may occur in individuals with **hypercoagulable states** (e.g., pancreatic adenocarcinoma). Before total occlusion, TIA suggests significant atherosclerotic disease.

3. **Embolic infarct**
   a. Emboli usually **occlude intracerebral arteries,** often producing an infarct in only part of a major cerebral artery.

   > Arterial occlusion frequently manifests as an abrupt, painless event accompanied by focal neurologic signs.

Brain anoxia caused by CO poisoning: produces multiple lesions in white matter

Thrombus: stationary clot

Thrombotic infarct: usually a pale infarct

Embolus: clot that travels

Embolic infarct: ischemic infarct

    b. **Cardiac emboli,** the **major cause of infarcts,** arise from mural thrombi or valvular heart disease

    c. **Atherosclerotic plaques** from the ascending aorta or carotids frequently shed emboli.

> Most **emboli** are sterile, but some may contain **bacteria** that may arise from acute or subacute endocarditis or lung infection.

    d. Cardiac and carotid emboli usually affect the **middle cerebral artery region.**

    e. Small emboli tend to affect most distal branches in border (watershed) zone between middle cerebral and anterior cerebral arteries.

> Ischemic infarcts (embolic or thrombotic) lead secondarily to hemorrhagic infarcts in up to three fourths of occurrences.

  4. **Watershed infarct**

    a. **Decreased brain perfusion pressure** can result from increased intracranial pressure (e.g., intracranial bleed after closed head injury).

    b. **Border zones** are the first regions to experience ischemia (see Fig. 3-4).

  5. **Multi-infarcts**

    a. **Vascular dementia** (multiple infarct dementia) is the second leading cause of dementia (Alzheimer disease is first).

    b. Likely causes: **vasculitis,** intravascular lymphoma, hypertension, and emboli

      • **Intravascular lymphoma** can produce multiple infarcts by local occlusion and is associated with vascular dementia.

C. **Intracranial hemorrhage**

  1. Cause: **rupture of any vessel in cranial cavity**

  2. **Classification**

    a. **Location:** epidural, subdural, subarachnoid, parenchymal, or intraventricular

    b. **Type** of ruptured vessel (e.g., cerebral artery, bridging vein, venous sinus)

    c. **Cause:** trauma, coagulation defect, degeneration, hypertension, or infection

> **Cranial computed tomography (CT) scan** is preferred technique for **differentiating hemorrhagic stroke from ischemic stroke.**

  3. **Intraparenchymal hemorrhage**

    a. **Causes:** amyloid angiopathy, brain tumor, blood dyscrasias, vascular malformation, and/or vasculitis

    b. Often associated with **hypertension**

      (1) **Hypertensive hemorrhage:** rupture of microaneurysm (e.g., Charcot-Bouchard aneurysm) that forms at bifurcation of small intraparenchymal arteries (lenticulostriate); aneurysm and surrounding brain tissue are destroyed.

    (2) **Lacunar infarcts:** necrotic foci 2 to 15 mm in diameter frequently found in deep areas of brain (i.e., basal ganglia, thalamus, internal capsule, cerebral white matter, and pons).
      • Often produce pure sensory or pure motor strokes

  c. **Prognosis**
    (1) **Hemorrhage** that spreads into **the ventricular system is almost always fatal.**
    (2) **Supratentorial hemorrhages** frequently lead to **progressive hemiplegias.**
    (3) **Initial mortality about 40%**
    (4) **Relatively good prognosis for initial survivors:** resolution of hematoma may be accompanied by a return of function.

4. **Subarachnoid hemorrhage**
  a. **Frequent cause: saccular** (berry, congenital) **aneurysm**
    (1) **Most frequent aneurysm** (95%)
    (2) Most are located along arterial circle and within anterior circulation
    (3) May compress cranial nerves

> Saccular aneurysms lead to subarachnoid hemorrhage, whereas microaneurysms bleed intraparenchymally.

  b. **Other causes:** atherosclerosis, infection, trauma, or rarely arteriovenous malformations
  c. **Signs and symptoms**
    (1) **Sudden, severe headache**
    (2) **Lower back pain:** sometimes more prominent than the headache
    (3) **Stiff neck** and **Kernig sign** are hallmarks (meningeal irritation).
    (4) Progression from alertness and lucidity to confusion, delirium, amnesia, lethargy, and coma; loss of consciousness implies grave prognosis.

Subarachnoid hemorrhage: "Worst headache of my life!"

  d. **Cerebral arteries** are prone to **vasospasm** following subarachnoid hemorrhage, leading to ischemic infarct.

> Of patients diagnosed with **stroke, four of five cases** are **caused by infarct.** Other causes are intracerebral hemorrhage and, less frequently, subarachnoid hemorrhage.

5. **Mixed hemorrhages**
  a. Involve **subarachnoid space** and brain **parenchyma**
  b. About 70% bleed into brain and subarachnoid space; 25% bleed into subarachnoid space alone.
  c. **Arteriovenous malformation** (AVM): usually produces mixed hemorrhage
    (1) Tangle of abnormal vessels where arteries connect directly to veins **without** intervening capillaries
    (2) About **90%** of AVMs are found in **cerebral hemispheres.**
    (3) In addition to bleeding, may "steal" blood, leading to transient ischemia

(4) Abnormal vessels separated by gliotic scar (evidence of repeated bleeds)

(5) **Signs and symptoms: may be asymptomatic;** unexplained seizures may be first sign of AVM.

D. **Hypertensive encephalopathy and vascular disease**

1. **Hypertensive encephalopathy**

   a. Associated with both **malignant hypertension** and **acute hypertension** (e.g., due to eclampsia and acute nephritis)

   b. **Signs and symptoms: headache,** drowsiness, vomiting, convulsions, progressing to stupor and coma

   c. If diastolic pressure rises above 130 mmHg, retinal exudate and hemorrhage with papilledema are seen; symptoms reverse if blood pressure is reduced.

2. **Hypertensive vascular disease:** associated with lacunar infarcts, slit hemorrhages (rupture of small penetrating arteries), and hypertensive encephalopathy

VII. **Vascular Compromise after Head Trauma**

A. **Epidural hematoma**

1. Likely source: **middle meningeal artery**
   - Meningeal arteries are within the dura and supply dura and skull, *not* the brain.

2. Likely cause: **skull fracture** in temporal region

> An epidural hematoma is a **life-threatening emergency** because the brain is compressed by the rapidly expanding mass.

B. **Subdural hematoma**

1. Likely source: **bridging veins** that drain venous blood from the brain to the superior sagittal sinus

2. Likely cause: **tear or rupture under stress**

   a. Rapid linear or angular acceleration or deceleration (e.g., from motor accidents) moves the brain relative to the skull, stretching bridging veins.

   b. Aging or prolonged alcohol use causes **brain atrophy,** which increases the distance between brain and skull.

> **Acute subdural** hematomas produce a rapidly expanding mass, constituting a life-threatening emergency. **Chronic subdural** hematomas frequently occur in elderly people and may leak slowly for several days before producing obtundation and other signs of impaired brain function.

Tearing of middle meningeal artery after skull fracture: epidural hematoma

Rapid acceleration–deceleration tears bridging veins: subdural hematoma

Neurocytology

I. **Neurons**
   A. **Function**
      1. Receive and integrate signals through **dendrites** and **soma**
      2. Communicate with other neurons and muscles through axons
   B. **Dendrites**
      1. Specialized to receive signals from other neurons; *not* **excitable** (i.e., do *not* have voltage-gated channels that support action potentials)
      2. Many processes extend from soma, each supporting hundreds of tapering branches.
      3. Invested with mushroom-shaped **dendritic spines** that can change shape with use and with some types of pathologies
      4. **Receptor proteins** in membrane **transduce** incoming neurochemical signals.
         a. Convert signals into passively conducted electrical signals
         b. May activate second-messenger pathways
   C. **Soma** (cell body, perikaryon)
      1. Receives signals from other neurons
      2. *Passively* integrates dendritic and somatic signals; *not* **excitable**
      3. **Contains all major types of cellular organelles**
         a. Golgi complex
         b. **Nissl substance:** abundant **rough endoplasmic reticulum** and free ribosomes support remodeling (synaptic plasticity) and constant secretory function (neurotransmitter release).
         c. Dispersed nuclear chromatin, reflecting high transcriptional activity
   D. **Axon hillock**
      1. **Specialized region** forming transition between soma and axon
      2. **Excitable membrane** (i.e., has voltage-gated Na^+ channels)
      3. Particularly **low threshold** for action potential generation
      4. High concentration of voltage-gated Na^+ channels makes hillock exquisitely sensitive to changes in membrane potential.
   E. **Axon**
      1. Thin process that extends through axon hillock from soma or proximal zone of a large dendrite to terminal region; can be more than 1 meter in length
      2. **Conducts individual action potentials** rapidly and efficiently over long distances to terminal regions of neuron
      3. Active conduction relies on **excitable membrane** containing voltage-gated Na^+ channels.

Myelinating cells:
oligodendrocytes (CNS),
Schwann cells (PNS)

4. Most axons are insulated with myelin derived from glial cells.
   a. **Oligodendrocytes** myelinate central nervous system (CNS) axons.
   b. **Schwann cells** myelinate peripheral nervous system (PNS) axons.
   c. **Nodes of Ranvier** are unmyelinated gaps and the only excitable region of the axon.
   d. Action potentials jump from node to node through **saltatory conduction.**
5. **C fibers** (smallest axons) are **unmyelinated**
   a. Frequently protected by "sleeves" formed by glial cells
   b. Excitable throughout their length
6. Cytoskeletal elements support extended, unique morphology and demanding transport requirements.

F. **Axon terminal**
   1. Communicates with target cells (i.e., other neurons or muscle cells)
   2. Contains **voltage-gated Ca^{2+}** channels but no voltage-gated Na^+ channels
   3. Passive spread of depolarization from axonal action potentials opens voltage-gated Ca^{2+} channels.
      • **Ca^{2+} entry** into axon terminal initiates cascade that results in **neurotransmitter release.**

G. **Variations on basic structure of neurons**
   1. **Sensory neurons** may rely on specialized elaborations or cells to transduce specific types of non-neural inputs (e.g., temperature, light, vibration).
   2. Small neurons may function without an excitable membrane.
      • Bipolar neurons of retina rely on **passive spread of electrical signals** from dendrites to terminal regions.

H. **Neuronal morphology** (Fig. 4-1)
   1. **Pseudounipolar neurons:** support general somatosensory input
      a. One main process extends from soma and bifurcates into peripheral and central branch; main process is formed from fusion of two processes.
      b. Primary sensory neurons in somatosensory chain, with cell bodies in dorsal root ganglia of spinal cord and trigeminal ganglion
   2. **Bipolar neurons:** serve special senses
      a. Two main processes extend from soma: one detects incoming signals; the other transmits information to the next neuron in sensory chain.
      b. **Primary sensory neurons** in pathways for **special senses**
         (1) *Do not* use action potentials in retina and olfactory system because bipolar neurons are small.
         (2) Use action potentials in **auditory and vestibular systems,** with cell bodies in inner ear and axons projecting to brainstem
   3. **Multipolar neurons:** most abundant form
      a. Many dendrites with one axon extending from soma.
      b. **Interneurons:** multipolar neurons with short axons that project locally
      c. **Projection neurons:** multipolar neurons supporting elongated axons that can project great distances

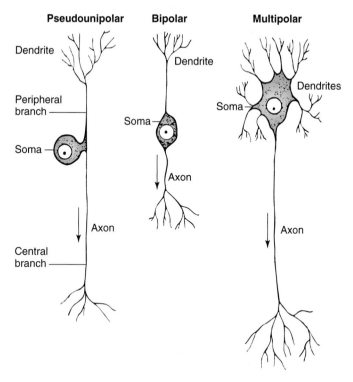

Pseudounipolar   Bipolar   Multipolar

Dendrite

Peripheral
branch

Soma

Central
branch

Axon

Dendrite

Soma

Axon

Soma

Dendrites

Axon

4-1: *Neuronal morphology. Arrows, Direction of action potential.*

    (1) **Upper motor neurons:** project from cerebral cortex and
        brainstem to lower motor neurons
    (2) **Lower motor neurons:** project to skeletal muscles
    (3) **Association neurons:** project from one gyrus or lobe to another
        within the same hemisphere

II. **Synapses**
  A. **Elements** (Fig. 4-2)
    1. **Presynaptic element:** source of information at synapse
    2. **Synaptic cleft:** physical gap between participating neurons
    3. **Postsynaptic element:** receives information through membrane
       receptors or gap junctions
    4. **Anatomic region** of a neuron **may function simultaneously** as
       presynaptic and postsynaptic element.
  B. **Types** (Fig. 4-3)
    1. **Chemical synapses**
      a. Chemical **neurotransmitters diffuse** across synaptic cleft and **bind
        to receptors on target cell**
      b. Allow subtle and specific transfer of information, depending on exact
        transmitters released presynaptically and exact postsynaptic receptors

Many pharmacologic
agents target chemical
synapses.

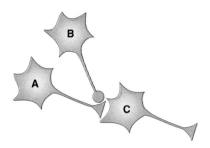

4-2: *Presynaptic and postsynaptic neurons. Neuron A forms an excitatory synapse on the soma of neuron C. Neuron B forms an inhibitory synapse on the terminal of neuron A. Thus, the terminal region of A is presynaptic to C and postsynaptic to B.*

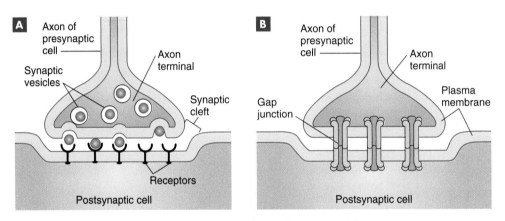

4-3: *Synapses. **A,** Chemical synapses rely on diffusion of neurochemical from presynaptic to postsynaptic membranes. **B,** Electrical synapses are points of physical communication between presynaptic and postsynaptic membranes that allow direct ionic current flow.*

     c. Allow for **integration** of information
     d. Presynaptic and postsynaptic neurons are **physically separated** by **synaptic cleft.**
     e. **Synaptic delay** (<1 msec) as transmitter molecules diffuse across synaptic cleft
  2. **Electrical synapses**
     a. Ions flow directly between cells.
     b. Allow for large numbers of cells to act as a syncytium (e.g., cardiac muscle fibers)
     c. Allow **rapid** communication with no synaptic delay
     d. Presynaptic and postsynaptic neurons are **physically connected** by **gap junctions** formed by **connexons.**

III. **Neuronal Cytoskeleton**
  A. **Microtubules** (Fig. 4-4)
    1. Composed of protofilaments consisting of alternating α- and β-tubulin subunits that confer polarity on tubule

Neurofilaments and microtubules: chief cytoskeletal elements in most mature nerve cells

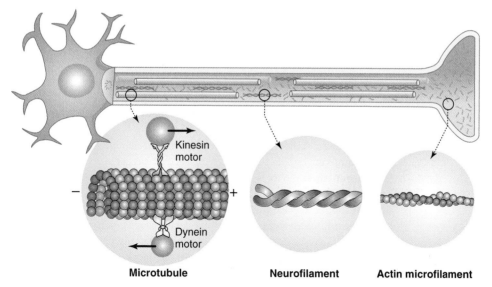

4-4: *Cytoskeletal elements of a neuron. Arrows, Direction of transport.*

2. **Exist in longitudinal arrays** in most dendrites and axons
   a. In dendrites, both orientations are found.
   b. In axons, "+" ends are away from soma.
3. **Provide tracks for axonal transport**
   a. **Kinesin** motor moves membrane-bound organelles in anterograde direction (toward "+" end) along microtubules.
   b. **Dynein** motor operates in retrograde direction (toward "−" end).
4. **Major structural framework** for neuronal growth, development, and axonal regeneration
   a. Stabilized by **microtubule-associated proteins** (MAP), including tau and MAP-2
   b. **Targeted by chemotherapeutic agents** (e.g., paclitaxel, vinblastine, and vincristine)

> Abnormalities in tau protein processing: hallmark of Alzheimer disease

B. **Neurofilaments**
   1. **Stabilize neuron shape**
   2. Major determinant of **axonal diameter**

> **Abnormal neurofilament aggregates** are histopathologic finding in neurodegenerative diseases including **amyotrophic lateral sclerosis** and **Parkinson disease.** Neurofilament and alpha-synuclein are major components in **Lewy bodies.**

C. **Actin microfilaments**
   1. Comprise two strands of globular actin monomer
   2. Homologous to thin filaments of striated muscle
   3. Found near microtubules and plasma membrane and are associated with presynaptic terminals, dendritic spines, and growth cones
   4. **Interact with extracellular matrix** and with other cells

D. **Collagen fibrils:** provide an extracellular framework for axons, although fibrils are *not* part of neuronal cytoskeleton

IV. **Axonal Transport**
A. **Fast anterograde transport** (see Fig. 4-4)
1. Moves vesicles and membrane-bound organelles away from cell body and toward axon terminal regions along microtubules using **kinesin motors**
2. **Component A** moves membrane proteins and neurotransmitters 200 to 400 mm/day.
3. **Component B** moves larger elements (e.g., mitochondria) 50 to 100 mm/day.
B. **Slow anterograde transport**
1. Moves **soluble proteins** (e.g., cytoskeletal proteins, neurofilament proteins, soluble neurotransmitter synthesizing enzymes, and proteins not membrane-bound or within organelles) 0.2 to 8 mm/day toward terminal regions.
2. Limits damaged axon regrowth to 1 to 4 mm/day.
C. **Retrograde axonal transport**
1. Moves vesicles, membrane-bound organelles, and peripherally endocytosed growth factors back to soma at a rate of 200 to 300 mm/day along microtubules using **dynein motors**
2. Allows peripheral cellular components to be degraded and recycled
3. Permits **pathogens** to **gain access to nerve cell body**
- **Rabies virus** is deposited in muscle of an animal bitten by a rabid host, and virus is taken up by nerve endings in muscle and transported centrally.

V. **Glia**
A. **Macroglia**
1. **Astrocytes**
a. Maintain stable brain environment and help transport nutrients to neurons
b. **Buffer** ions in extracellular space, particularly K^+, and help remove chemical transmitters released by active neurons
c. **End-feet** surround brain capillaries, take up glucose, and promote formation of **blood–brain barrier.**
d. During neuronal damage, can proliferate and **phagocytose dying neurons**
e. **Radial glia:** guide migration of neurons, direct outgrowth of axons in the developing brain
f. **Fibrous astrocytes:** found in white matter
g. **Protoplasmic astrocytes:** found in gray matter
2. **Oligodendrocytes** (Fig. 4-5)
a. A single oligodendrocyte myelinates segments of many CNS axons.
b. Destroyed in **slow viral diseases,** including progressive multifocal leukoencephalopathy

---

Regrowth of damaged axons: depends on slow transport to supply cytoskeletal materials

Glioblastoma multiforme: high-grade (i.e., very malignant) astrocytoma; the most common primary brain tumor

Oligodendroglioma: rare tumor of cortical white matter, frequently leading to seizures

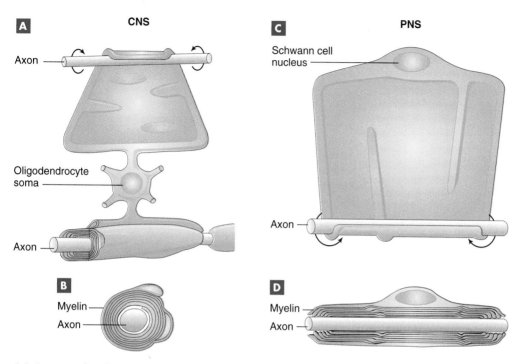

4-5: *Formation of myelin.* **A,** *In the central nervous system (CNS), an oligodendrocyte myelinates portions of several neurons.* **B,** *Cross section of myelinated axon.* **C,** *In the peripheral nervous system (PNS), a Schwann cell myelinates a portion of only one neuron.* **D,** *Longitudinal section of myelinated axon. Arrows, Direction of myelination.*

3. **Schwann cells**
   a. A **single** Schwann cell myelinates one segment of a single axon
   b. **Secrete growth factors** critical to regeneration of damaged PNS axons
   c. **Loss of myelin** characterizes several **neuropathies,** including acute **inflammatory demyelinating polyneuropathy (Guillain-Barré syndrome).**

B. **Microglia**
   1. Arise from monocytes derived from bone marrow
   2. Migrate into brain during development and **become resident microglia**
   3. Transformed into **activated microglia** to phagocytose dying cells in response to damage within CNS

> **Toxic environment** generated by dying microglia may be direct cause of CNS involvement and **dementia associated with human immunodeficiency virus type 1 (HIV-1) infection.**

C. **Ependymal cells**
   1. Non-neuronal cells within CNS
   2. **Choroid epithelial cells:** specialized ependymal cells that produce cerebrospinal fluid (CSF)

Acoustic neuroma: Schwann cell tumor of CN VIII

Microglia: susceptible to HIV-1 infection

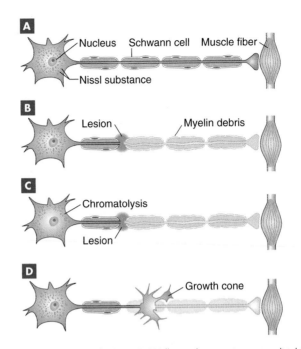

4-6: *Neuronal degeneration.* **A,** *Normal neuron.* **B,** *Wallerian degeneration occurs distal to a point of severe axonal damage.* **C,** *Chromatolysis follows.* **D,** *Reinnervation of target may occur within the peripheral nervous system.*

3. Most ependymocytes have cilia and/or microvilli at apical processes that beat to move CSF.
4. **Tanycytes** move selected molecules from blood to CSF.

> **Ependymomas** develop in the fourth ventricle in children and in filum terminale in adults.

VI. **Degeneration**
   A. **Wallerian degeneration** (Fig. 4-6)
     1. Axonal degeneration distal to point of severe axonal damage
     2. Nerve terminal fills with clumps of neurofilaments and disrupted mitochondria.
     3. Contact with postsynaptic membrane is lost, and axon segment distal to injury withdraws.
     4. Glial cells invade and phagocytose debris.
   B. **Proximal degeneration**
     1. Severe axonal damage may cause **chromatolysis** within soma: cell body swells, nucleus moves to side of soma, rough endoplasmic reticulum disintegrates
     2. **Neuron may survive:** if neuron successfully reinnervates or if axotomy does not damage all terminals, chromatolysis may reverse.

3. **Neuron may die:** neurons without functional terminal frequently undergo apoptosis.

C. **Anterograde transneuronal degeneration:** when a neuron dies, downstream synaptic target neurons may die.

D. **Retrograde transneuronal degeneration:** when a neuron dies, upstream synaptic partners may die.

VII. **Axonal Regeneration**

A. **May occur in PNS**

1. Growth cones **sprout** from proximal axon stump (see Fig. 4-6D).
2. **Schwann cells** and extracellular elements of remaining distal stump produce chemotropic factors that promote axon regrowth.
3. Axons may reinnervate muscles, although target specificity may not be perfect.
4. Some functional motor control of denervated muscle returns.

B. **Actively inhibited within CNS**

1. Oligodendrocytes actively **inhibit neurite outgrowth.**
2. Reactive astrocytes cause **glial scarring,** which interferes with nerve regrowth.
3. Fewer chemotropic factors are available in CNS.

Axon regrowth following damage: occurs in PNS; inhibited in CNS

Neurophysiology and Synaptic Interactions

I. **Basic Electrical Concepts**
- Neurons use the movement of ions across and along the membranes to receive and integrate incoming signals, to rapidly transmit information, and to pass that information to other cells.
  A. **Current (I)**
     1. **Charge** flowing past a single point
     2. In neurons, involves **cations** such as K^+, Na^+, and Ca^{2+} and **anions** such as Cl^-.
  B. **Potential difference**
     1. Work required to separate electrical charges
     2. Measured *between* two points in millivolts
     3. A neuron with **resting membrane potential** of $-70\,mV$ has a difference of $70\,mV$ between the electrical potential outside its membrane and the electrical potential inside its membrane, with the inside being the more electrically negative.
  C. **Conductance (g)**
     1. Extent to which a given pathway allows charge to flow
     2. **Inverse of resistance (R): $g = 1/R$**
     3. A membrane with **few open ion channels** has **low conductance** (and high resistance), whereas a membrane with many open channels has high conductance (and low resistance).
     4. Resistive current is produced as ions flow through membrane channels.
  D. **Ohm's law**
     1. Expresses relationship among potential difference (voltage), current, and conductance (or resistance)
     2. $V = I/g$ **(or $V = IR$)**
  E. **Capacitance (C)**
     1. Measure of separation and storage of charge
     2. **Cell membrane** is an **excellent capacitor;** it consists of two sheets of conductive material (membrane proteins and cytoplasmic ions) separated by a good insulator (lipid bilayer).
     3. **Capacitive current** results as charges accumulate on either side of a capacitor; capacitor is fully charged when it can accept and store no more charges.

Myelin: ↓ membrane capacitance and speeds membrane depolarization

II. Membrane Potentials and Signal Conduction

A. Equilibrium potential

1. Potential at which an ion's flux down its **concentration gradient** exactly balances flux down its **electrical gradient**
2. Described by **Nernst equation**

For cation X^+:

$$E_{X^+} = 61 \log \frac{[X^+]_{out}}{[X^+]_{in}}$$

For anion X^-:

$$E_{X^-} = -61 \log \frac{[X^-]_{out}}{[X^-]_{in}}$$

where

$$E = \textbf{equilibrium potential (mV)}$$

3. Determined for an ion by **concentration gradient** of that ion across cell membrane
4. Does not indicate there is *no* movement of ions, but indicates that there is no *net* movement of ions
5. Not a fixed property of an ion; varies with cell type
   - K^+ equilibrium potential in muscle cells may be $-100\,mV$, whereas it is closer to $-90\,mV$ in most neurons.

B. Resting membrane potential (RMP)

1. **Steady-state** membrane potential
   a. Results primarily from constant net flux of K^+ ions out of the neuron and smaller net flux of Na^+ into the neuron
   b. Depends on action of **Na^+/K^+ ATPase** pump that maintains both K^+ and Na^+ concentration gradients
   c. Normally, does not change with minor perturbations, such as action potential generation
2. **Goldman-Hodgkin-Katz equation** is used to calculate resting membrane potential:

$$V_m = \frac{RT}{F} \ln \frac{P_{K^+}[K^+]_{out} + P_{Na^+}[Na^+]_{out} + P_{Cl^-}[Cl^-]_{in}}{P_{K^+}[K^+]_{in} + P_{Na^+}[Na^+]_{in} + P_{Cl^-}[Cl^-]_{out}}$$

   - V_m = resting membrane potential
   - R = universal gas constant
   - T = temperature (in degrees Kelvin)
   - F = Faraday constant
   - P = permeability coefficient

3. **Resting membranes** are **most permeable to K^+**, so resting membrane potential is determined primarily by **K^+ gradient.**
4. **Changes in ion concentrations** affect resting membrane potential, which may have significant clinical impact.

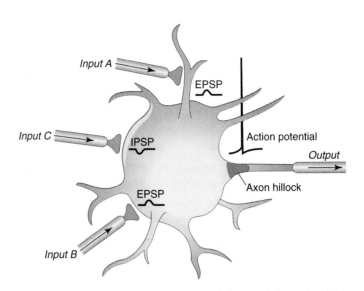

5-1: *Graded potentials. Synaptic inputs to a neuron cause graded potentials. Inputs A and B cause excitatory postsynaptic potentials (EPSP); input C causes an inhibitory postsynaptic potential (IPSP). If sufficient excitatory inputs are present to depolarize the axon hillock to threshold, that region of membrane will generate an action potential, as shown. Note that figure is not drawn to scale; action potential amplitude could easily be 20 times greater than EPSP.*

Intravenous K⁺-based
solutions: cause cardiac
fibrillation and death

    a. Infusion of K^+-based, rather than Na^+-based, solutions decreases K^+ gradient, causing K^+ equilibrium potential and RMP to become more positive.

    b. **Lethal injection with KCl** depolarizes excitable cardiac tissues, causing fibrillation.

C. **Graded potentials** (Figs. 5-1 and 5-2)

    1. Brief (milliseconds) **hyperpolarizations or depolarizations** caused by opening or closing of a select population of ion channels

    2. "Graded" because larger incoming signal affects more channels, causing a larger-amplitude change in membrane potential

    3. Move across membrane surface by **electrotonic** (passive) conduction

    4. **Signal amplitude** diminishes as depolarizing wave travels from source.

    5. **End-plate potentials** occur at motor end plate when **acetylcholine** released from the nerve terminals binds with muscle receptors to open Na^+/K^+ channels.

    6. **Receptor** or **generator potentials** occur at the sensory region of primary sensory neurons that are exposed to an adequate stimulus.

    7. **Excitatory postsynaptic potentials** (EPSPs) are produced at **dendrites** and **somas** in response to excitatory neurotransmitters.

    8. **Inhibitory postsynaptic potentials** (IPSPs) are produced at **dendrites** and **somas** in response to inhibitory neurotransmitters.

    9. **Temporal summation** occurs when a second graded potential arrives in time to build on the first, creating a larger graded potential (Fig. 5-3).

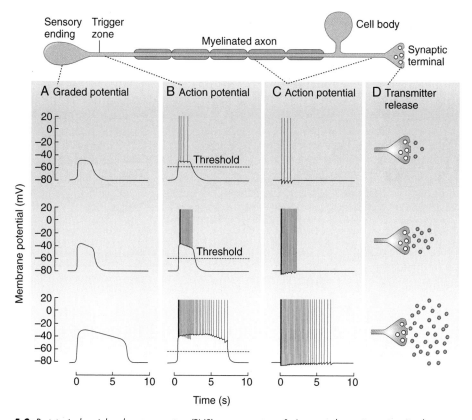

5-2: *Prototypical peripheral nervous system (PNS) sensory neuron. **A,** Larger or longer incoming stimulus causes larger or longer graded potential. **B,** Larger graded potentials are coded as increased action potential frequency, whereas longer graded potentials cause a longer train of action potentials. **C,** Action potentials carry information from the source to the terminal region without signal degradation. In PNS sensory neurons, the source is the trigger zone; in central nervous system neurons, the axon hillock is the source. **D,** Neurotransmitter release increases as terminal depolarization increases.*

10. **Spatial summation** occurs when two graded potentials arrive simultaneously on a region of a neuron and add together (Fig. 5-4).
11. **Passively conducted signals** (i.e., without action potential) are common to specialized receptor cells (e.g., retinal rods and cones, inner ear hair cells) and small neurons (e.g., olfactory bipolar neurons, retinal bipolar neurons, and retinal horizontal cells).

D. **Action potential** (Fig. 5-5)
   1. Generated by **excitable membrane,** containing **voltage-gated ion channels**
      a. Na⁺ channel opening depolarizes membrane.
         • Channels respond in a probabilistic fashion to membrane potential. At more depolarized membrane potentials, the probability that a given channel will be "open" is higher.
      b. K⁺ channel opening accelerates repolarization of membrane.

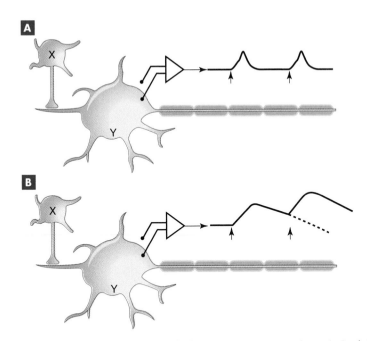

5-3: *Temporal summation.* **A,** *Neuron X excites a dendrite on neuron Y two times (arrows). Graded potentials can be measured some distance away. However, because the time constant of the membrane is short, the first excitatory postsynaptic potential (EPSP) has died before the second arrives, and they do not add.* **B,** *Time constant of the membrane is longer, so the first EPSP has not died before the second arrives. The second EPSP builds on the first, causing a larger depolarization.*

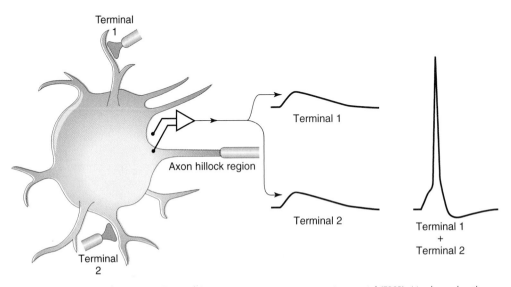

5-4: *Spatial summation. Terminal 1 causes an excitatory postsynaptic potential (EPSP). Membrane length constant is large enough to allow the EPSP to reach the axon hillock. Similarly, terminal 2 causes an EPSP to reach the axon hillock. Neither alone is sufficient to take the hillock to threshold. However, when the EPSPs from terminals 1 and 2 arrive simultaneously at the hillock, they add, and the resulting depolarization is large enough to bring the axon hillock to threshold.*

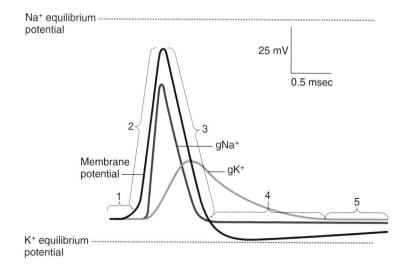

Na⁺ equilibrium potential

25 mV

0.5 msec

2 3

gNa⁺

Membrane potential

gK⁺

1 4 5

K⁺ equilibrium potential

5-5: *Ionic basis of the action potential. (1) At rest, few leak channels are open, and conductance is low. However, many more K⁺ channels than Na⁺ channels are open, and membrane potential is much closer to K⁺ equilibrium potential than to Na⁺ equilibrium potential. (2) Depolarization is due to rapid opening of many voltage-gated Na⁺ channels, causing a dramatic increase in gNa⁺. (3) Early repolarization is due to the combined effects of automatic closing of voltage-gated Na⁺ channels plus recruitment of voltage-gated K⁺ channels. (4) The hyperpolarizing afterpotential is due to delayed closing of voltage-gated K⁺ channels. The increased gK⁺ due to the combined effects of K⁺ leak channels plus voltage-gated K⁺ channels moves membrane potential even closer to K⁺ equilibrium potential. (5) As voltage-gated K⁺ channels close, the membrane returns to resting state.*

   2. **All-or-none** if a membrane depolarizes to **threshold**
   3. **Actively transmitted** over long distances from cell body to nerve terminal **without signal degradation**
   4. **Refractory periods prevent a second action potential** during the first action potential.
      a. During **absolute refractory period** (immediately after action potential), neuron cannot produce another action potential.
      b. During **relative refractory period** (after absolute refractory period), only a strong stimulus will induce an action potential.
   5. Action potentials do not add; rather, information is coded in the frequency and pattern of action potentials.
   6. Large transient inward and outward currents generated during an action potential require energy-consuming pumps (Na⁺/K⁺ ATPase) to maintain necessary ion gradients.

III. **Myelination**
  A. **Myelin**
   1. **Electrical insulation** surrounding axons (see Fig. 4-5)
   2. **Increases membrane resistance** of axons
      a. Increased membrane resistance increases length constant, which allows current generated by action potentials to travel further.

b. Increased length constant allows **nodes of Ranvier** to be spaced far apart on an axon.

3. **Decreases membrane capacitance** by increasing charge separation
   a. Decreased membrane capacitance decreases membrane time constant, allowing membrane to charge and discharge more rapidly.
   b. Rapid membrane charging allows for faster conduction of action potentials.

4. Most peripheral nervous system (PNS) axons of at least 1 μm diameter and most central nervous system (CNS) axons of at least 0.25 μm are myelinated.

B. **Nodes of Ranvier**
1. **Segments of excitable membrane** that interrupt myelination every 0.5- to 1.0-mm intervals
2. Allow for **saltatory** ("jumping") **conduction**
   a. Neurons **conserve energy** by producing action potentials only at nodes.
   b. Increases rate of action potential conduction
3. **Voltage-gated Na⁺ channels** stabilized at nodes
4. **Voltage-gated K⁺ channels** stabilized adjacent to nodes

> Demyelination (e.g., from **multiple sclerosis**) leads to redistribution of voltage-gated channels throughout length of axon.

C. **Schwann cells**
1. **Supply myelin to PNS**
2. Each supplies a portion of only one axon.
3. **Acute inflammatory demyelinating neuropathy** (Guillain-Barré syndrome)
   a. Most common immune-mediated disorder to affect peripheral myelin
   b. Frequent presentation: **weakness ascending** rapidly from **legs to arms** and finally to **face, without sensory involvement.**
   c. **Progression:** may be less than 2 weeks from first signs of weakness to respiratory insufficiency requiring ventilatory support
4. Some **diabetic neuropathies** cause peripheral demyelination.
   a. May affect sensory, motor, or autonomic systems or a combination
   b. **Signs: stocking-and-glove distribution** of sensory loss
5. **Peroneal muscular atrophy** (Charcot-Marie-Tooth disease)
   a. Family of **genetic** disorders affecting **peripheral myelin**
   b. **Progression:** slow, causing muscle weakness and mild sensory loss
   c. **Signs: "stork-like legs," clumsiness,** and eventual difficulty with fine motor skills

D. **Oligodendrocytes** (see Fig. 4-5)
1. Glia responsible CNS myelination
2. One oligodendrocyte provides myelin to up to at least 40 different axons.
3. **Multiple sclerosis**
   a. **Inflammatory progressive disorder** destroying central myelin
   b. Multiple lesions disseminated in space and time, commonly periventricular, viewed on magnetic resonance imaging (Fig. 5-6)

Acute inflammatory demyelinating neuropathy: rapid onset, ascending PNS disorder

Diabetes mellitus: damages peripheral myelin and axons

Multiple sclerosis: destroys CNS myelin, causing sensory and motor deficits

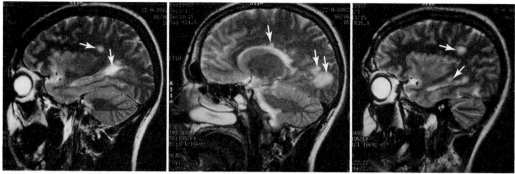

| Left hemisphere | Midline | Right hemisphere |

5-6: *Multiple sclerosis demonstrated by magnetic resonance imaging. Arrows, Multiple demyelinating plaques.*

    c. **Cause:** unknown, but genetic susceptibility, autoimmunity, and viral infections have been implicated.

    d. **Frequent presentation**
       (1) **Third or fourth decade** of life
       (2) Incidence is slightly higher in **women.**

    e. **Signs and symptoms**
       (1) **Blurry or sudden loss of vision:** optic neuritis, frequent initial finding
       (2) **Ataxia and scanning speech:** cerebellar involvement
       (3) **Urinary incontinence, muscle weakness,** and **paresthesias:** demyelination of long tracks
       (4) **Jerky eye movements: internuclear ophthalmoplegia** from pontine demyelination in **medial longitudinal fasciculus**

IV. **Synaptic Transmission**
  A. **Electrical synapses** (Fig. 5-7)
    1. **Rapid** but limited communication
    2. Membranes of the presynaptic and postsynaptic neurons contain connexons formed by specialized proteins that link across the space, separating the cells.
    3. Connexons form a **gap junction** (aqueous pore of communicating cytoplasm).
    4. No delay and minimal modification of signal, because flow of ions between cells is direct
  B. **Chemical synapses** (Fig. 5-8)
    1. **Slower than electrical** but allow for more **complex** signaling
      a. **Release of neurotransmitter** from presynaptic terminal **requires calcium,** which enters through voltage-dependent calcium channels.
      b. Voltage-dependent calcium channels open as action potentials depolarize the terminal (see Fig. 5-2).

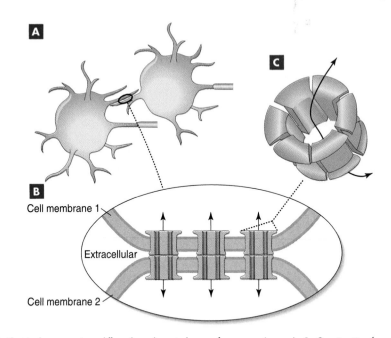

5-7: Electrical synapse. Ions diffuse through central pore of connexon (arrows). **A,** Gap junction forms between dendrites of two neurons. **B,** Gap junction. **C,** Connexon.

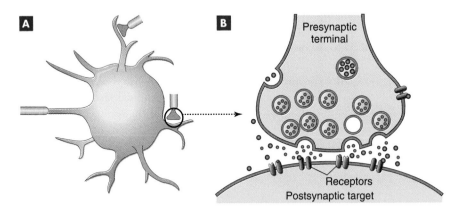

5-8: Chemical synapse. **A,** Axon terminal forms chemical synapse on dendrite of another neuron. **B,** Two neurotransmitters (gray and green dots) are released by presynaptic terminal. One (green) has postsynaptic effect. The other (gray), by binding both to postsynaptic receptors and presynaptic autoreceptors, can affect both postsynaptic target and activities of the presynaptic terminal.

    c. **Synaptic cleft:** space between presynaptic axon terminal and postsynaptic membrane through which transmitter diffuses

    d. **Postsynaptic responses** depend on **receptor.**

2. **Direct gating:** ligand-gated receptors

    a. Binding of neurotransmitter opens or closes an ion channel within the receptor.

    b. Result of **ligand-gated channel activation** is a rapid change in postsynaptic membrane potential (EPSP or IPSP).

    c. Several **neurotransmitters** can activate directly gated channels, including **glutamate, acetylcholine,** γ-aminobutyric acid **(GABA), glycine,** and serotonin.

3. **Indirect gating:** non–channel-linked receptors

    a. **Binding of neurotransmitter** activates second-messenger pathways by way of guanosine triphosphate–binding (G proteins).

    b. **Signal transduction pathways** activated by second messengers may have multiple and lasting effects.

    c. **Second-messenger pathways:** cyclic adenosine monophosphate, phosphoinositide, and prostaglandin

Benzodiazepines: potentiate chloride conductance through GABA receptors within CNS

Nonsteroidal anti-inflammatory drugs (aspirin and indomethacin): inhibit prostaglandin formation

Neurochemistry

I. **Substrates for Central Nervous System Metabolism**
   A. **Carbohydrates**
      1. **Glucose**
         a. Primary source for energy in the brain
            (1) Energy generated through **aerobic oxidation**
            (2) During **prolonged starvation** and in neonates, brain can use **ketone bodies** as energy source.
         b. Levels in the brain depend on levels in the blood and **uptake across the blood–brain barrier.**
         c. Crosses blood–brain barrier by **insulin-independent facilitated diffusion**
         d. **Hypoglycemia**
            (1) Brain glycogen stores are small (about 10% of muscle)
            (2) Glycogen levels in the brain vary directly with plasma glucose levels.
            (3) Repeated episodes of hypoglycemia **damage neurons.**
   B. **Amino acids**
      1. **Neutral amino acids** (histidine, isoleucine, leucine, methionine, phenylalanine, tryptophan, tyrosine, and valine) and **precursor L-dopa compete for transport across blood–brain barrier.**
      2. **Small neutral amino acids** (alanine, glycine, and proline): synthesized in the brain
      3. **Basic and acidic amino acids:** transported into the brain
      4. **Glutamate, aspartate, glutamine,** and γ-aminobutyric acid (GABA)
         a. Synthesized in the brain
         b. High content in the brain relative to rest of body
         c. Pharmacologically active as **neurotransmitters**
         d. **Glutamate, aspartate** and GABA are metabolic intermediates as well as neurotransmitters.
            • Glutamate and aspartate use a slow transporter to cross blood–brain barrier.
      5. **Dietary sources** affect neurotransmitter availability through competition for transporters.
         a. Large neutral amino acids, such as tyrosine (catecholamine precursor) and tryptophan (serotonin precursor), share a common transporter
         b. **Dietary proteins** contain small amounts of tryptophan, which allow other large neutral amino acids to out-compete it for the uptake transporter.

Breast-feeding infant's brain: uses ketone bodies because mother's milk has high fat content

Hypoglycemia: can induce seizures

High-protein diet: reduces levels of tryptophan in the brain

TABLE 6-1:
Pharmacology of the Cholinergic System

Terminal	Preganglionic	Postganglionic Parasympathetic	CNS	CNS
	N_G M_1	M_2	M_1 M_2	N
Target	Autonomic ganglion	Smooth or cardiac muscle	CNS	CNS
Receptor type	Nicotinic	Muscarinic	Muscarinic	Nicotinic
Example of action	Excite postganglionic neuron	Decrease cardiac output ($\downarrow$heart rate, $\downarrow$ contractility)		May enhance memory; weak analgesic; linked to rare genetic form of epilepsy
Agonist	Nicotine	Muscarine	Muscarine Others under development for treatment of pain	Nicotine Others under development for treatement of Alzheimer disease, etc.
Antagonist	Trimethaphan (e.g., vasodilation to counter hypertensive crisis)	Atropine (e.g., to relax smooth muscle and as an anticholinesterase antidote)	Scopolamine (e.g., CNS depression and amnesia)	NA

    c. **Dietary carbohydrates** reduce plasma levels of all large neutral amino acids except tryptophan; facilitated tryptophan uptake increases synthesis of serotonin.

C. **Lipids**
    1. Function as **chemical messengers** (e.g., steroid hormones and eicosanoids)
    2. Structural membrane component of **myelin**
    3. Three categories: **cholesterol, sphingolipids,** and **glycerophospholipids**
      a. Cholesterol is only sterol in the brain in significant levels.
      b. Major structural lipids: cerebroside (a sphingolipid) and cholesterol
    4. **Genetic defects** in sphingolipid degradation cause Niemann-Pick, Gaucher, and Tay-Sachs diseases.

Niemann-Pick disease: defective cholesterol transport

II. **Metabolic Diseases**
- Deficiencies in carbohydrate, amino acid, and lipid metabolism can impair cerebral function.
  A. **Phenylketonuria** (PKU)
     1. Inborn error of metabolism affecting 1 in 20,000 infants
     2. **Lack of phenylalanine hydroxylase** leads to **increased phenylalanine** and **decreased tyrosine**
     3. Phenylalanine metabolites (e.g., phenylpyruvic acid) damage central nervous system (CNS) myelin, **impairing brain function.**
     4. **Signs and symptoms:** marked irritability, severe vomiting, seizures, musty odor, and eventual **mental retardation;** progressive disorder
     5. **Treatment:** restricted dietary phenylalanine
  B. **Tay-Sachs disease**
     1. Lipid-storage disease transmitted as **autosomal recessive** trait
     2. **Deficiency of hexosaminidase** found in lysosomes involved in ganglioside degradation
     3. **Lipids and proteins accumulate** in membranous cytoplasmic bodies.
     4. Incidence is about 1 in 3,000 in eastern and central European (Ashkenazi) Jews
     5. **Signs and symptoms:** seizures, vision and hearing loss, mental retardation, and eventual paralysis; progressive disorder.
     6. **Death** often occurs **within 3 to 5 years.**

> Excessive excretion of neutral amino acids (tryptophan) in the urine caused by defective absorption from the intestine and reabsorption from the kidney can cause mental retardation, headache, gait disorders, and fainting.

III. **Small-Molecule Neurotransmitters**
  A. **Metabolism**
     1. Synthesized at terminal region and packaged into small synaptic vesicles
     2. Inactivated by reuptake into terminals after release or degraded in synaptic cleft
     3. Repackaged, allowing sustained synaptic activation
  B. **Acetylcholine** (Fig. 6-1)
     1. **Neurotransmitter** of specific regions in the brain, including basal forebrain, and of effector neurons that project from CNS into peripheral nervous system
        a. Lower motor neurons projecting to neuromuscular junction
        b. Sympathetic and parasympathetic preganglionic neurons
        c. Parasympathetic postganglionic neurons
     2. Synthesized in terminals from acetyl coenzyme A and from choline by choline acetyltransferase
     3. Degraded into acetyl coenzyme A and choline in synaptic cleft by **acetylcholinesterase.**
     4. **Choline is reuptaken** into terminal for recycling into acetylcholine. **Reuptake** is blocked by **hemicholinium.**

Cholinesterase inhibitors: ↑ acetylcholine concentration at synapses; treat Alzheimer disease and myasthenia gravis

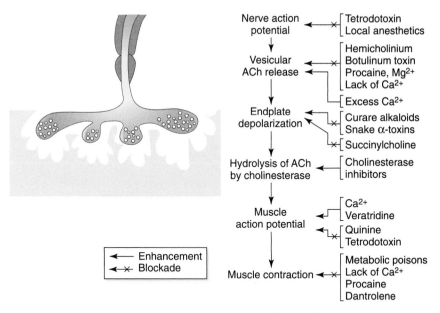

6-1: *Pharmacology of motor end plate. ACh, acetylcholine.*

C. **Biogenic amines: catecholamines**

1. **Dopamine** (Fig. 6-2)

   a. Sources: mesencephalic **substantia nigra** and ventral tegmental area

   b. Rate-limiting step for synthesis is **conversion of tyrosine to L-dopa** in the nerve terminal by **tyrosine hydroxylase.**

   c. **L-Dopa**

      (1) Converted to dopamine by L-dopa decarboxylase

      (2) **Carbidopa blocks conversion** of L-dopa **to dopamine** in the periphery, thus increasing the availability of L-dopa for conversion into dopamine in the brain.

      (3) Used in the treatment of **Parkinson disease**

   d. **Inactivation:** by reuptake into terminals

      (1) **Reuptake** is **blocked by cocaine.**

      (2) **Methylphenidate,** a dopamine transporter blocker, is effective in treatment of **attention deficit hyperactivity disorder.**

   e. **Degradation:** by monoamine oxidase (MAO; intraneuronal) and catechol-*O*-methyltransferase (COMT; extraneuronal)

   f. **Metabolite: homovanillic acid** (HVA)

      (1) Reflect activity of the dopamine systems

      (2) Cerebrospinal fluid (CSF) levels can be used to assess disease state (e.g., Parkinson and Huntington diseases and schizophrenia).

Cocaine: blocks reuptake of catecholamines

L-Dopa: crosses the blood–brain barrier; dopamine does not

Parkinson disease: ↓ HVA levels can be detected in the CSF.

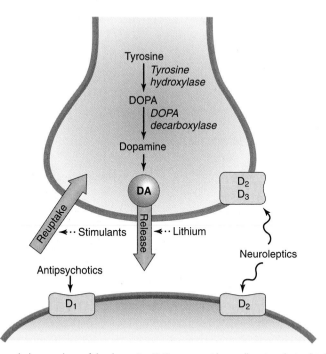

6-2: *Chemistry and pharmacology of the dopamine (DA) synapse. Almost all antipsychotics bind to the D_2 receptor, and some bind to the D_1 receptor.*

  g. **Lithium**
   (1) **Interferes with dopamine neurotransmission** presynaptically and postsynaptically
   (2) Used in the treatment of bipolar disorder and severe aggression
  h. **Agonists:** bromocriptine, ropinirole, and pramipexole
 2. **Norepinephrine** (Fig. 6-3)
  a. **Sources: locus ceruleus,** lateral tegmental nuclei of brainstem, and most **postganglionic sympathetic neurons**
  b. Shares cytoplasmic synthetic pathway with dopamine
  c. **Conversion** of dopamine to norepinephrine by **dopamine-β-hydroxylase** occurs within vesicles in nerve terminal.
  d. **Inactivation is** by **reuptake** into terminals and is **blocked by cocaine.**
  e. **Degradation is** by MAO (intraneuronal) and **catechol-*O*-methyltransferase** (extraneuronal)
  f. **Metabolites**
   (1) **3-Methoxy-4-hydroxyphenylglycol (MHPG):** found in CSF
   (2) **Vanillylmandelic acid:** found in urine, index of sympathetic function
  g. **Agonists:** ephedrine, phenylephrine, and propranolol
 3. **Epinephrine**
  a. Synthesized primarily in **adrenal medulla**

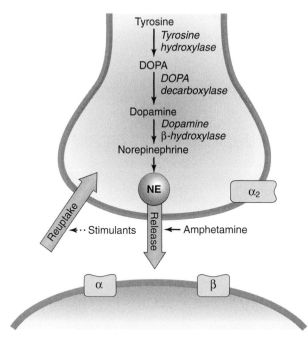

6-3: *Chemistry and pharmacology of the norepinephrine (NE) synapse.*

    b. Phenylethanolamine *N*-methyltransferase (PNMT) converts norepinephrine to epinephrine.

    c. At high concentrations may activate norepinephrine receptors

D. **Biogenic amines: indolamines**

  1. **Serotonin** (5-hydroxytryptamine) (Fig. 6-4)

    a. Synthesized primarily in brainstem **raphe nuclei**

    b. Rate-limiting step for synthesis is conversion from tryptophan by **tryptophan hydroxylase**

    c. **Inactivation**

      (1) By reuptake into nerve terminals

      (2) **Serotonin reuptake inhibitors** (SRIs) increase serotonin synaptic activity.

    d. **Degradation:** by MAO

      (1) Most serotonin is converted to 5-hydroxyindole acetic acid (5-HIAA).

      (2) **MAO inhibitor antidepressants** potentiate both catecholaminergic and serotonergic transmission.

  2. **Histamine**

    a. Diffusely distributed within CNS

    b. Rate-limiting enzyme for synthesis: histidine decarboxylase

E. **Amino acid neurotransmitters**

  1. **Glutamate** (Fig. 6-5)

    a. Acts through **ligand-gated channel receptors** to mediate fast excitatory transmission in CNS and through G-protein–coupled

Toxic epinephrine side effect: cardiac arrhythmias

↑ Urinary 5-HIAA: indicates carcinoid syndrome

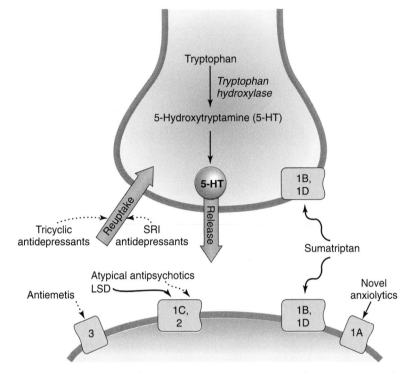

6-4: *Chemistry and pharmacology of the serotonin (5-HT) synapse. 5-HT, 5-hydroxytryptamine; LSD, lysergic acid diethylamide; SRI, serotonin reuptake inhibitor; 1A, 1B, 1C, 1D, 2, and 3, are receptor subtypes.*

(metabotropic) receptors to mediate slower and more complex responses.

    b. **Inactivation:** uptake by glia followed by conversion to glutamine and return to the neuron terminal where it can be converted to glutamate

    c. Excessive extraneuronal glutamate is **excitotoxic,** triggering **apoptosis.**

2. **GABA** (Fig. 6-6)

    a. Major **inhibitory** CNS neurotransmitter

    b. Synthesized from glutamate by **glutamic acid decarboxylase**

    c. **Inactivation:** by reuptake into nerve terminals (for reuse) and by glia

    d. **Valproate,** an anticonvulsant used to **control seizures,** increases GABA concentration by stimulating glutamic acid decarboxylase and inhibiting degradative enzymes.

3. **Glycine**

    a. **Inhibitory** neurotransmitter in brainstem and spinal cord used by Renshaw cells (inhibitory neurons responsible for recurrent inhibition)

    b. **Receptor:** direct ligand-gated Cl⁻ channel

Poststroke: Glutamate excitotoxicity causes neuronal cells to undergo apoptosis.

Altered GABA function: basal ganglia disorders, seizures, schizophrenia, and sleep disorders

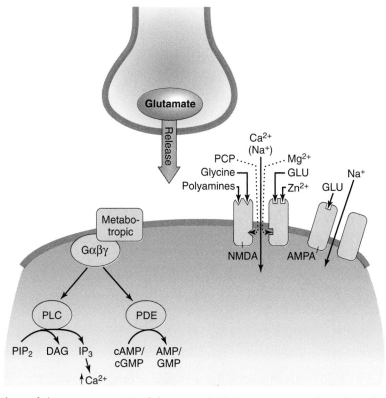

6-5: *Classes of glutamate receptors. N-methyl-D-aspartate (NMDA) receptor is primarily a calcium channel. Aminohydroxymethylisoxazole propionate (AMPA) receptor is a ligand-gated sodium channel. Metabotropic receptors are coupled to G protein (G), and each is coupled to a different second messenger system. AMP, adenosine monophosphate; cAMP, cyclic AMP; DAG, diacylglycerol; GMP, guanosine monophosphate; cGMP, cyclic GMP; IP$_3$, inositol 1,4,5-triphosphate; PCP, phencyclidine; PDE, phosphodiesterase; PIP, phosphatidylinositol phosphate; PLC, phospholipase C.*

Strychnine is a glycine receptor antagonist. Tetanus toxin is carried to inhibitory interneurons and prevents release of GABA and glycine. Both release motor neurons from inhibitory modulation, resulting in excess motor activity, muscle spasm, and potentially respiratory failure and death.

IV. **Neuroactive Peptides**
  A. **Metabolism**
    1. Synthesized in cell body
    2. More than one neuroactive peptide may be formed from a larger precursor molecule (e.g., proenkephalin gives rise to methionine-enkephalin, leucine-enkephalin and several extended enkephalins).
    3. Packaged into **large dense-core vesicles**
    4. **Can be depleted** at the terminal under sustained high-frequency stimulation

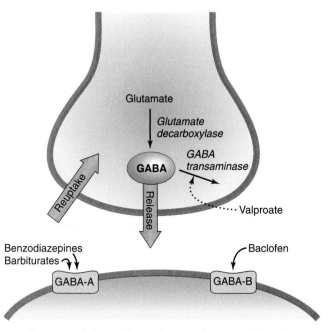

6-6: Chemistry and pharmacology of the γ-aminobutyric acid (GABA) synapse.

    5. Neuroactive peptides and small-molecule neurotransmitters are frequently **co-localized** at terminals.
    6. Often coupled to second messengers and frequently **modulate actions of small neurotransmitters** with which they are co-released
  B. **Common neuroactive peptides**
    1. **Tachykinins: substance P,** substance K, and neurokinins A and B
    2. **Secretins:** secretin, **vasoactive intestinal peptide,** and growth hormone–releasing hormone
    3. **Insulins:** insulin and insulin-like growth factors I and II
    4. **Pituitary peptides:** arginine vasopressin and oxytocin
    5. **Peptides** related to **pancreatic polypeptide:** neuropeptide Y
    6. **Opioids:** methionine and leucine **enkephalin, β-endorphin,** and dynorphin
    7. **Other small molecules:** angiotensin II, calcitonin gene-related peptide, cholecystokinin, corticotropin-releasing factor, and somatostatin

V. **Recently Identified Nontraditional Neurotransmitters**
  A. **Nitric oxide**
    1. Produced as a gas with a short duration of action
    2. Can act as a **retrograde** neurotransmitter because it can be produced in the postsynaptic neuron and diffuse to the presynaptic terminal
    3. Functions include **relaxation of blood vessels** and synaptic plasticity.
  B. **Anandamide**
    1. **Cannabinoid** receptor ligand

2. Fatty acid amide that is cleaved from a membrane-bound phospholipid precursor

VI. **Neurotransmitter Receptors**
   A. **General features**
      1. **Allow neurons to communicate using chemical signals**
         a. **Membrane spanning proteins** located on dendrites, soma, and terminals
         b. Bind ligands with high specificity
      2. **Determine response of neurons**
         a. **Inhibitory receptors**
            (1) Frequently located on soma
            (2) Decrease likelihood that neuron will produce an action potential
            (3) May inhibit by **hyperpolarizing** the neuron
         b. **Excitatory receptors**
            (1) Frequently located on dendrites
            (2) Increase likelihood that neuron will produce an action potential
            (3) Generally cause membrane **depolarization**
         c. **Modulatory receptors**
            (1) Located on terminals
            (2) Do *not* affect excitability of neuron, but can affect amount of neurotransmitter released by local terminal
      3. **May be regulated by activity**
         a. Activity can stabilize receptors in a membrane.
         b. **Down-regulation:** increased activity sometimes decreases receptor number.
         c. **Up-regulation:** decreased activity sometimes increases receptor number.
   B. **Classes**
      1. **Ionotropic receptors**
         a. **Direct-gated** (ligand-gated) channel receptors
         b. Ion channels opened or closed by neurotransmitter binding
         c. Electrical response is **fast** and of **short duration**
      2. **Metabotropic receptors**
         a. **Indirect-gated receptors** (channels linked to second messengers) or **receptors linked to G proteins**
         b. **Effects of activation**
            (1) Opens or closes membrane channels, causing a slow and long electrical response
            (2) Initiates intracellular enzyme cascades
            (3) Amplifies signal
            (4) Interacts with other second-messenger pathways
            (5) **Modifies gene transcription**
   C. **Cholinergic receptors**
      1. **Nicotinic subtypes:** neuromuscular junction, at autonomic preganglionic synapses, some CNS synapses

> The nicotinic acetylcholine receptor is the target of immune response in **myasthenia gravis.**

   2. **Muscarinic subtypes:** parasympathetic postganglionic synapses (on target organs), some CNS synapses.
D. **Dopaminergic receptors** (see Fig. 6-2)
   1. Two families: D_1 (D_1, D_5) and D_2 (D_2, D_3, D_4)
   2. **Treatment of Parkinson disease:** increase availability of dopamine to striatal dopamine receptors
   3. **Treatment of schizophrenia:** block mesolimbic and cortical dopamine receptors (especially D_2 subtypes)

> Newer **atypical antipsychotics** effectively target mesolimbic dopamine receptors and spare basal ganglia receptors, thus avoiding **tardive dyskinesia.**

E. **Adrenergic receptors** (see Fig. 6-3)
   1. α **and** β; α_2 is the major CNS subtype.
   2. **Activation** of CNS receptors may **increase blood pressure** and **heart rate** independent of effects at peripheral adrenergic receptors.
   3. Additional effects of receptor activation: **elevated mood** and **increased wakefulness** and **attention**

Antidepressant effects of SRIs: reflect activated serotonin autoreceptors and ↑ activity of serotonergic synapses

F. **Serotonergic receptors** (see Fig. 6-4)
   1. About **20 serotonin receptor subtypes,** including receptors linked by second messengers and ligand-gated channels (e.g., K^+)
   2. Serotonin release strongly regulated by autoreceptors, which are found on the presynaptic terminal; autoreceptor activation limits further neurotransmitter release.

Antihistamines: sedate by blocking hypothalamic histamine receptors

G. **Histamine receptors** (see Fig. 6-5)
   1. Family of receptors (H_1, H_2, H_3) located in CNS, peripheral nervous system (PNS), bronchial smooth muscle, gastric mucosa, cardiac tissue, and mast cells
   2. **Multiple actions**
      a. Mediate response to inflammation and tissue damage in the nervous system
      b. Activate pain and itch receptors in periphery
      c. Promote **acid secretion** in stomach
      d. **Hypothalamic histamine receptor activation** leads to increased **wakefulness** and **suppressed appetite**
H. **Glutamate receptors**
   1. Located throughout the brain and expressed by both neurons and glia
   2. **Ionotropic:** ligand-gated cation channels, activated rapidly (milliseconds)
      a. **NMDA** (*N*-methyl-D-aspartate) **receptors**
         (1) Calcium channels that are Mg^{2+} and glycine dependent
         (2) Functions in **synapse development** and plasticity, including **long-term potentiation** and **depression**

      b. **AMPA** (aminohydroxymethylisoxazole propionate) receptors
        (1) Cation channels
        (2) Ampakines increase AMPA channel activity, improve cognitive function.
      c. **Kainate receptors**
        (1) Cation channels
        (2) Activation has been associated with temporal lobe seizure induction
    3. Metabotropic receptors: see section VI.B.2

I. **GABA receptors** (see Fig. 6-6)

    1. **GABA$_A$**
      a. Direct-gated Cl$^-$ channel
      b. **Benzodiazepines** (e.g., diazepam) bind to GABA$_A$ receptors.
      c. Agonists include muscimol; antagonists include bicuculline.
    2. **GABA$_B$**
      a. **Linked to G protein;** inhibits K$^+$ permeability, decreasing Ca^{2+} influx
      b. Agonists include **baclofen,** which acts as a muscle relaxant to prevent spasticity.

J. **Cannabinoid receptors**

    1. **Three known types: CB$_1$** (CNS and PNS), **CB$_2$** (PNS), **CB$_3$** (CNS)
    2. Activation associated with neural protection against excitotoxicity (e.g., modulating Ca^{2+} influx through the NMDA receptor/channel) and with **endogenous analgesia.**
    3. **Cannabinoids** can **modulate** (inhibit) **pain transmission** by binding to peripheral (dorsal root ganglion) and central (dorsal horn of the spinal cord) cannabinoid receptors.

K. **Drug–receptor interactions**

    1. **Mimetics** mimic a neurotransmitter effect.
    2. **Agonists** bind and activate receptor.
    3. **Antagonists** bind and prevent activation of receptor.
    4. **Reuptake into terminal** is a common method of neurotransmitter inactivation in CNS.
      a. May potentiate effects of neurotransmitter in synapse
      b. May decrease further neurotransmitter availability

VII. **Neurotoxins**

    A. **Botulinum toxin** (clostridial neurotoxin)
      1. Produced by bacterium *Clostridium botulinum*
      2. **Blocks neuromuscular and autonomic transmission** by blocking acetylcholine release
      3. **Cleaves proteins** needed for vesicle fusion at peripheral cholinergic nerve endings
      4. In **adults,** most frequently contracted by **ingesting improperly canned food**
      5. Prevalence high in **infants** younger than 1 year: botulinum spores can grow in the infant intestine, releasing toxin.
      6. Wound botulism occurs if bacteria infects wound.

GABAergics: seizure disorder treatment; benzodiazepine treats anxiety and causes sedation

Neurotoxins: exert presynaptic or postsynaptic effects

Botulinum: most lethal toxin known

Infants <1 year: susceptible to botulinum poisoning from spores found in honey

7. **Signs and symptoms of toxicity**
    a. **Descending paralysis:** blurred vision; difficulties with speech, swallowing, and breathing; dry mouth; muscle weakness in arms and legs
    b. **Death** by paralysis of respiratory muscles
8. Therapeutic use: **controls focal muscle spasms** (e.g., cervical dystonia)

B. **Tetanus toxin** (clostridial neurotoxin)
    1. Produced by bacterium *Clostridium tetani*
    2. Spores are ubiquitous but require anaerobic conditions to germinate: deep puncture wounds supply appropriate conditions.
    3. **Released into CNS** after retrograde transport by peripheral nerves; taken up by inhibitory neurons
    4. **Cleaves proteins** needed for vesicle fusion (synaptobrevin), **preventing release of inhibitory neurotransmitter** (GABA and glycine)
    5. **Signs and symptoms:** muscle spasms and tetanus from loss of motor neuron inhibition

C. **α-Latrotoxin** (black widow spider venom)
    1. Releases massive amounts of neurotransmitters at neuromuscular junction until neurotransmitter stores are depleted
    2. **Signs and symptoms**
        a. Hyperexcitability, muscle spasms, and rigidity followed by loss of neuromuscular transmission, paralysis
        b. Death by asphyxiation; less than 1% of cases are fatal

D. **Tetrodotoxin**
    1. Blocks voltage-gated Na^+ channels
    2. Lethal quantities in **puffer fish** (served as sushi or sashimi)
    3. **Signs and symptoms:** numbness, paralysis, and possible respiratory failure

7 CHAPTER

Sensory Systems

I. **Sensory Receptors**
   A. **Function**
      1. **Monitor environment**
         a. **Exteroceptors** detect inputs originating outside the body (e.g., auditory and visual inputs, vibration).
         b. **Interoceptors** detect internal body functions (e.g., blood, pH) and organ states (e.g., distention of intestines).
         c. **Proprioceptors** detect body **position** or **movement** (e.g., muscle, joint, and vestibular receptors).
      2. **Transduce mechanical, chemical, thermal, and electromagnetic energy into electrochemical signals**
      3. **Code stimulus attributes:** modality, intensity, duration, location
   B. **Modality**
      1. Quality or type of stimulus
      2. Coded by "labeled lines" (e.g., stimuli that excite receptors designed to detect vibration are interpreted centrally as vibration), whereas stimuli that excite cold thermoreceptors are interpreted centrally as cold sensation
      3. **Somatic sensation modalities** (all spinal and many cranial nerves): touch-pressure, flutter-vibration, temperature, pain, itch, proprioception, and visceral distention
      4. **Special sensation modalities** (one or more cranial nerves): olfactory (CN I), visual (CN II), gustatory (CN VII, CN IX, and CN X), auditory (CN VIII), and vestibular (CN VIII)
   C. **Intensity**
      1. Increasing stimulus intensity causes larger receptor potential and is coded as **higher frequency of action potentials** from a single sensory neuron.
      2. Increasing stimulus intensity recruits additional receptors and is coded as **increased number of active sensory neurons.**
   D. **Duration**
      1. **Sensory adaptation:** receptor no longer responds to repeated or prolonged stimulus.
         a. **Slowly adapting receptors** detect maintained stimuli such as constant pressure, touch, or temperature.
         b. **Rapidly adapting receptors** detect changing stimuli (on/off) and support detection of moving stimuli and flutter-vibration.

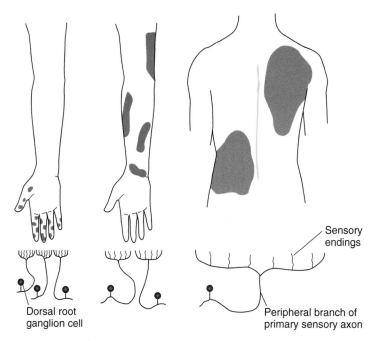

Sensory
endings

Dorsal root
ganglion cell

Peripheral branch of
primary sensory axon

7-1: Two-point discrimination thresholds showing differential sensitivity on the body.

2. **Perceptual adaptation:** relies on changing response of cortical neurons despite continued activation of sensory receptor

E. **Location**

1. **Receptive field of a neuron:** cutaneous region or spatial distribution of a stimulus that will excite that particular sensory neuron.

   a. **Two-point discrimination:** ability to distinguish two closely spaced tactile stimuli

   b. **Two-point threshold** is smallest distance between two stimuli at which they can be perceived as two stimuli rather than one (Fig. 7-1).

      (1) Small receptive fields (e.g., fingertips) have high receptor density, supporting a two-point threshold as small as 2 mm.

      (2) Large receptive field (e.g., skin of back) has low receptor density, supporting a two-point threshold that may exceed 40 mm.

2. **Dermatome:** area of skin innervated by one spinal nerve (Fig. 7-2)

   a. **Segmental sensory loss** suggests damage to sensory root.

   b. Adjacent sensory roots innervate overlapping dermatomes so that loss of one spinal nerve does not completely eliminate sensation from that body segment.

F. **Abnormal (pathologic) sensation**

1. **Anesthesia:** complete loss of sensation

2. **Hypesthesia:** partial loss of sensation

3. **Hyperesthesia:** heightened sensation or tenderness

Dermatomal landmarks: T4 (nipples) and T10 (umbilicus)

Dermatomal overlap: greater for fine touch than for pain/temperature

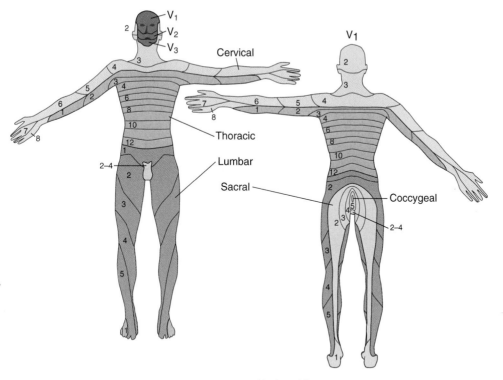

7-2: *Dermatomes of body and face.*

4. **Paresthesia:** abnormal sensation frequently associated with a buzzing or tingling quality
5. **Analgesia:** loss of pain sensation
6. **Hyperalgesia:** increased pain sensation in response to painful stimuli
7. **Allodynia:** pain sensation in response to normally nonpainful stimuli
8. **Athermia:** loss of temperature sensation
9. **Hyperpathia:** increased sensitivity to touch, resulting in pain

Vitamin B$_{12}$ deficiency: demyelination of long spinal cord tracts causes paresthesias

II. **Cutaneous and Subcutaneous Receptors** (Fig. 7-3)
  A. **Touch-pressure mechanoreceptors**
    1. **Tactile meniscus** (Merkel corpuscles), in superficial glabrous skin, provides stimulus localization and respond to steady skin indentation.
    2. **Ruffini corpuscles,** in deeper dermis in subcutaneous hairy and glabrous skin, respond to steady indentation, stretch and stroking of skin.
    3. **Free endings** respond to strong pressure.
  B. **Flutter mechanoreceptors**
    1. **Hair follicle receptors,** in hairy skin, detect velocity of hair movement.
    2. **Tactile** (Meissner) corpuscles, in superficial glabrous skin, detect low-frequency vibration and movement.

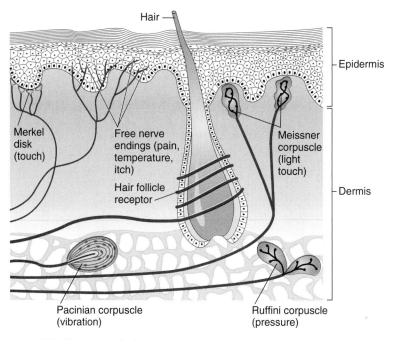

Hair

Epidermis

Merkel
disk
(touch)

Free nerve
endings (pain,
temperature,
itch)

Meissner
corpuscle
(light
touch)

Hair follicle
receptor

Dermis

Pacinian corpuscle
(vibration)

Ruffini corpuscle
(pressure)

7-3: *Cutaneous and subcutaneous sensory receptors and associated structures.*

C. **Vibration mechanoreceptors**
  • **Lamellated (pacinian) corpuscles,** in hairy and glabrous skin, are sensitive to high frequency vibration.
D. **Thermoreceptors**
  1. **Cold receptors** are spontaneously active from 12°C to 37°C and again above 45°C **(paradoxical cold).**
  2. **Warm receptors** are spontaneously active from 25°C to 45°C and peak around 37°C.
  3. Pain fibers are activated above 45°C.
E. **Nociceptors**
  1. **Mechanical:** sensitive to pricking and crushing; acute pain
  2. **Thermal:** sensitive to heat above 45°C
  3. **Polymodal:** sensitive to mechanical, thermal, chemical pain; slow burning pain

III. **Muscle and Joint Receptors**
  A. **Muscle spindle** (Fig. 7-4)
    1. Located within body of muscle
    2. Responds to **muscle stretch** and contributes to detection of **muscle length**
    3. Supplies sensory input for myotatic **(deep tendon) reflexes** via large, myelinated type Ia and type II axon fibers
    4. Receives motor innervation from **gamma motor neurons** that **adjust spindle sensitivity** to muscle stretch

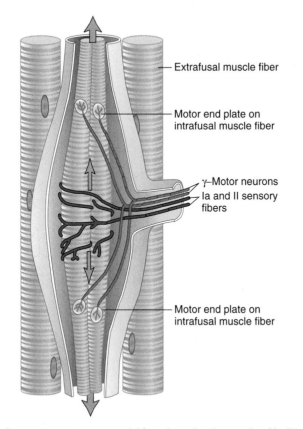

Extrafusal muscle fiber

Motor end plate on
intrafusal muscle fiber

γ–Motor neurons
Ia and II sensory
fibers

Motor end plate on
intrafusal muscle fiber

7-4: *Muscle spindle. Large arrows, passive stretch of annulospiral endings produced by lengthening of the relaxed muscle. Small arrows, active stretch of annulospiral endings produced by activity of fusimotor nerve fibers.*

    B. **Golgi tendon organ** (Fig. 7-5)
       1. Located within tendon
       2. Responds to strong **muscle contraction** and contributes to detection of **muscle tension.**
       3. Supplies sensory input for inverse myotatic reflexes via large, myelinated type Ib axon fibers
    C. **Lamellated (pacinian) corpuscles** detect vibration and contribute to position sense
    D. **Free nerve endings** detect tissue-damaging stresses and protect joints

IV. **Somatic Sensation: Posterior (Dorsal) Column–Medial Lemniscal System (DCML)**
    A. **Origin:** sensory receptors in skin, joints, and muscles supplied by large, fast conducting myelinated fibers (Aβ)

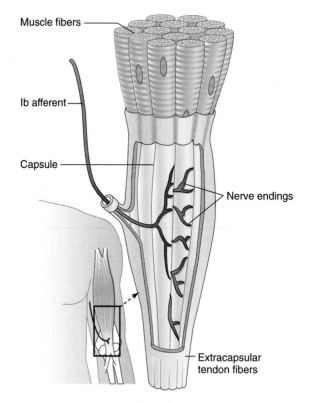

Muscle fibers

Ib afferent

Capsule

Nerve endings

Extracapsular
tendon fibers

7-5: Golgi tendon organ.

B. **Course** (Fig. 7-6)
1. Fibers from **legs** and **lower trunk** ascend in **fasciculus gracilis** of spinal cord posterior columns to terminate in **nucleus gracilis** of caudal medulla.
2. Fibers from **upper trunk** and **arms** ascend in **fasciculus cuneatus** of spinal cord posterior columns to terminate in **nucleus cuneatus** of caudal medulla and upper cervical spinal cord.
3. Nucleus gracilis and nucleus cuneatus project axons that cross to contralateral medulla as internal arcuate fibers and ascend through medulla, pons, and midbrain as **medial lemniscus.**
4. Fibers of medial lemniscus terminate in **ventral posterolateral nucleus (VPL)** of thalamus.
5. VPL projects axons through posterior limb of the **internal capsule** to **somatosensory cortex** (somatotopically organized).

C. **Function:** carries **fine touch, vibration, and proprioception** from arms, legs, and trunk

D. **Testing function**
1. **Vibration:** tuning fork

Testing proprioception by assessing joint position effectively tests DCML.

Testing for vibration has limited clinical value in adults older than 60 years.

> The ability to sense vibration diminishes with age.

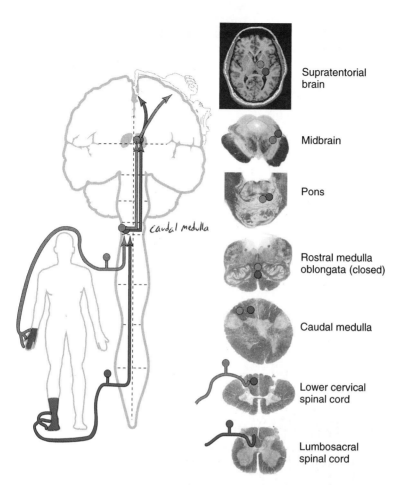

Supratentorial brain

Midbrain

Pons

Rostral medulla oblongata (closed)

Caudal medulla

Lower cervical spinal cord

Lumbosacral spinal cord

Caudal medulla

7-6: *Posterior column-medial lemniscal system and cortical projections.*

2. **Position sense (proprioception):** awareness of limb position with eyes closed

> Hold digit (e.g., a toe) by sides, not top and bottom, to test position sense.

3. **Light touch:** wisp of cotton

E. **Testing complex sensations** requiring intact DCML and somatosensory cortex

1. **Perception:** sandpaper and cloth test (roughness and texture)
2. **Topognosis:** figure writing on palm
3. **Stereognosis:** recognition of objects by palpation

> Identify the "head side" of a coin with eyes closed.

Romberg sign: loss of position sense and hallmark of posterior column damage

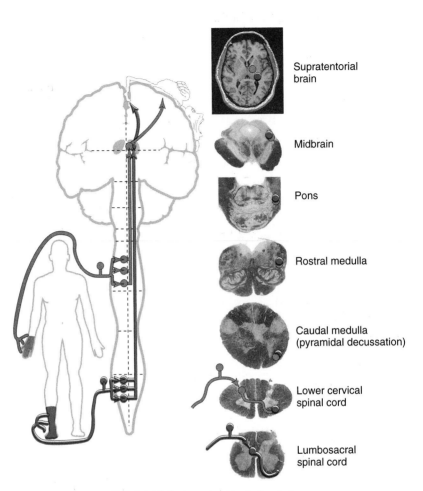

Supratentorial
brain

Midbrain

Pons

Rostral medulla

Caudal medulla
(pyramidal decussation)

Lower cervical
spinal cord

Lumbosacral
spinal cord

7-7: *Spinothalamic tract and cortical projections.*

4. **Two-point discrimination:** discrimination of simultaneously applied
   punctate stimuli
5. **Deep pressure:** weight discrimination

V. **Somatic Sensation: Spinothalamic Tract**
   A. **Origin:** sensory receptors in skin, joints, and muscles supplied by small
      myelinated (Aδ) and unmyelinated (C) fibers.
   B. **Course** (Fig. 7-7)
      1. Fibers enter spinal cord at all levels, divide into ascending and
         descending branches to form **dorsolateral fasciculus** (Lissauer tract),
         and synapse in **posterior horn (substantia gelatinosa)**
      2. **Axons of pain transmission neurons** cross to contralateral spinal cord
         via **anterior white commissure** and ascend through spinal cord,
         medulla, pons, and midbrain as **spinothalamic tract** of anterolateral
         system.

3. Fibers of spinothalamic tract terminate in **VPL** of thalamus.
4. VPL projects axons through posterior limb of the **internal capsule** to reach **somatosensory cortex** (somatotopically organized).

C. **Function:** carries **pain and temperature** from arms, legs, and trunk
D. Two additional pain pathways ascend as part of the anterolateral system.

1. **Spinoreticular tract**
   a. Carries pain and crude touch sensations to brainstem reticular formation, which projects via nonspecific relay nuclei of thalamus to all regions of cortex.
   b. **Reticular activating system** ascends from central core of brainstem to wide areas of the cortex and is required for **arousal of higher CNS centers.**

2. **Spinomesencephalic tract**
   a. Carries pain, temperature, and crude touch sensations to midbrain reticular formation
   b. Activates the intrinsic analgesia system of midbrain periaqueductal gray (PAG)
   c. Important for emotional response to pain

E. **Cordotomy:** surgical sectioning of spinothalamic tract
1. Provides immediate relief of **intractable pain** (e.g., from pancreatic cancer)
2. Pain usually returns after several months; reasons are unknown.
   a. Uncrossed spinothalamic or spinomesencephalic fibers may contribute to return of pain.
   b. Some pain input may be carried through posterior column system.
   c. **Neuropathic pain** may be major source of returning pain (see section VII, E)

F. **Testing function**
1. **Pain:** pinprick
2. **Temperature:** warm and cold vials

> Posterior column and spinothalamic tract: both carry touch; examining touch has little clinical value

VI. **Trigeminothalamic system**
A. **Function:** trigeminal nerve afferents carry sensation from three non-overlapping segments of face (ophthalmic, V_1; maxillary, V_2; mandibular, V_3) to three trigeminal nuclei (Fig. 7-8; see also Fig. 7-2 and Chapter 11).

B. **Main (pontine) trigeminal nucleus**
1. Receives **fine touch and vibration** from face via three branches of trigeminal nerve
2. Projects axons that cross to join contralateral medial lemniscus and terminate in **ventral posteromedial nucleus (VPM) of thalamus.**
3. **Testing function**
   a. **Vibration:** tuning fork
   b. **Fine (light and discriminative) touch:** wisp of cotton

C. **Spinal trigeminal nucleus**
1. Receives **pain and temperature** from face through trigeminal, facial, glossopharyngeal, and vagus nerves

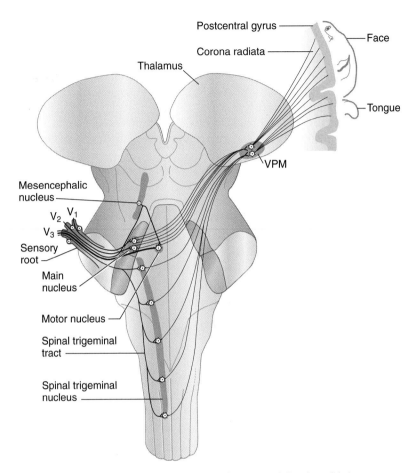

7-8: *Trigeminothalamic system. VPM, ventral posteromedial nucleus of thalamus.*

2. Projects axons that cross to join contralateral spinothalamic pathway and terminate in VPM.
3. **Testing function**
   a. **Pain:** pinprick
   b. **Temperature:** warm and cold vials

D. **Mesencephalic trigeminal nucleus**
   1. Contains cell bodies of axons of the mandibular branch (V_3) of the trigeminal nerve that carry **proprioceptive** input. (All other cell bodies of trigeminal nerve axons are located in trigeminal ganglion of PNS.)
   2. Projects axons to neurons of trigeminal motor nucleus
   3. **Testing function:** jaw-jerk reflex

E. **VPM of thalamus**
   1. Relays fine touch and pain and temperature input from contralateral face
   2. Projects axons through genu of internal capsule to reach somatosensory cortex.

Lesion involving genu of internal capsule: affects head while sparing lower body

VII. **Visceral Sensation and Referred Pain**
   A. **Physiologic sensations**
      1. Adequate stimulus is related to normal visceral functioning
         a. Bladder fullness (sensory input for reflexive bladder emptying)
         b. Pulmonary irritation (triggering cough)
         c. Blood pressure (baroreceptor-mediated reflex)
         d. Chemoreceptors (sensory input for respiratory control)
      2. Detected by mechanoreceptors and specialized baroreceptors and chemoreceptors
      3. Carried in axons that are **bundled with parasympathetic fibers** and enter CNS through CN IX, CN X, and sacral spinal roots
   B. **Pain sensations**
      1. Adequate stimulus is potentially tissue damaging
         a. Excessive distention or traction
         b. Ischemia
         c. Presence of released neurochemicals that activate free nerve endings (e.g., prostaglandins, bradykinin)
      2. Detected by free nerve endings
      3. Carried in small myelinated (Aδ) and unmyelinated axons that are **bundled with sympathetic fibers** and enter spinal cord at T1 to L2
      4. **Viscerosomatic pain**
         a. **Origin:** linings of body cavities, including pleura, peritoneum, and mesentery
         b. Provoked when visceral inflammation extends to involve abdominal wall adjacent to inflamed viscera
         c. Frequently localizable

         > Acute appendicitis pain is initially periumbilical and migrates to the lower right quadrant following rupture.

      5. **Cardinal signs of visceral disease**
         a. Pain, hyperalgesia, and hyperesthesia
         b. Autonomic reflexes: sweating, piloerection, or vasomotor changes
         c. Somatic reflexes: muscular rigidity
         d. Pain poorly localized, frequently referred to midline, and often accompanied by nausea, malaise, and sweating
   C. **Referred pain** (Fig. 7-9)
      1. Pain sensation arising from a visceral structure can cause pain perception localized to predictable cutaneous regions.
      2. Pain is referred to dermatomes supplied by the same posterior roots that carry visceral afferents to spinal cord (dermatomal rule)

      Gallbladder inflammation: may be referred as right shoulder pain

      > Pain from a **myocardial infarct** radiates from the chest down the ulnar aspect of the left arm. Primary afferents from the left arm and heart converge on the same second-order neurons. Experience has "taught" the brain to interpret input from these neurons as originating from the arm.

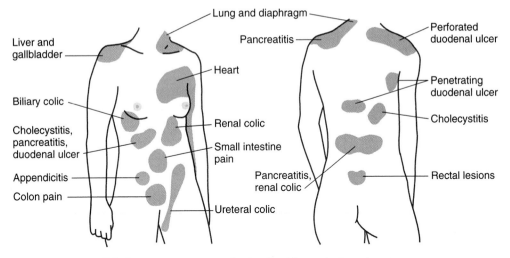

7-9: *Cutaneous representation of pain referred from major internal structures.*

VIII. **Pain Processing**
- A. **Peripheral nerve endings**
  1. **Peripheral sensitization**
     a. Repeated mechanical stimulation can cause nociceptors that were unresponsive to become responsive.
     b. **Bradykinin, serotonin, histamine, and prostaglandins** at site of peripheral tissue injury activate or sensitize nociceptors.
     c. Activated nociceptors releases **substance P** from sensory nerve endings; substance P increases release of histamine from mast cells; histamine activates nociceptors.

> Topical **capsaicin** (red pepper extract) causes acute intense pain followed by extended analgesia (months) by suppressing synthesis and release of substance P. Effects are mediated through a capsaicin (vanilloid) receptor located on primary pain afferents. Capsaicin receptors are also activated by noxious heat.

  Capsaicin application: intense heat followed by analgesia

  2. **Mechanisms of analgesia**
     a. Endogenous **cannabinoids** (e.g., anandamide) bind to receptors on peripheral nociceptive endings as well as central terminals in posterior horn of spinal cord.
     b. Cyclooxygenase-2 **(COX-2)** inhibitors block production of prostaglandins and reduce pain transmission in several chronic inflammatory conditions (e.g., osteoarthritis)

  Pain of chronic arthritis: can be treated with COX-2 inhibitors

- B. **Primary afferent terminals** within posterior horn of spinal cord
  1. **Increased activation** following tissue damage
     a. **Wind-up**
        (1) Repetitive activation of C fibers increases activity of spinal pain transmission neurons.

       (2) Dependent on release of glutamate and subsequent activation of NMDA glutamate receptors

       (3) Can produce lasting changes in posterior horn neurons that resemble changes seen during long-term potentiation in cortical neurons

  b. **Central sensitization**

       (1) Repetitive activation of C fibers decreases threshold and increases receptive field size of spinal pain transmission neurons

       (2) Activated nociceptor C fibers release **glutamate** and **substance P** from terminals in spinal cord posterior horn.

          (a) **Substance P** acts as a modulator to extend activity of glutamate at synapse.

          (b) Released glutamate stimulates AMPA receptors, activating ascending pain pathways.

       (3) Excessive activation of NMDA receptors can also cause hyperexcitability of posterior horn neurons.

  c. **Complex regional pain syndromes, type 1 and 2**

       (1) Continuous, burning pain, changes in skin temperature, changes in skin and bone, and tissue edema

       (2) Includes **reflex sympathetic dystrophy** (type 1) and **causalgia** (type 2)

       (3) Follows damage to major peripheral nerve trunk

       (4) **Cause unknown,** with both peripheral and central sensitization implicated

       (5) Symptoms may be decreased or eliminated after **partial sympathetic block.**

2. **Mechanisms of analgesia**

  a. **Gate control theory** (Fig. 7-10)

       (1) Neurons in posterior horn receive convergent input from small myelinated and unmyelinated nociceptive fibers (Aδ and C) and large myelinated sensory fibers (Aβ).

       (2) Small fibers activate posterior horn neurons that transmit pain centrally ("open the gate").

       (3) Large myelinated fibers activate interneurons that inhibit neurons in posterior horn that transmit pain ("close the gate").

       (4) **Transcutaneous electrical nerve stimulation** (activates large myelinated fibers that overlap area of pain input to "close the gate") is based on the gate control theory.

  b. **Intrinsic analgesic system** (endogenous pain control system) (see Fig. 7-10)

       (1) Electrical stimulation of the midbrain **PAG** produces analgesia without affecting fine touch.

       (2) PAG activates **serotonergic neurons** in medullary **raphe nuclei**

       (3) Raphe nuclei project to **enkephalin interneurons** in spinal cord posterior horn.

Pain sensation: may be increased or attenuated by disease

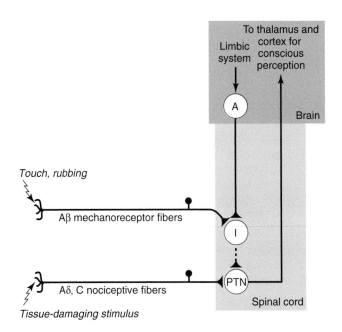

7-10: *Endogenous analgesia systems. Nociceptors (Aδ and C fibers) excite pain transmission neurons (PTN). Large, myelinated mechanoreceptors (Aβ fibers) excite inhibitory (e.g., enkephalinergic) interneurons (I) that inhibit pain transmission at the first synapse. Pain transmission neurons (anterolateral system) project to thalamus with collaterals to brainstem. Limbic cortex contributes to activation of periaqueductal gray intrinsic analgesia circuitry. Periaqueductal gray projects to medullary raphe, which project to posterior horn to inhibit pain transmission.*

(4) **Enkephalin** interneurons inhibit presynaptic nociceptor terminals and posterior horn pain transmission neurons.

> **Morphine** suppresses input from pain fibers; this can be reversed by the opioid antagonist naloxone.

C. **Thalamus and cortex**
1. VPL and VPM process and relay localizable pain information from the spinothalamic tract to primary somatosensory cortex.
2. Nonspecific relay nuclei and intralaminar nuclei process and relay pain information from the reticulospinal tract to most areas of the cortex, including the **cingulate gyrus** and **insular cortex** of the limbic system.

> The cingulate gyrus and insular cortex have been implicated in the emotional component to pain.

3. **Thalamic pain: spontaneous, burning, neuropathic pain that can follow damage to the VPL nucleus of the thalamus.**

> In **thalamic syndrome,** the patient experiences thalamic pain, loss of sensation, and sensory ataxia on the contralateral side of the body

4. Impulses reaching thalamus create awareness of pain, whereas cortex is necessary for appreciation of pain intensity and localization of pain sensation.

> Distraction, suggestion, or strong emotion may reduce the level of pain awareness.

D. **Neuropathic pain**
  1. Continuous, intractable, frequently excruciating, burning pain with or without peripheral nerve damage
  2. Results from damage to sensory pathways, not from nociceptor activation

> Management of neuropathic pain is difficult. Conventional treatments (e.g., nonsteroidal anti-inflammatories) may be ineffective. Antidepressants and anticonvulsives can be useful.

E. Chronic pain
  1. Pain lasting at least 3 months
  2. **Major causes:**
     a. Pain accompanying a structural disease
     b. Pain of psychophysiologic origin; frequently representing adaptation to a previous structural disease
     c. Pain with psychiatric implications (rare)
  3. Causes structural or functional changes within pain-processing circuitry extending from spinal cord to limbic cortex

> **Phantom limb** after amputation may result from plasticity changes in VPL and VPM neurons and from changes in cortical processing of sensory input.
>
> **Rheumatoid arthritis and fibromyalgia** feature aspects of chronic pain.

8

Motor Systems

I. **Neuronal Cell Types**

A. **Lower motor neurons**

Lower motor neurons: innervate muscles

1. Neurons with cell bodies in **brainstem** and **spinal cord** that innervate muscles
2. Receive input from sensory systems (e.g., for reflex activity) and cortical and brainstem upper motor neurons
3. **Motor unit: one lower motor neuron** (α-motor neuron), **its axon** and all **extrafusal muscle fibers** innervated by terminal branches of axon
4. **Final common pathway:** motor unit through which all other components of motor system must act

Damaged lower motor neurons: cause weakness or flaccid paralysis

5. **Damage to motor unit** (e.g., from polio, amyotrophic lateral sclerosis) causes **paresis (weakness)/flaccid paralysis, hyporeflexia/areflexia, fasciculations, and fibrillations** (Table 8-1)

    a. **Fasciculation:** contraction of complete motor units; visible as twitching through skin.

    > Fasciculations can be provoked in normal individuals in response to excess caffeine consumption, stress, and sleep deprivation.

    b. **Fibrillation:** contraction of individual muscle fibers that cannot be seen; **must be measured by electromyography.**

    > Complete loss of motor neurons to a muscle causes neurogenic atrophy within weeks.

B. **Upper motor neurons** (Fig. 8-1)

Upper motor neurons: synapse with lower motor neurons in brainstem or spinal cord

1. Neurons with cell bodies in **cortex** and **brainstem** that project to lower motor neurons
2. **Direct activation pathways**

    a. Project from cortex to lower motor neurons in brainstem **(corticobulbar tract)** or spinal cord **(corticospinal tract)**
    b. Facilitate **voluntary** activity, particularly **skilled movements**
    c. **Damage causes Babinski** sign and **paresis/paralysis of voluntary movements,** especially **fine skilled movements,** with preservation of other motor activity (e.g., segmental reflexes)

3. **Indirect activation** (nonpyramidal) **pathways**

    a. Project from specific nuclei in brainstem **(tectospinal, rubrospinal, reticulospinal, and vestibulospinal tracts)** to lower motor neurons

Lower Motor Neuron Lesion	Lesion Limited to Corticospinal Tract	Upper Motor Neuron Lesion
Paralysis	Paresis	Paralysis or paresis
Flaccidity	Flaccidity	Spasticity*
Hyporeflexia/reflexia	Hyporeflexia	Hyperreflexia*
No clonus	No clonus	Clonus*
No reflexes	Babinski sign	Babinski sign
Depends on motor neurons affected	Absence of abdominal reflexes	Absence of abdominal reflexes
Fasciculations	No fasciculations	No fasciculations
Marked neurogenic atrophy	Possible disuse atrophy	Possible disuse atrophy

TABLE 8-1:
Signs of Damage to Lower and Upper Motor Neurons and Corticospinal Tract

*During *initial* phase of *acute* upper motor neuron damage, expect flaccid paralysis.

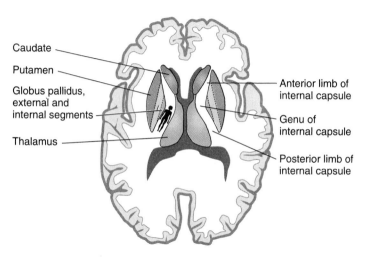

8-1: *Horizontal section through cerebral hemispheres showing internal capsule in relation to thalamus and components of the basal ganglia. Small human figure superimposed on internal capsule, somatotopic organization of upper motor neuron axons traveling through internal capsule.*

of spinal cord that integrate supporting musculature during voluntary movements

b. Facilitate spinal reflexes involved with balance, posture, equilibrium, and gait

c. **Damage causes spastic paralysis, hyperreflexia, clasp-knife rigidity** (see section VIII, C), and **ankle clonus**

C. **Local interneurons**
  1. Project locally within spinal cord and brainstem
  2. Integrate inputs from upper motor neurons and from sensory neurons
  3. Modulate lower motor neuron activities
  4. May be excitatory or inhibitory
     • Inhibitory neurotransmitters: **glycine** and **GABA** (γ-aminobutyric acid)

Tetanus toxin: causes uncontrolled sustained muscle contraction by blocking glycine interneurons

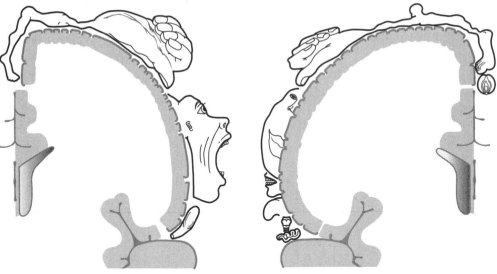

Primary motor cortex   **Primary sensory cortex**

8-2: Homunculus for primary motor and sensory cortices.

II. **Corticospinal (Pyramidal) Tract**
   A. **Origin**
      1. **Pyramidal cells** in frontal (motor and premotor areas) and parietal cortex
         • Largest pyramidal cells in **precentral gyrus** (Betz cells) give rise to about 3% of the corticospinal tract.
      2. Primary motor areas of cortex are **somatotopically** organized (Fig. 8-2).
   B. **Course**
      1. Passes through corona radiata, posterior limb of internal capsule, cerebral peduncle, base of pons, and medullary pyramids

      > Lesion to medullary pyramids can damage corticospinal tracts while sparing other motor pathways.

      2. Most fibers (about 90%) cross in caudal medulla at pyramidal decussation to enter the lateral funiculus of the spinal cord and descend as the lateral corticospinal tract.
         • **Pyramidal decussation:** transition between the medulla and the spinal cord
   C. **Function**
      1. Controls voluntary movement, in particular involving distal extremities
      2. **Stimulation of motor cortex** causes **complex movements** resulting from inhibition of extensor motor neurons and facilitation of flexor motor neurons.
      3. Corticospinal control can be interrupted by damage in the cerebral cortex, subcortical white matter, internal capsule, brainstem, and spinal cord (Table 8-2; see also Table 8-1)

Corticospinal system: maintains a flexor bias to enable fine skilled movements

TABLE 8-2:
Signs and Symptoms Following Lesions at Various CNS Levels

SITE	SIGNS AND SYMPTOMS
Lateral convexity of cortex	**Motor** Paralysis of contralateral lower face **Sensory** Loss of sensation in contralateral face
Medial cortex	**Motor** Paralysis of contralateral leg **Sensory** Loss of sensation in contralateral leg
Genu of internal capsule	**Motor** Paralysis of contralateral lower face **Sensory** Loss of sensation in contralateral face
Posterior limb of internal capsule	**Motor** Paralysis of contralateral lower leg **Sensory** Loss of sensation in contralateral lower leg
Midbrain cerebral peduncle	**Motor** Paralysis of contralateral leg, arm, tongue, lower face, and ipsilateral eye (eye down and out, dilated pupil, ptosis)
Pontine base	**Motor** Paralysis of contralateral leg, arm, tongue, and ipsilateral eye on lateral gaze
Medial medulla	**Motor** Paralysis of contralateral leg and arm and ipsilateral tongue **Sensory** Loss of sensation (discriminative touch, vibration, proprioception) in contralateral body
Spinal cord (hemisection)	**Motor** Spastic paralysis of ipsilateral body below lesion Flaccid paralysis of ipsilateral body at level of lesion **Sensory** Loss of sensation (discriminative touch, vibration, proprioception) in ipsilateral body below lesion Loss of sensation (pain, temperature) in contralateral body below lesion

4. **Effects of damage**
   a. **Motor cortex: loss of fine skilled movements** in distal limb muscles; control of gross movement of arms and legs is retained.
   b. **Cortical white matter or internal capsule:** corticospinal (pyramidal) and nonpyramidal systems are simultaneously affected.
      (1) Initial signs: **flaccid paralysis** and **hyporeflexia/areflexia,** appearance of **Babinski** sign ("up-going toes")
      (2) Late signs (days to weeks after initial lesion): hypertonia, hyperreflexia, loss of superficial reflexes and persistence of Babinski sign
   c. **Medullary pyramids:** paresis or flaccid paralysis, hyporeflexia, **Babinski** sign, and loss of superficial reflexes
      • Signs of lesion to medullary pyramids do *not* fit classic presentation of upper motor neuron lesion because only the corticospinal tracts are damaged and nonpyramidal pathways are spared.
   d. **Damage to brain (i.e., rostral to pyramidal decussation) affects contralateral body.**
   e. **Damage to spinal cord affects ipsilateral body.**

Damaged medullary pyramids: flaccid paresis, hyporeflexia, Babinski sign.

III. **Corticobulbar Tract**
   A. **Origin: pyramidal cells** in frontal (motor and premotor areas) and parietal cortex
   B. **Course** (Fig. 8-3)
      1. Passes through corona radiata, genu of internal capsule, and cerebral peduncle in association with corticospinal tract
      2. Descends near corticospinal tract, so a lesion frequently affects both corticospinal and corticobulbar systems
      3. Axons innervate both ipsilateral and contralateral brainstem lower motor neurons with two important **exceptions:** lower face and tongue
   C. **Function**
      1. Controls voluntary movement involving muscles of head and neck, which are innervated by cranial nerves (see Chapter 11)
      2. Fibers distribute **bilaterally** to cranial nerve lower motor neurons with the following exceptions.
         a. **Facial motor nucleus (CN VII):** motor neurons innervating muscles of lower face (motor neurons in inferior portion of nucleus) receive only contralateral innervation from corticobulbar tracts; motor neurons innervating muscles of forehead (motor neurons in superior portion of nucleus) are under bilateral cortical control.

Damaged corticobulbar fibers: paresis of contralateral lower face; forehead is preserved

> Damage to corticobulbar fibers results in weakness to the contralateral lower face but not the upper face.

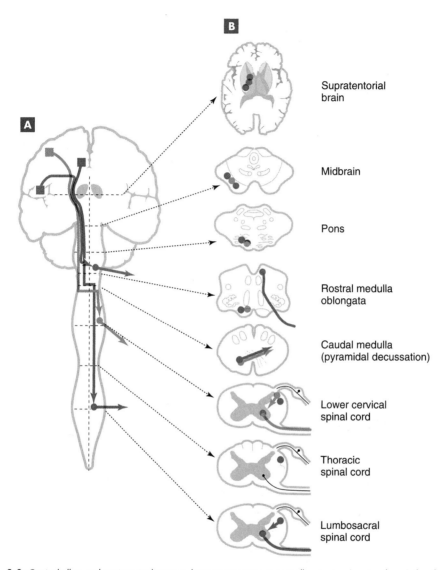

B

Supratentorial
brain

Midbrain

Pons

Rostral medulla
oblongata

Caudal medulla
(pyramidal decussation)

Lower cervical
spinal cord

Thoracic
spinal cord

Lumbosacral
spinal cord

A

8-3: *Corticobulbar and corticospinal tracts to lower motor neurons controlling tongue (gray pathway), hand (light green pathway), and lower leg (dark green pathway).* **A,** *Approximate location of upper motor neuron pools within cortex (squares), pathway taken by each upper motor neuron axon (arrows), and location of each lower motor neuron pool (circles).* **B,** *Horizontal sections through brain and spinal cord showing location of upper motor neuron axons at each level.*

b. **Hypoglossal (CN XII):** motor neurons innervating tongue receive only contralateral innervation from corticobulbar fibers.

CN XII lesion: tongue deviates to weak side on protrusion

> Damage to corticobulbar fibers results in weakness to the contralateral tongue; on protrusion, the tongue deviates to weak side (i.e., tongue deviates away from lesion).

IV. **Rubrospinal Tract**
   A. **Origin:** red nucleus in midbrain
   B. **Course:** descends as crossed pathway in lateral brainstem and intermingled with lateral corticospinal tract in lateral funiculus of spinal cord
   C. **Function:** facilitates flexor musculature (inhibits extensor musculature) for **skilled voluntary movements** in arm

Flexor bias in arms in decorticate rigidity: damage above midbrain

> Arm flexion seen in **decorticate rigidity** stems from unopposed activity of intact rubrospinal tract. No known clinical syndromes are associated with selective damage to this tract.

V. **Vestibulospinal Tract**
   A. **Lateral vestibulospinal tract**
      1. **Origin:** lateral vestibular nucleus in medulla
      2. **Course:** descends as uncrossed pathway in anterior funiculus of spinal cord
      3. **Function: facilitates extensor musculature** (inhibits flexor musculature) and controls (trunk) musculature involved with **posture and equilibrium**

Extensor bias in decerebrate rigidity: damage extending to pons

> Upper and lower extremity extension seen in **decerebrate rigidity** stems in part from unopposed activation of lateral vestibulospinal tract.

   B. **Medial vestibulospinal tract**
      1. **Origin:** medial vestibular nucleus in medulla
      2. **Course:** descends bilaterally in anterior funiculus of spinal cord
      3. **Function:** with medial longitudinal fasciculus, mediates reflexes of vestibular system, including **eye movement** and **position of head and neck**

VI. **Reticulospinal Tracts**
   A. **Pontine (medial) reticulospinal tract**
      1. **Origin:** pontine reticular nuclei that are under cortical control
      2. **Course:** descends as uncrossed pathway in anterior funiculus in spinal cord
      3. **Function:** facilitates **posture** and extensor (antigravity) muscle tone
   B. **Medullary (lateral) reticulospinal tract**
      1. **Origin:** medullary pontine nucleus
      2. **Course:** descends bilaterally in anterior funiculus in spinal cord
      3. **Function:** inhibits posture and extensor (antigravity) muscle tone and facilitates flexor muscle tone

VII. **Tectospinal Tracts**
   A. **Lateral tectospinal tract**
      1. **Origin:** neurons in tectum of midbrain
      2. **Course:** descends bilaterally in anterior funiculus of spinal cord

3. **Function: pupillary (dilation) reflex** to darkness mediated by sympathetic nervous system

B. **Medial tectospinal tract**
   1. **Origin:** neurons in superior colliculus
   2. **Course:** descends as crossed fibers to cervical cord
   3. **Function: reflex orienting movements of head and neck**

VIII. **Reflexes**
   A. **Overview**
      1. **Function**
         a. Form the basis of stereotypical motor outputs
         b. Regulate muscle tone, tailoring contractile state of muscle to load conditions
      2. **Input:** muscle spindles, Golgi tendon organs, and cutaneous and subcutaneous somatosensory receptors
      3. **Output:** lower motor neuron activation of skeletal muscles
      4. **Damage to sensory or motor limb of reflex arc:** hyporeflexia or areflexia
      5. **Damage to upper motor neuron:** hyperreflexia and Babinski sign
      6. **Myotatic and inverse myotatic reflexes:** necessary to maintain upright posture but not sufficient; descending influences from upper motor neurons are also required.

      A quadriplegic cannot sit upright without external support.

   B. **Myotatic (muscle stretch) reflex (deep tendon reflex)** (Fig. 8-4)
      1. Monosynaptic
      2. Detects muscle stretch through muscle spindle and counters with muscle contraction
      3. More pronounced in **extensors** (antigravity) than flexors
      4. **Quadriceps** (knee jerk reflex)
         a. **Sensory limb:** tapping patellar tendon causes rapid quadriceps stretch and muscle spindle activation, activating Ia and group II afferents that project to spinal cord.
         b. **Motor limb:** spindle afferents excite lower motor neurons to quadriceps, causing quadriceps contraction.
      5. Known clinically as **deep tendon reflex** (Table 8-3) because tendon tap is used to stretch muscle in clinical setting; tendon is not actually part of reflex

      Deep tendon reflexes are lost with complete lesions of lower motor neuron and are increased (hyperreflexia) with upper motor neuron lesions. Ankle clonus is an expression of hyperreflexia.

   C. **Inverse myotatic reflex** (Fig. 8-5)
      1. Multisynaptic
      2. Detects muscle contraction through Golgi tendon organ and counters with muscle relaxation

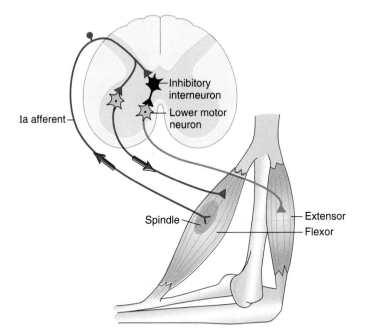

8-4: *Biceps reflex. Myotatic reflex (deep tendon reflex) tested at the elbow. Arrow, sensory input and motor output.*

TABLE 8-3:
Routinely Tested
Deep Tendon
Reflexes

Reflex	Test, Response, and Spinal Roots Tested
Biceps	Biceps contracts and elbow flexes when thumb is placed on biceps tendon and is tapped (C5–C6) (see Fig. 8-4).
Brachioradialis	Elbow flexes and forearm supinates when brachioradialis tendon is tapped (C5–C6).
Triceps	Elbow extends slightly when triceps tendon is tapped (C6–C8).
Quadriceps (knee jerk)	Knee extends when patellar tendon is tapped (L3–L4).
Triceps surae (ankle jerk)	Foot plantar-flexes when calcanal (Achilles) tendon is tapped (L5, S1–S2).

3. **Biceps contraction**
   a. **Sensory limb:** stretches Golgi tendon organs, activating Ib afferents that project to spinal cord
   b. **Motor limb:** Ib afferents inhibit lower motor neurons to biceps (via interneurons)
4. **Clasp-knife rigidity**
   a. Caused by **upper motor neuron damage**
   b. Passive manipulation of arm is met with strong resistance because stretch reflex activation is excessive. Resistance then fades, and the joint moves freely.
   c. Fading resistance is due to sudden domination of inverse myotatic reflex on the same muscles.

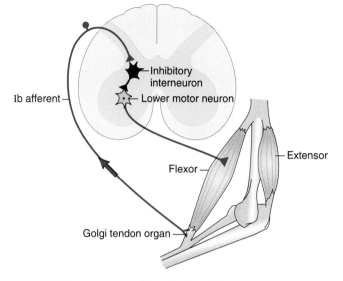

8-5: *Inverse myotatic reflex at the elbow. Arrow, sensory input.*

D. **Flexion withdrawal and crossed extensor**
1. Multisynaptic with bilateral spinal involvement
2. Mediates withdrawal of limb from painful stimuli and extension of contralateral limb
3. Crossed part of the reflex is less pronounced in the arms but is used in the legs.

> Flexion withdrawal reflex is normally suppressed by upper motor neuron input unless sensory input is sufficiently painful. Thus, an individual will not fall when all weight is put on one leg. With upper motor neuron damage, reflex may be elicited with more benign sensory inputs.

E. **Superficial reflexes**
1. **Abdominal reflex:** cutaneous stimulation of any abdominal quadrant causes contraction of that musculature (i.e., umbilicus "jumps" to stimulated quadrant).
2. **Cremasteric reflex:** downward stroking of superior, medial thigh causes contraction of cremasteric muscle with retraction of ipsilateral scrotum and testicle.

Superficial reflexes: lost with damage to either lower or upper motor neurons

9

Basal Ganglia

I. **Structure**
   A. A group of nuclei of varied origin that act as a functional unit; nuclei of telencephalic origin are basal to the overlying cerebral cortex; the rest are deeper within the central nervous system (CNS).
   B. **Corpus striatum** (telencephalic origin) (Figs. 9-1 and 9-2)
      1. **Neostriatum** (striatum)
         a. **Caudate nucleus** is **C**-shaped, following lateral ventricle.
         b. **Putamen**
         c. **Caudate-putamen connections** give region a striated appearance.
      2. **Globus pallidus:** external and internal segments
      3. **Lentiform** (lenticular) **nucleus:** putamen and globus pallidus
   C. **Subthalamic nucleus** (diencephalic origin): located inferior to thalamus
   D. **Substantia nigra** (mesencephalic origin)
      1. Located in anterior mesencephalon
      2. Consists of substantia nigra pars compacta and substantia nigra pars reticulata
      3. Separated from globus pallidus by internal capsule

II. **Function**
   A. Plan, initiate, and maintain **voluntary motor activities**
   B. **Regulatory role** in other cortical activities
      1. Voluntary control of **eye movements**
      2. **Cognitive** and **emotional function**
      3. Procedural **learning** underlying **routine behaviors** ("habits")
   C. **Damage**
      1. **Negative signs:** loss of motor function
         a. **Akinesia:** lack of movement, an inability to initiate movement
         b. **Bradykinesia:** abnormal slowing of movement
         c. **Micrographia:** decreased size of handwriting, an early expression of bradykinesia
         d. **Postural and gait abnormalities:** flexed trunk, neck, and limbs; loss of righting reflexes; festinating gait
         e. **Masked facies** (**reptilian stare,** parkinsonian facies): masklike facial expression with infrequent eye blinks

Basal ganglia damage: Abnormal motor function may include negative and positive signs.

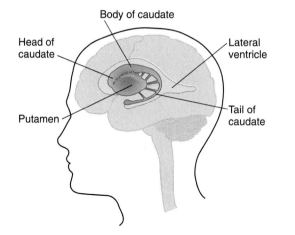

9-1: *Neostriatum, lateral view. Note relationship of caudate to lateral ventricle and relationship of putamen to caudate.*

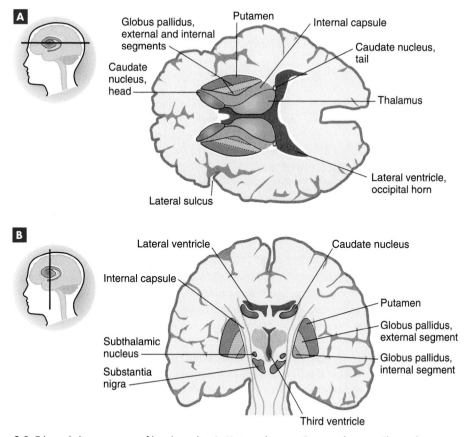

9-2: *Telencephalic components of basal ganglia.* **A,** *Horizontal section;* **B,** *coronal section. The caudate forms part of the lateral wall of the lateral ventricle. The internal capsule separates the caudate and putamen and also the lentiform nucleus and thalamus. Note proximity of diencephalic subthalamic nucleus and mesencephalic substantia nigra to the telencephalic caudate nucleus, putamen, and globus pallidus. The internal capsule separates the subthalamic nucleus and globus pallidus.*

2. **Positive signs:** new motor activities or an inability to suppress unwanted motor function
   a. **Athetosis:** slow, sinuous, purposeless movements
      (1) Often in fingers, hands, face, tongue, and throat
      (2) Can include lip smacking and grimacing
   b. **Dystonia:** persistent form of one movement of athetosis resulting in sustained muscle contractions that produce postural abnormality
   c. **Chorea** (choreiform movements): rapid, arrhythmic, jerky, involuntary movements, especially involving distal musculature
   d. **Ballismus:** violent flinging of a limb or limbs

> Hemiballismus, a unilateral ballismus, appears in the body contralateral to stroke damage to one subthalamic nucleus

Hemiballismus: lesion of contralateral subthalamic nucleus

   e. **Resting tremor:** rhythmic (3–6 Hz) oscillating motor output, frequently in hands ("pill-rolling" tremor), but may appear in other muscle groups and even as a vocal tremor
   f. **Rigidity:** hypertonus of skeletal muscles felt as increased resistance to passive muscle stretch
      (1) Often more pronounced in flexors; may be described as "stiffness"
      (2) Independent of rate of movement, unlike resistance felt with spasticity
         (a) **Lead-pipe rigidity:** uniform throughout movement
         (b) **Cogwheel rigidity:** rhythmic ratchet-like variation in resistance to passive muscle stretch
   g. **Tics**
      (1) **Motor:** neck stretching, eye blinking, facial twitches
      (2) **Vocal:** grunting, sniffing, throat clearing
   h. **Dyskinesia:** general term that includes resting tremor, athetosis, chorea, and ballismus

III. **Circuits**
   A. Best-understood basal ganglia circuit loop subserves control of voluntary movement and involves motor-related areas of cortex. Other loops subserve cognitive, emotional, and visceral functions.
   B. **Input** (excitatory, glutamate) **to basal ganglia**
      1. From **cortex** (motor, premotor, supplementary motor, sensorimotor)
      2. Directed to **neostriatum**
   C. **Output** (inhibitory, γ-aminobutyric acid [GABA]) **from basal ganglia**
      1. To thalamus (ventromedial, ventrolateral, dorsomedial nuclei)
      2. Arising from substantia nigra, pars reticulata, and globus pallidus, internal segment
   D. **Output** reflects **balance between two pathways** (Fig. 9-3).
      1. **Direct pathway**
         a. Cortex → neostriatum → substantia nigra, pars reticulata, and globus pallidus, internal segment → thalamus → cortex
         b. **Increases cortical activation**

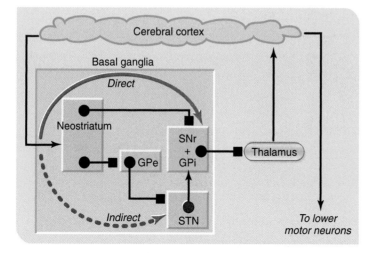

9-3: *Direct and indirect pathways. Black lines ending in arrowheads,* excitatory projections; *black lines ending in boxes,* inhibitory projections. *GPe, globus pallidus, external segment; GPi, globus pallidus, internal segment; SNr, substantia nigra pars reticulata; STN, subthalamic nucleus.*

    2. **Indirect pathway**
       a. Cortex → neostriatum → globus pallidus, external segment → subthalamic nucleus → substantia nigra, pars reticulata, and globus pallidus, internal segment → thalamus → cortex
       b. **Decreases cortical activation**

IV. **Neurotransmitters** (Fig. 9-4).
  A. **GABA:** major neurotransmitter within basal ganglia
    1. Striatal medium spiny projection **neurons** of direct pathway use GABA coupled with **substance P.**
    2. Striatal medium spiny projection **neurons** of indirect pathway use GABA coupled with **enkephalin.**
    3. Medium striatal aspiny interneurons are GABAergic
  B. **Glutamate**
    1. **Caudate** and **putamen** receive glutamate from the cortex.
    2. Glutamate excitotoxicity may be involved in degeneration seen in the neostriatum in **Huntington disease.**
    3. **Subthalamic nucleus,** the only non-GABAergic nucleus within the basal ganglia, sends glutamatergic projections to the substantia nigra, pars reticulata, and globus pallidus, internal segment.
  C. **Dopamine**
    1. Mesencephalic **substantia nigra, pars compacta,** projects to neostriatum through nigrostriatal pathway
       a. **Excites direct** path through dopamine D_1 receptors
       b. **Inhibits indirect** path through dopamine D_2 receptors
    2. Degeneration of dopamine neurons of substantia nigra, pars compacta, underlies **Parkinson disease.**

Parkinson disease: Degeneration of substantia nigra causes loss of dopamine to caudate and putamen.

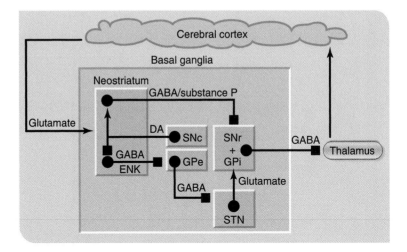

9-4: *Major neurotransmitters used by neurons projecting between component nuclei of the basal ganglia. Projections ending in arrowheads,* excitatory; *projections ending in boxes,* inhibitory. *DA, dopamine; ENK, enkephalin; GABA, γ-aminobutyric acid; GPe, globus pallidus, external segment; GPi, globus pallidus, internal segment; SNc, substantia nigra pars compacta; SNr, substantia nigra pars reticulata; STN, subthalamic nucleus.*

    3. **Typical antipsychotics target D$_2$ receptors** of the limbic system but affect striatal D$_2$ receptors equally, causing **tardive dyskinesia.**

    4. **Atypical antipsychotics,** with less effect at D$_2$ receptors, **cause fewer side effects** (e.g., tardive dyskinesia).

  D. **Acetylcholine**

    1. Found in large aspiny striatal interneurons

    2. Disturbances in balance between acetylcholine and dopamine in the neostriatum may be important in basal ganglia disorders, especially **Huntington disease.**

V. **Hyperkinetic and Hypokinetic Disorders**

  A. **Hyperkinetic** (Fig. 9-5)

    1. Balance of activity shifts toward direct pathway.

    2. Inhibitory output to thalamus is reduced.

    3. Thalamic output to cortex is poorly regulated.

    4. **Dyskinesias:** Ballismus, chorea, athetosis, hemiballismus

> **Huntington disease** features degeneration of medium spiny striatal projection neurons with sparing of spiny and aspiny striatal interneurons.

  B. **Hypokinetic** (Fig. 9-6)

    1. Balance of activity shifts toward indirect pathway.

    2. Substantia nigra, pars reticulata, and globus pallidus, internal segment, are released from inhibition.

    3. Inhibitory output to thalamus is increased.

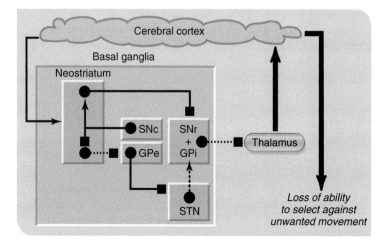

9-5: *Hyperkinetic disorders. Loss of indirect pathway leads to hyperkinetic basal ganglia disorders. Broken line, decreased activity in pathway. Thick line, increased activity in pathway. GPe, globus pallidus, external segment; GPi, globus pallidus, internal segment; SNc, substantia nigra, pars compacta; SNr, substantia nigra, pars reticulata; STN, subthalamic nucleus.*

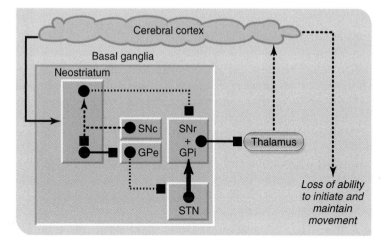

9-6: *Hypokinetic disorders. Loss of direct pathway leads to hypokinetic basal ganglia disorders. Broken line, decreased activity in pathway. Thick line, increased activity in pathway. GPe, globus pallidus, external segment; GPi, globus pallidus, internal segment; SNc, substantia nigra, pars compacta; SNr, substantia nigra, pars reticulata; STN, subthalamic nucleus.*

4. Thalamic inputs to cortex decreases.
5. **Bradykinesia** or **akinesia**

> **Parkinson disease** features degeneration of substantia nigra, pars compacta, and dopaminergic projection neurons, with resultant shift of balance from direct to indirect pathway.

VI. **Parkinson Disease**
   A. **Degeneration of dopaminergic neurons of the substantia nigra pars compacta (SNc)**
      1. More than 70% of these neurons may be lost before clear clinical signs emerge.
      2. **Lewy bodies** (eosinophilic cytoplasmic inclusion bodies) are seen in SNc neurons
   B. **Risk factors:**
      1. **Environmental causes:** herbicides and pesticides
      2. **Genetic predisposition** to both early- and late-onset forms
      3. **Age**
         a. Occurs in roughly 1% of adults older than 50 years
         b. Rate of associated dementia increases with age, approaching 80% beyond age 80 years.
         c. Less common early-onset form develops before 50 years of age.

TRAP: **T**remor (resting), **R**igidity, **A**kinesia/ bradykinesia, **P**ostural instability. At least three of these are required for diagnosis of Parkinson disease.

   C. **Signs**
      1. **Resting tremor**
      2. **Rigidity** and stiffness
      3. **Bradykinesia** or **hypokinesia,** including masked facies
      4. **Postural instability:** postural changes, including flexed posture and loss of postural reflexes leading to festinating gait
      5. Behavioral changes, including depression and dementia
   D. **Pharmacotherapies**
      1. **Dopamine agonists** replace the dopamine lost to neurodegeneration.
      2. **L-dopa** (levadopa), a dopamine precursor that crosses the blood–brain barrier, is **mainstay of treatment.** Co-administration of **carbidopa** prevents peripheral conversion of L-dopa to dopamine, which does not cross the blood–brain barrier.
      3. **Monoamine oxidase type B (MAO-B) inhibitors** slow the breakdown of dopamine.
   E. **Surgical treatment**
      1. **Pallidotomy** and **thalamotomy:** ablate discrete regions within basal ganglia nuclei and related thalamic nuclei to relieve specific symptoms, such as tremor and bradykinesia.
      2. **Deep brain stimulation (DBS):** inhibits discrete regions of basal ganglia and related thalamic nuclei. Because it is reversible and adjustable, DBS is replacing some ablative surgeries.
      3. **Dopamine restoration** has been attempted with dopamine tissue transplantation to neostriatum.

Genetic tests predict Huntington disease; chorea and behavioral changes leading to dementia determine onset.

VII. **Huntington Disease**
   A. **Autosomal dominant** neurodegenerative disorder resulting from expansion of the **CAG trinucleotide** repeat on chromosome 4, coding for huntingtin protein
      1. **Striatal neurodegeneration** seen on computed tomography and magnetic resonance imaging as **severely atrophied caudate** with concomitantly enlarged lateral ventricles

2. **Adult onset** most common, **typically third or fourth decade**
3. Uncommon: affects less than 0.01% of most populations

B. **Signs**
1. Changes in mental status, including irritability, depression, and eventual **dementia**
2. Choreoathetosis

C. **Treatment:** symptomatic, using antipsychotics and antidepressants

VIII. Other Disorders

A. **Parkinson-plus syndromes:** collection of neurodegenerative disorders resembling Parkinson disease but not responding to standard treatments for Parkinson disease.
   1. **Multiple system atrophy:** several degenerative disorders believed to be variations of one disorder.
      a. **Features:** adult onset, progressive, Parkinson-like signs, cerebellar signs and autonomic dysfunction, and glial cytoplasmic inclusions
      b. **Olivopontocerebellar atrophy:** primarily affects speech, balance, and coordination
      c. **Striatonigral degeneration:** bradykinesia and rigidity predominate.
      d. **Shy-Drager syndrome:** multiple system atrophy with postural hypotension
   2. **Progressive supranuclear palsy:** severe postural and gait instability and vertical (downward) gaze palsy are common; neurofibrillary tangles are seen within basal ganglia, brainstem, and cerebellar nuclei.

B. **Wilson disease** (hepatolenticular degeneration)
   1. Genetically induced **disruption of copper metabolism** affecting children and adults
      a. Copper deposits cause lesions in many brain regions, including most basal ganglia
   2. **Signs** reflect neurologic and hepatic abnormalities.
      a. Behavioral and emotional changes, ranging from anger and depression to psychoses
      b. Motor abnormalities including **chorea, athetosis, tremor**
      c. **Kayser-Fleischer ring** (golden brown or green ring encircling cornea) is a hallmark but not pathognomonic
   3. **Treatment:** copper chelating agents, such as penicillamine

C. **Tardive dyskinesia**
   1. **Iatrogenic** disorder resulting as **side effect of typical antipsychotic drugs** that target D_2 receptor
   2. **Signs:** varied dyskinesia, including athetosis and chorea
      a. **Face:** grimacing, lip smacking, and blinking
      b. **Body:** uncontrolled arm and leg movements and finger activity
   3. **Treatment:** atypical antipsychotics that are less active at D_2 receptors and produce fewer side effects

D. **Dystonia**
   1. **Cause unknown**
   2. **Signs:** sustained muscle contractions causing abnormal, twisted posture

a. **Cervical dystonia** (spasmodic torticollis): cramping of neck muscles affecting position of head and neck

b. **Blepharospasm:** cramping of eyelids, possibly forcing eyes shut uncontrollably

3. **Treatment:** botulinum toxin administered directly to region of neuromuscular junction to limit release of acetylcholine

E. **Tourette syndrome**

Obsessive-compulsive disorder and attention-deficit hyperactivity disorder (ADHD): frequent with Tourette syndrome

1. Probable **genetic component,** may lead to disinhibition of specific basal ganglia circuits

a. More common in males

b. Manifests before age 10 years

2. **Signs**

a. **Motor tics** can range from brief jerks of which the patient is unaware to complex movements.

b. **Vocal tics** such as throat clearing. Coprolalia occurs in less than 10% of cases.

3. **Treatment** varies with expression and may address dopaminergic, serotonergic, and noradrenergic systems.

10

Cerebellum

I. **Anatomy**
  A. Divided into **three lobes** separated by **primary and posterolateral fissures** (Fig. 10-1)
    1. **Anterior lobe** (paleocerebellum)
      a. Involved in maintaining **posture, muscle tone,** and **lower limb coordination** during "reflexive" movements (e.g., walking)
      b. Susceptible to damage from **alcohol abuse**
    2. **Posterior lobe** (neocerebellum)
      a. Involved in maintaining **posture** and **muscle tone** in the trunk and distal extremities
      b. Separated from anterior lobe by **primary fissure**
      c. **Cerebellar tonsils** are part of the inferior posterior lobe.
    3. **Flocculonodular lobe** (archicerebellum)
      a. Involved in maintaining **balance** and **eye movements** related to **vestibulo-ocular reflex**
      b. Separated from body of cerebellum by **posterolateral fissure**
      c. Direct bidirectional communication with vestibular system
  B. **Cerebellar cortex:** divided functionally into three zones (Figs. 10-2 and 10-3)
    1. **Vermis**
      a. Receives proprioceptive inputs from ipsilateral body and from contralateral motor cortex
      b. Communicates through fastigial nucleus to brainstem nuclei (vestibular and reticular) and to contralateral cerebral cortex through thalamus
      c. **Coordinates musculature of head and face** and **axial musculature** important to posture, balance, and locomotion through **medial descending motor systems** (medial reticulospinal and vestibulospinal tracts)
    2. **Intermediate zone**
      a. Receives proprioceptive inputs from ipsilateral body and from contralateral motor cortex.
      b. Communicates through globose and emboliform nuclei to brainstem reticular nuclei and to contralateral cerebral cortex through thalamus
      c. **Controls distal limb musculature** and **posture, balance,** and **locomotion** through **lateral descending motor systems** (lateral reticulospinal and vestibulospinal tracts)
    3. **Lateral hemisphere**
      a. Receives input from contralateral premotor, somatosensory, and association cortices

> Lumbar puncture in the presence of increased intracranial pressure can cause tonsillar herniation.

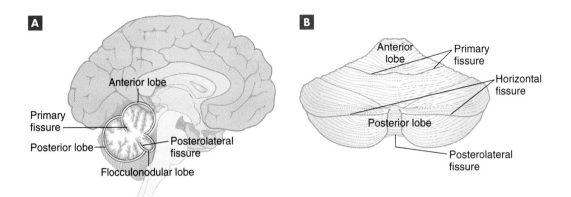

10-1: *Cerebellum.* **A,** *Midsagittal section.* **B,** *Posterior view. Primary fissure separates anterior and posterior lobes. Posterolateral fissure separates posterior and the flocculonodular lobes.*

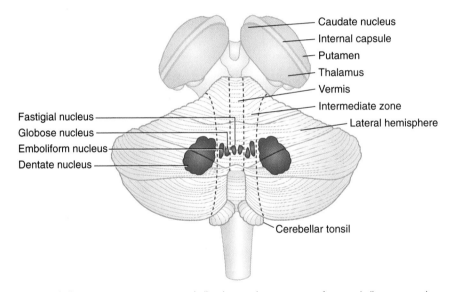

10-2: *Cerebellar cortex, posterior view. Cerebellar deep nuclei receive input from cerebellar cortex and send outputs to brainstem and thalamus. Vermis sends outputs via fastigial nuclei. Intermediate zone projects to the globose and emboliform (interposed) nuclei. Lateral hemispheres project to the dentate nucleus.*

      b. Communicates through dentate nucleus to contralateral targets, including red nucleus, and to contralateral cerebral cortex through thalamus

      c. Involved in planning of **spatial** and **temporal aspects** of **voluntary movement**

    C. **Cerebellar cortex:** three layers and five cell types (Fig. 10-4)

      1. **Molecular layer**

        a. **Basket cells:** GABAergic interneurons

        b. **Stellate cells:** GABAergic interneurons

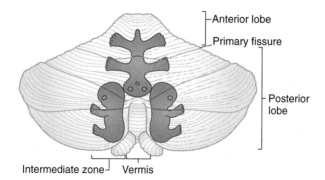

10-3: *Reflection of the body on the cerebellar cortex. Vermis is important for axial musculature and, therefore, for gait, posture, and balance. Note contribution of the intermediate zone in distal control.*

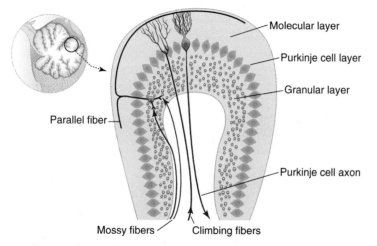

10-4: *Major cell types and layers of the cerebellar cortex. Each climbing fiber synapses on several Purkinje cells, although each Purkinje cell is contacted by only one climbing fiber. Each mossy fiber contacts granule cells. Each parallel fiber in the molecular layer contacts dendritic arbors of many Purkinje cells. Purkinje cells are the only output neurons of the cerebellum.*

   2. **Purkinje cell layer**
      a. **Purkinje cells:** GABAergic projection neurons with large, planar dendritic arbor extending into molecular layer
      b. Only **output neurons** of cerebellar cortex, with axons terminating on neurons of deep cerebellar nuclei or directly on neurons in lateral vestibular nucleus
   3. **Granular layer**
      a. **Granule cells**
         (1) Glutamatergic neurons; **only excitatory neurons** of cerebellar cortex
         (2) Axons extend into molecular layer, where they split into **parallel fibers** that run at right angles to Purkinje cell dendritic planes
         (3) Each granule cell may contact several hundred Purkinje cells.

       b. **Golgi cells:** large GABAergic interneuron

D. **Deep nuclei:** four pairs in white matter below cortex (see Fig. 10-2)

    1. **Fastigial nucleus**

       a. Receives input from Purkinje cells of vermis

       b. Projects to vestibular and reticular nuclei in brainstem and to contralateral cerebral cortex through thalamus

    2. **Globose** and **emboliform nuclei**

       a. Receive input from Purkinje cells of intermediate zone

       b. Projects to contralateral red nucleus and to contralateral cerebral cortex through thalamus

    3. **Dentate nucleus**

       a. Receives input from Purkinje cells in the lateral cerebellar hemispheres

       b. Projects to contralateral red nucleus and to contralateral cerebral cortex through thalamus

II. **Function**

  A. **Coordinates motor output**

    1. Compares motor programs encoded in cerebral cortex with actual ongoing movements

       a. Makes adjustments to movements as they occur

       b. **Temporal coordination** of motor outputs and **timing**

       c. **Spatial coordination** of motor outputs and **targeting**

    2. Maintains **normal muscle tone**

    3. Regulates **balance** and **equilibrium**

    4. **Coordinates eye movements**

  B. **Stores motor memories** for new motor skills and patterns

> Cerebellar damage may decrease muscle tone **(hypotonia).** This leads to **pendular reflexes** due to loss of damping of limb movement during deep tendon reflex activation.

III. **Neuronal Circuits**

  A. **Inputs** (Fig. 10-5)

    1. From **spinal cord:** spinocerebellar tracts transmit limb position, joint angles, muscle length, and muscle tension communicate to cerebellum through several tracts.

       a. **Posterior spinocerebellar tract**

         (1) Afferents from **lower limb** and trunk synapse in posterior thoracic nucleus, which extends from T1 to L2.

         (2) Axons from dorsal thoracic nucleus ascend ipsilaterally in lateral funiculus of spinal cord, and enter cerebellum through inferior cerebellar peduncle as **mossy fibers.**

       b. **Anterior spinocerebellar tract**

         (1) Afferents from **lower limb** and trunk tract synapse in posterior thoracic nucleus.

         (2) Axons from posterior thoracic nucleus ascend contralaterally to pons and then cross to enter ipsilateral cerebellum through superior peduncle as **mossy fibers.**

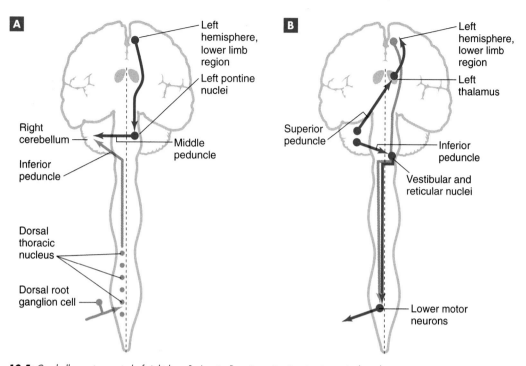

10-5: *Cerebellar motor control of right leg.* **A,** *Inputs. Proprioceptive input enters spinal cord, synapses in the posterior (dorsal) thoracic nucleus, and is directed, via inferior cerebellar peduncle, to right cerebellum (light green arrows). Left hemisphere, lower limb region, communicates via left pontine nuclei to right cerebellum via middle cerebellar peduncle (dark green arrows).* **B,** *Outputs. Right cerebellum communicates via superior peduncle to left thalamus and left cortex (upper dark green arrows). Left motor cortex communicates via corticospinal tracts to lower motor neurons in right lumbosacral spinal cord (light green arrow). Right cerebellum communicates via inferior peduncle with reticular and vestibular nuclei (lower dark green arrows). Reticulospinal and vestibulospinal pathways communicate to lower motor neurons and interneurons in right lumbosacral spinal cord.*

   c. **Cuneocerebellar tract**
     (1) Afferents from **upper limb** and trunk enter spinal cord, ascend ipsilaterally in cuneate fasciculus within posterior funiculus of spinal cord, and synapse in lateral cuneate nucleus in posterior caudal medulla.
     (2) Axons from lateral cuneate nucleus enter cerebellum through inferior cerebellar peduncle as **mossy fibers.**
  2. From **vestibular system**
    a. Some vestibular primary afferents project directly to flocculonodular lobe as **mossy fibers**
    b. Most vestibular input arises from brainstem vestibular nuclei and enters cerebellum through the inferior peduncle as **mossy fibers.**
  3. From **cerebral cortex**
    a. Massive corticopontine pathway from premotor, motor, somatosensory, and association cortices projects to pontine nuclei.

b. **Pontocerebellar tracts** project from pontine nuclei to contralateral cerebellum, entering through contralateral middle cerebellar peduncle as **mossy fibers.**

4. From **inferior olivary nucleus**

a. Input from cerebral cortex, red nucleus, cerebellum, and spinal cord

b. Axons cross midline and enter contralateral cerebellum through inferior cerebellar peduncle as **climbing fibers.**

B. **Output**

1. To **contralateral cortex**

a. Exit through superior peduncles

b. Relayed primarily through contralateral ventral lateral thalamic nucleus

2. To **contralateral red nucleus** (midbrain)

a. Exit through superior peduncles

b. Modulates upper body flexor tone through the rubrospinal tract

3. To **bilateral vestibular nuclei** (pons and medulla)

a. Exit through inferior peduncles

b. Modulates balance and equilibrium through vestibulospinal tracts

4. To **bilateral reticular nuclei** (pons and medulla)

a. Exit through inferior peduncles

b. Modulates posture through the reticulospinal tracts

Cerebellar signs:
ipsilateral to lesion

DANISH: **D**ysmetria,
Ataxia, **N**ystagmus,
Intention tremor,
Scanning speech,
Hypotonia

IV. **Signs of Cerebellar Damage** (Table 10-1)

A. **Unilateral lesion** of hemisphere or peduncles causes **ipsilateral movement disorder.**

B. **Ataxia** (not unique to cerebellar disorders): loss of coordination of voluntary movement

C. **Dysmetria:** inability to properly measure distance in motor activities ("past-pointing")

D. **Dysdiadochokinesia:** inability to perform rapid, alternating movements

E. **Asynergia** and **dyssynergia:** jerky, irregular, arrhythmic movement during planned motor activity (e.g., reaching for a target) caused by loss of muscle coordination

F. **Cerebellar gait** (ataxic gait): wide-based, unsteady, and irregular

• Common for individual to veer toward side of lesion

• Typically seen in **anterior lobe syndrome**

1. **Swaying** and **instability** when standing with feet together

> **Romberg sign:** can stand with feet close together and eyes open, but unstable and swaying after eyes are closed. Ability to stand with feet close together indicates cerebellar output is intact. Instability with eyes closed indicates a loss of proprioceptive input from the lower limbs to cerebellum (e.g., caused by vitamin B_{12} deficiency).

2. **Dysarthria** (not unique to cerebellar disorders): slowed, slurred speech reflecting loss of cerebellar coordination of muscles of speech production

3. **Scanning speech:** words, phrases, or sentences are broken into syllables of equal or unpredictable stress

Scanning speech:
cerebellar sign of
multiple sclerosis

TABLE 10-1:
Summary of
Cerebellar
Structure and
Function

Component	Connections	Syndrome
Flocculonodular lobe (derives from archicerebellum)	*Input:* from vestibular nerve and vestibular nuclei *Output:* to vestibular nuclei directly and via fastigial nuclei	Gait disturbance, head rotation, nystagmus, disturbance in station (eyes open or closed)
Vermis, intermediate zone (derives from paleocerebellum)	*Input:* from spinocerebellar tracts and brainstem nuclei receiving spinal input (reticular formation, inferior olivary nucleus) *Output:* to brainstem nuclei giving rise to bulbospinal paths (reticular formation, lateral vestibular nucleus, and red nucleus) via fastigial nuclei and interposed nuclei (globose and emboliform)	Gait disturbance, rigidity in animal models
Hemispheres (derive from neocerebellum)	*Input:* from corticopontocerebellar pathway; indirect connections from cerebral cortex through inferior olivary nucleus and reticular formation *Output:* to ventrolateral nucleus of thalamus via dentate nucleus; thalamic projections to motor cortex	Hypotonia, pendular knee jerk, disturbance in station, weakness, delay in starting and stopping muscular contractions, disturbances in rate of voluntary movements, dysmetria, decomposition of movement, dysdiadochokinesia speech disturbance, gait disturbance, intention tremor

    a. Reflects a loss of timing coordination from the cerebellum
    b. Observed after damage to vermis
G. **Hypotonia**
    1. Caused by loss of cerebellar influence on stretch reflexes
    2. **Hyporeflexia** may occur
    3. Tests of deep tendon reflexes can yield **pendular reflexes.**
H. **Intention** (action) **tremor:** slow, rhythmic (2- to 3-Hz) tremor caused by hypotonia of limb-girdle muscles
    1. **Occurs at the end of a planned movement** (during target acquisition); not present at rest or initial stages of movement, in contrast to **resting tremor of Parkinson disease.**
    2. Especially prominent in fine-control movements; may extend to head, trunk, upper limb

V. **Causes of Cerebellar Damage**
  A. **Wernicke-Korsakoff syndrome**
    1. Caused by malnutrition leading to **thiamine deficiency,** most often after **chronic alcohol use**

Signs of cerebellar damage: gait ataxia, limb ataxia, and hypotonia

Prevention of Wernicke encephalopathy: Thiamine must be administered with glucose.

Chronic alcohol abuse: gait ataxia without limb ataxia

2. Degeneration occurs in the anterosuperior cerebellar vermis, mammillary bodies, and dorsomedial thalamus.
   • Orange mammillary bodies due to hemorrhage
3. **Wernicke syndrome (acute phase):** gait ataxia, horizontal and vertical nystagmus and ophthalmoplegias (diplopia, strabismus), and confusion
4. **Korsakoff's psychosis (chronic phase):** severe anterograde and retrograde **amnesia with confabulation**

B. **Alcoholic cerebellar degeneration**
   1. Superior vermis more affected than hemispheres
   2. Often correlated with **malnutrition**
   3. **Gait ataxia without limb ataxia**

C. **Cerebellar hemorrhage**
   1. May be only hours from onset to irreversible coma
   2. **Signs:** vomiting (consistent with many parenchymal hemorrhages, in contrast to infarcts) and ataxia

D. **Friedreich ataxia**
   1. Gradual onset in first, second, or third decade of life
   2. Involves **spinocerebellar tracts, posterior columns,** and **lateral corticospinal** tracts
   3. **Trinucleotide repeat** (GAA) in frataxin gene on chromosome 9
   4. **Signs and symptoms: gait disturbances,** dysarthria, sensory loss in limbs, pyramidal signs, and possible areflexia

E. **Lateral medullary syndrome**
   1. Damage to lateral medulla and cerebellum resulting from **occlusion of vertebral or posterior inferior cerebellar artery**
   2. **Signs and symptoms:** analgesia and thermanesthesia affecting ipsilateral face and contralateral body, dysphagia, dysarthria, ipsilateral Horner syndrome, nystagmus, vertigo, loss of taste from ipsilateral tongue

F. **Multiple sclerosis** (see Chapter 5, section II, D)

G. **Tumors** that increase intracranial pressure
   1. **Medulloblastoma:** embryonic tissue in posterior cerebellum; frequently occurs in children
   2. **Ependymoma:** in wall of fourth ventricle
   3. **Choroid plexus papilloma** commonly within fourth ventricle (adult) or lateral ventricle (children)
   4. **Hemangioblastoma** of cerebellum

Cranial Nerves

I. **CN I: Olfactory**
   A. **Sensory:** smell
   B. **Anatomy**
      1. Bipolar sensory neurons in olfactory neuroepithelium project through cribriform plate to synapse in olfactory bulb (Figs. 11-1 and 11-2, Table 11-1).
      2. Central projections from olfactory bulb run in olfactory tract to piriform cortex in medial temporal lobe.
   C. **Signs of damage:** partial or complete loss of **smell and taste**

> If accompanied by any visual disturbance, partial or complete loss of sense of smell can indicate a **compression injury** by an orbital or skull-based tumor.
> **Olfactory groove meningioma** (Foster-Kennedy syndrome) can cause ipsilateral anosmia, blindness in the ipsilateral eye, and contralateral papilledema.
> **Olfactory hallucinations** can be aura preceding temporal lobe epilepsy ("uncinate fits").

Test olfaction after head trauma, if frontal lobe lesion suspected, and when taste is diminished.

II. **CN II: Optic** (see Chapter 12)
   A. **Sensory:** vision and visual reflexes
   B. **Anatomy**
      1. **Retina**
         a. **Rods:** function in dim light for monochromatic vision
         b. **Cones:** work in bright light for color vision
         c. **Bipolar cells:** transmit rod and cone signal to ganglion cells
         d. **Retinal ganglion cells:** project to thalamus
      2. **Projection to thalamus**
         a. **Optic nerve:** axons of retinal ganglion cells leave the retina.
         b. **Optic chiasm:** retinal ganglion cell axons as they redistribute from left and right eye to carry left visual field of both eyes to right hemisphere and vice versa
         c. **Optic tract:** retinal ganglion cell axons carrying one visual field from both eyes to contralateral **lateral geniculate nucleus (LGN) of thalamus**
   C. **Signs of damage**
      1. **Retina:** partial or complete loss of vision in ipsilateral eye

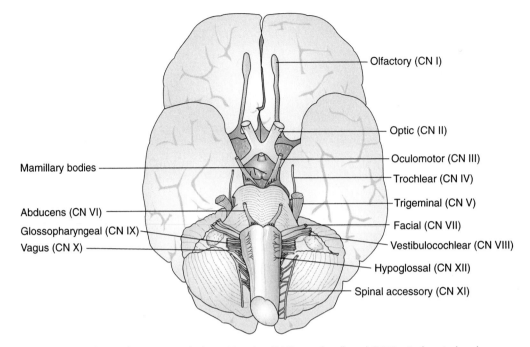

Olfactory (CN I)

Optic (CN II)

Oculomotor (CN III)

Trochlear (CN IV)

Trigeminal (CN V)

Facial (CN VII)

Vestibulocochlear (CN VIII)

Hypoglossal (CN XII)

Spinal accessory (CN XI)

Mamillary bodies

Abducens (CN VI)

Glossopharyngeal (CN IX)

Vagus (CN X)

11-1: *Each cranial nerve exiting the brain. Note that CN IV exits dorsally and CN XI exits the spinal cord.*

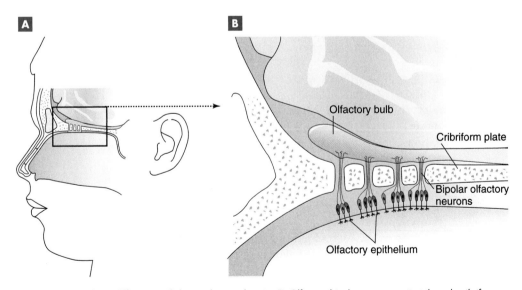

A

B

Olfactory bulb

Cribriform plate

Bipolar olfactory neurons

Olfactory epithelium

11-2: A, *Olfactory epithelium within nasal cavity.* **B,** *Olfactory bipolar neurons project through cribriform plate.*

TABLE 11-1:
Origin and
Function of Cranial
Nerves

Cranial Nerve	Origin	Function
CN I, Olfactory	Olfactory mucosa	Smell
CN II, Optic	Ganglion cells of retina	Vision
CN III, Oculomotor	Oculomotor nucleus	Extraocular muscles: superior rectus, inferior rectus, medial rectus, inferior oblique, superior levator palpebrae
	Edinger-Westphal nucleus	Accommodation for near vision: pupillary sphincter and ciliary muscles
CN IV, Trochlear	Trochlear nucleus	Extraocular muscle: superior oblique
CN V, Trigeminal	Trigeminal ganglion	General sensation: scalp, face, upper and lower jaws, oral cavity, nasal cavity, eye
	Trigeminal motor nucleus	Muscles of mastication plus mylohyoid, anterior digastric, tensor tympani, tensor veli palatini
CN VI, Abducens	Abducens nucleus	Extraocular muscle: lateral rectus
CN VII, Facial	Facial nucleus	Muscles of facial expression plus stylohyoid, posterior digastric, stapedius
	Superior salivatory nucleus	Secretomotor to lacrimal gland, submandibular and sublingual salivary glands, small glands of oral and nasal cavities
	Geniculate ganglion	Taste from anterior two thirds of tongue
	Geniculate ganglion	Visceral sensation
	Geniculate ganglion	Somatic sensation: external ear and tympanic membrane
CN VIII, Vestibulocochlear	Vestibular ganglion	Equilibrium
	Spiral ganglion	Hearing
CN IX, Glossopharyngeal	Nucleus ambiguus	Stylopharyngeus
	Inferior salivatory nucleus	Secretomotor to parotid salivary gland
	Inferior glossopharyngeal ganglion	Taste from posterior third of tongue
	Inferior glossopharyngeal ganglion	Visceral sensation: pharynx and posterior third of tongue; visceral reflexes
	Superior glossopharyngeal ganglion	Somatic sensation: tympanic membrane and middle ear
CN X, Vagus	Nucleus ambiguus	Muscles of pharynx, larynx, and soft palate excluding stylopharyngeus but including palatoglossus
	Dorsal motor nucleus	Cardiac muscle, smooth muscle, and glands of thorax and abdomen
	Inferior vagal ganglion	Taste over epiglottis
	Inferior vagal ganglion	Visceral sensation and reflexes
	Superior vagal ganglion	Somatic sensation: external auditory canal and dura
CN XI, Spinal accessory	Accessory nucleus in spinal cord	Sternocleidomastoid and trapezius
CN XII, Hypoglossal	Hypoglossal nucleus	Intrinsic and extrinsic muscles of tongue except palatoglossus

Handwritten annotation at right of CN V row: exits upper lateral pons → middle cerebellar peduncle junction

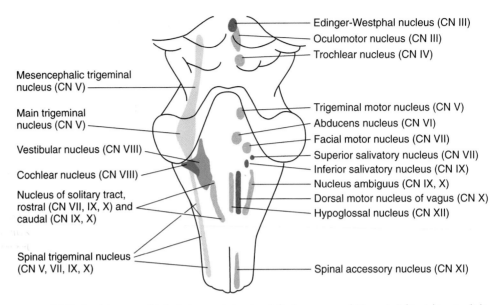

Edinger-Westphal nucleus (CN III)
Oculomotor nucleus (CN III)
Trochlear nucleus (CN IV)

Mesencephalic trigeminal nucleus (CN V)

Main trigeminal nucleus (CN V)

Vestibular nucleus (CN VIII)

Cochlear nucleus (CN VIII)

Nucleus of solitary tract, rostral (CN VII, IX, X) and caudal (CN IX, X)

Spinal trigeminal nucleus (CN V, VII, IX, X)

Trigeminal motor nucleus (CN V)
Abducens nucleus (CN VI)
Facial motor nucleus (CN VII)
Superior salivatory nucleus (CN VII)
Inferior salivatory nucleus (CN IX)
Nucleus ambiguus (CN IX, X)
Dorsal motor nucleus of vagus (CN X)
Hypoglossal nucleus (CN XII)

Spinal accessory nucleus (CN XI)

11-3: *Cranial nerve nuclei. Brainstem, posterior view. Left, six sensory nuclei (green); right, eight motor (light gray) and four parasympathetic (dark gray) nuclei. The cranial nerve through which each motor nucleus projects and the cranial nerve(s) that carry sensory input to each sensory nucleus are indicated.*

2. **Optic nerve**
   a. Partial or complete loss of vision in ipsilateral eye
   b. Loss of pupillary light reflex

   > Partial or complete loss of the direct and consensual light reflex **(afferent pupillary defect)** is frequently an early sign in multiple sclerosis that reflects inflammation of the optic nerve.

3. **Optic chiasm**
   a. **Lateral chiasm** (e.g., from aneurysm of internal carotid artery): ipsilateral nasal field anopsia
   b. **Central chiasm** (e.g., from tumor or aneurysm of anterior communicating artery): bitemporal hemianopsia
4. **Optic tract:** homonymous contralateral hemianopsia

III. **CN III: Oculomotor**
   A. **Motor:** eye movement, lid retraction, pupil constriction
   B. **Motor component** (Figs. 11-3 and 11-4, Table 11-2)
      1. **Anatomy: oculomotor nucleus** in medial midbrain sends axons that emerge from anterior midbrain, medial to cerebral peduncles
      2. **Function:** controls most eye movement (superior rectus, inferior rectus, medial rectus, and inferior oblique) and raises eyelid (levator palpebrae superioris)

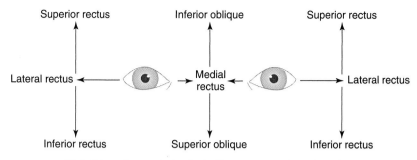

11-4: *Extraocular muscles involved with eye movement in each quadrant.*

TABLE 11-2:
Function of Cranial Nerve Nuclei

Nuclei	Cranial Nerves	Function
Motor		
Oculomotor nucleus	CN III	Extraocular muscles: superior rectus, inferior rectus, medial rectus, inferior oblique, superior levator palpebrae
Trochlear nucleus	CN IV	Extraocular muscle: superior oblique
Trigeminal motor nucleus	CN V	Muscles of mastication
Abducens nucleus	CN VI	Extraocular muscle: lateral rectus
Facial motor nucleus	CN VII	Muscles of facial expression
Nucleus ambiguus	CN IX, CN X	Muscles of speech and swallowing
Accessory nucleus	CN XI	Muscles to turn head, tilt chin
Hypoglossal nucleus	CN XII	Tongue
Autonomic (Parasympathetic)		
Edinger-Westphal nucleus	CN III	Pupil constriction, lens thickening
Superior salivatory nucleus	CN VII	Tearing, salivation
Inferior salivatory nucleus	CN IX	Salivation
Dorsal motor nucleus of vagus	CN X	Control all thoracic viscera and all abdominal viscera to splenic flexure of colon
Sensory		
Olfactory bulb	CN I	Smell
Retinal ganglion cells	CN II	Vision
Trigeminal nucleus		
Mesencephalic	CN V	Proprioception
Main (pontine)	CN V	Fine touch, vibration
Spinal	CN V, VII, IX, X	Pain, temperature, crude touch
Nucleus of solitary tract		
Rostral	CN VII, IX, X	Taste
Caudal	IX, X	Homeostasis (blood pressure, blood gases)
Cochlear nucleus	CN VIII	Hearing
Vestibular nucleus	CN VIII	Balance

C. **Autonomic (parasympathetic) component**
   1. **Anatomy: Edinger-Westphal nucleus** in medial midbrain **projects to ciliary ganglion,** which innervates pupillary constrictor and ciliary muscles
   2. **Function:** pupillary constriction (**miosis**) and accommodation (**lens thickening**)
D. **Signs of damage:** eye down and out, pupil dilation (mydriasis), eyelid droop (ptosis)

CN III compression: eye down and out, pupil dilated, eyelid drooped

CN III ischemia from diabetes: extraocular muscle palsy with pupil sparing

> A dilated and unresponsive pupil is an early sign of oculomotor nerve compression from a temporal lobe herniation because the parasympathetic fibers are affected first.
>
> Vascular lesions to nerve frequently affect eye movement with pupil sparing.

IV. **CN IV: Trochlear**
   A. **Motor:** depresses and extorts eye (superior oblique)
   B. **Anatomy: trochlear nucleus** in medial midbrain sends **axons that emerge from posterior midbrain**
   C. **Signs of damage: diplopia** when gaze directed **down and in,** frequently with head tilt to "good" eye

CN IV lesion: difficulty walking down steps because of double vision

V. **CN V: Trigeminal**
   A. **Mixed:** sensation from face; control of bite and chewing (Fig. 11-5)
   B. **Motor component**
   1. **Anatomy: trigeminal motor nucleus** (masticator nucleus) in pons projects through **mandibular branch** (V_3).
   2. **Function:** innervates muscles of mastication (masseter, temporalis, and pterygoid)

> The **jaw-jerk reflex** is a monosynaptic stretch reflex that relies on input from muscle spindles through the mandibular branch of the trigeminal nerve, which relays through the mesencephalic trigeminal nucleus to the trigeminal motor nucleus.

   C. **Sensory component**
   1. **Anatomy:** three branches with cell bodies in trigeminal ganglion that enter lateral pons at level of middle cerebellar peduncle
   2. **Function:** transmits fine touch, pressure, vibration, pain, temperature, proprioception from skin, muscle, and joints of face
   3. **Ophthalmic branch** (V_1): sensory innervation from upper face, including conjunctiva, cornea, forehead, eyelid, bridge of nose, dura, and vasculature of anterior brain
   4. **Maxillary branch** (V_2): sensory innervation from cheeks, nasal cavity, and upper jaw
   5. **Mandibular branch** (V_3)
      a. Sensory innervation from lower jaw, teeth, gums, anterior two thirds of tongue, external auditory meatus, and external tympanic membrane

Corneal reflex tests CN V (sensory) and CN VII (motor).

Headache pain: may arise from activation of trigeminal nerve endings within brain vasculature

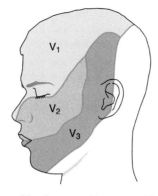

11-5: *Regions of face and head innervated by trigeminal branches V_1, V_2, and V_3.*

    b. Proprioception (stretch receptors) from lower jaw
6. **V_1, V_2, and V_3 sensory fields do not overlap.**

> **Herpes zoster virus,** which may remain latent in the **trigeminal ganglia** for years, may reemerge in ophthalmic branch to cause corneal scarring.
>
> **Herpes simplex virus,** which may also remain latent in the **trigeminal ganglia,** can course through the trigeminal branches that innervate the dura and vasculature on the base of the brain, causing herpes simplex encephalitis. The same virus traveling through V_2 or V_3 can cause cold sores.

D. **Sensory nuclei**
  1. **Mesencephalic trigeminal nucleus**
    a. Nucleus located in lateral midbrain; only sensory nucleus containing primary sensory neuron cell bodies; all other primary sensory cell bodies are in peripheral ganglia.
    b. Receives **proprioceptive information** from jaw (V_3)
    c. Projects to trigeminal motor nucleus to form sensory arm of monosynaptic jaw jerk reflex arc
  2. **Main (pontine) trigeminal nucleus**
    a. Nucleus located in lateral pons
    b. Receives **fine discriminative touch** and **vibration** from V_1, V_2, and V_3
    c. Sends central projections (ventral trigeminothalamic tract) across midline to join contralateral medial lemniscus and project to ventral posteromedial nucleus of thalamus (VPM)
    d. Sends minor projection (dorsal trigeminothalamic tract) to ipsilateral VPM
  3. **Spinal trigeminal nucleus**
    a. Nucleus located in caudal lateral pons to rostral spinal cord
    b. Receives **pain, temperature,** and crude **touch** from V_1 to V_3 (through spinal trigeminal tract) and minor components from glossopharyngeal and vagus nerves

c. Sends central projections across midline to join spinothalamic tract and project to VPM.

E. **Signs of damage to trigeminal system**
1. **Lower motor neuron damage:** unilateral bite weakness
2. **Upper motor neuron damage:** minimal effect, because of bilateral cortical control
3. **Trigeminal neuralgia** (tic douloureux)
   a. Frequently caused by **pressure from a blood vessel** (e.g., anterior inferior cerebellar artery or superior cerebellar artery)

   > Microvascular decompression (separation of the nerve and blood vessel with a Teflon plate) has been used to treat this disorder.

   b. Often precipitated by **activating trigger zone** (e.g., chewing or touching nose or cheek)
   c. Excruciating, intermittent (<1 minute duration), **lancinating pain,** most often in distribution of V_2 or V_3, which may cause **facial grimace**
   d. **No sensory loss**

Pain of trigeminal neuralgia: relieved by surgical ablation of spinal trigeminal tract

VI. **CN VI: Abducens**
A. **Motor: abducts** eye movement (lateral rectus)
B. **Anatomy:** abducens nucleus in posterior medial pons
C. **Signs of damage**
1. **Paralysis of lateral gaze** with possible medial deviation of affected eye
2. Damage to peripheral nerve paralyzes lateral gaze in ipsilateral eye
3. Damage at base of pons paralyzes lateral gaze in ipsilateral eye and contralateral body.
4. Damage to nucleus region paralyzes lateral gaze in both eyes because lateral gaze center is damaged.

CN VI: longest cranial nerve run in subarachnoid space and susceptible to increased intracranial pressure

VII. **CN VII: Facial**
A. **Mixed:** facial expression, touch, taste, tearing, salivation, and damping loud noises
B. **Motor component**
1. **Anatomy:** motor nucleus located in posterior medial pons sends axons that **wrap around abducens nucleus** before exiting anterolateral pons in cerebellopontine angle.
2. **Function**
   a. Innervates muscles of facial expression
   b. Innervates stapedius muscle of middle ear

   > Loud, low-frequency noise activates the **stapedial reflex** to contract the muscle, which damps the sound.

C. **Autonomic (parasympathetic) component**
1. **Anatomy:** superior salivatory nucleus in dorsal posterior pons projects to postganglionic cell bodies in pterygopalatine and submandibular ganglia

Dorsal pontine lesion: ipsilateral facial and lateral gaze paralysis.

Facial nerve makes a face!

2. **Function**
   a. **Pterygopalatine ganglion** innervates lacrimal glands for **tearing** (and palatal, pharyngeal, nasal mucous glands)
   b. **Submandibular ganglion** innervates submandibular and sublingual glands and mucous glands of oral cavity for **salivation**

D. **Sensory component**
   1. **Touch** from external ear carried in **intermediate nerve,** with cell bodies in geniculate ganglion, projects to spinal trigeminal nucleus
   2. **Taste** from anterior two thirds of tongue carried in **chorda tympani,** with cell bodies in geniculate ganglion, projects to nucleus of solitary tract

Front of Tongue: Trigeminal Feels, Facial Tastes FT TF FT!

E. **Signs of damage**
   1. **Lower motor neuron (Bell palsy)**
      a. Paralysis of ipsilateral face, upper and lower
      b. Ipsilateral hyperacusis
      c. Ipsilateral loss of salivation and tearing
      d. Ipsilateral loss of taste in anterior two thirds of tongue
   2. **Upper motor neuron**
      a. Paralysis of contralateral lower face
      b. **Forehead unaffected,** because of bilateral cortical control (Fig. 11-6)

VIII. **CN VIII: Vestibulocochlear** (see Chapter 13)
   A. **Sensory:** balance and hearing
   B. **Anatomy:** central projection from inner ear (basilar membrane of cochlea and labyrinth) courses through **internal acoustic meatus** to brainstem cochlear and vestibular nuclei.

   An **acoustic neuroma** on either the facial or vestibulocochlear nerve affects hearing and control of facial muscles because both nerves pass through the restricted space of the internal acoustic meatus.

Tumor near internal acoustic meatus: ipsilateral facial paralysis with vertigo and ipsilateral sensorineural hearing loss

   C. **Function of auditory component**
      1. **Hair cells at base** of basilar membrane respond to **high-frequency** input.
      2. **Hair cells at apex** of basilar membrane respond to **low-frequency** input.
   D. **Function of vestibular component**
      1. **Hair cells of static labyrinth** (utricle and saccule) respond to head position in space (e.g., **gravity**).
      2. **Hair cells of kinetic labyrinth** (semicircular canals) respond to rotational movements (e.g., **head turning**).
   E. **Sensory nuclei**
      1. **Cochlear nucleus**
         a. Dorsolateral nucleus located at pontomedullary junction
         b. Sends bilateral outputs through lateral lemniscus to inferior colliculus and then to medial geniculate nucleus of thalamus

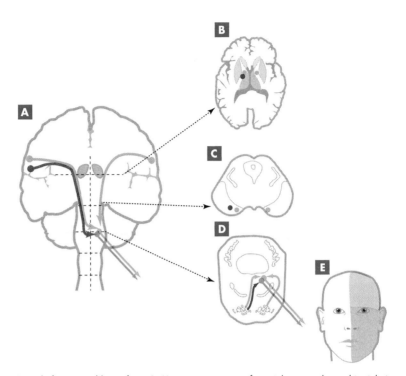

11-6: *Control of upper and lower face.* **A,** *Upper motor neurons from right cortex descend in right internal capsule and cross to innervate upper (green) and lower (gray) portions of facial motor nucleus in left pons. Upper motor neurons from left cortex descend in left internal capsule to innervate only upper portion of left facial motor nucleus (green).* **B,** *Horizontal section through hemispheres showing upper motor neuron axons in right and left internal capsule.* **C,** *Transverse section through midbrain showing upper motor neuron axons in right and left cerebral peduncles.* **D,** *Transverse section through pons showing upper motor neuron axons as they reach lower motor neurons in facial motor nucleus.* **E,** *Upper face is controlled bilaterally from the cortex; lower face is controlled only from the contralateral cortex.*

      2. **Vestibular nucleus**
         a. Four-part nucleus extending through dorsolateral pons and medulla
         b. Projects to ocular motor nuclei through medial longitudinal fasciculus and the spinal cord through medial vestibulospinal tract
  F. **Signs of damage**
      1. **Cochlea damage: loss of pure tonal hearing**
      2. **Labyrinth damage:** transient **vertigo** and **nystagmus**
      3. **Vestibulocochlear nerve damage: tinnitus, high-frequency hearing loss,** difficulty with speech comprehension, **loss of stapedial reflex, vertigo** with nystagmus toward an irritative lesion or away from a destructive lesion

 IX. **CN IX: Glossopharyngeal**
  A. **Mixed:** speech and swallowing, cardiovascular and respiratory control
  B. **Motor component**
      1. **Anatomy: nucleus ambiguus** in lateral medulla

    2. **Function:** innervates stylopharyngeus, which elevates pharynx for **speech and swallowing**
- C. **Autonomic (parasympathetic) component**
  1. **Anatomy:** inferior salivatory nucleus in dorsal medulla synapses on postganglionic cell bodies in otic ganglion
  2. **Function:** stimulates **salivation** from parotid gland
- D. **Sensory component**
  1. **Touch, pressure, pain, and temperature** from posterior oral cavity (pharynx, soft palate, and posterior third of tongue), with cell bodies in **superior glossopharyngeal ganglion,** projects to **spinal trigeminal nucleus**
  2. **Blood pressure and blood gases** from carotid sinus and carotid body, with cell bodies in **inferior glossopharyngeal ganglion,** projects to **caudal nucleus of solitary tract**
  3. **Taste** from posterior third of tongue, with cell bodies in **inferior glossopharyngeal ganglion,** projects to **rostral nucleus of solitary tract**
- E. **Signs of damage**
  1. **Lower motor neuron:** may involve vagus nerve
     - a. **Dysarthria and dysphagia**
     - b. Ipsilateral loss of **gag reflex**
  2. **Upper motor neuron:** little effect because of bilateral cortical control

> Gag reflex tests CN IX (sensory) and CN X (motor).

X. **CN X: Vagus**
- A. **Mixed:** speech and swallowing; parasympathetic control of visceral organs in thoracic cavity and abdomen to the level of the transverse colon
- B. **Motor component**
  1. **Anatomy: nucleus ambiguus** in lateral medulla
  2. **Function:** innervates pharynx, larynx, upper esophagus, levator veli palatini, which **elevates soft palate,** and palatoglossus, which elevates tongue and constricts fauces
- C. **Autonomic (parasympathetic) components**
  1. **Anatomy:** dorsal motor nucleus in dorsal medulla (see Chapter 14)
  2. **Function:** parasympathetic control to organs of body extending through rostral third of transverse colon

> Stimulating ear canal: can cause vomiting, coughing, and fainting because CN X is activated

- D. **Sensory component**
  1. **Touch, pressure, pain, and temperature** from external ear and ear canal, infratentorial dura, and tympanic membrane (**vomiting reflex**), with cell bodies in **superior vagal ganglion,** projects to **spinal trigeminal nucleus**
  2. **Touch** from pharynx, larynx, trachea, esophagus, and thoracic and abdominal viscera, with cell bodies in **inferior vagal ganglion,** projects to brainstem reticular neurons
  3. **Taste** from epiglottis, with cell bodies in **inferior vagal ganglion,** projects to **rostral nucleus of solitary tract**
- E. **Signs of damage**
  1. **Lower motor neuron:** may involve glossopharyngeal nerve
     - a. Dysarthria and dysphagia

b. Ipsilateral loss of **gag reflex**

c. **Bilateral lesion not compatible with life**

2. **Upper motor neuron:** minimal effect because of bilateral cortical control

XI. **CN XI: Spinal Accessory**

A. **Motor**

1. Innervates sternocleidomastoid, which **tilts chin** and **rotates head to opposite side**

2. Innervates trapezius, which **shrugs shoulder**

B. **Anatomy:** cell bodies in spinal segments C1–C6 project through spinal roots; axons ascend in peripheral nervous system (PNS), pass through foramen magnum, and exit cranial cavity through jugular foramen.

C. **Signs of damage**

1. **Lower motor neuron:** difficulty in turning head to contralateral side with ipsilateral shoulder droop

2. **Upper motor neuron:** no signs because of bilateral cortical control

XII. **CN XII: Hypoglossal**

A. **Motor:** innervates ipsilateral hypoglossus to **control ipsilateral tongue protrusion**

B. **Anatomy:** hypoglossal nucleus in dorsomedial medulla sends axons that emerge from anterior medulla as rootlets between medullary pyramids and inferior olive.

C. **Signs of damage**

1. **Lower motor neuron:** tongue deviates to side of lesion.

2. **Upper motor neuron:** tongue deviates to side opposite lesion.

UMN or LMN lesion of CN XII: tongue deviates to weak side on protrusion

> Each hypoglossal nerve directs the tongue to opposite side. After damage, the **tongue deviates toward its weak side** on protrusion, that is, toward a lower motor neuron lesion and away from an upper motor neuron lesion.

XIII. **Brainstem Syndromes Affecting Multiple Cranial Nerves** (Tables 11-3 to 11-9)

TABLE 11-3:
Posterior Inferior Cerebellar Artery Syndrome (Lateral Medullary, or Wallenberg, Syndrome)

Likely cause: infarct of posterior inferior cerebellar artery or vertebral artery

Site of Lesion	Signs and Symptoms
Spinal trigeminal tract and nucleus	Loss of pain, ipsilateral face
Spinothalamic tract	Loss of pain, contralateral body
Nucleus ambiguus/CN IX, X	Difficulties with speech (dysarthria) and swallowing (dysphagia) Loss of ipsilateral gag reflex Hiccups
Descending sympathetic control	Ipsilateral Horner syndrome: pupil constriction (miosis), narrowed palpebral fissure (ptosis), lack of sweating (anhidrosis)
Vestibular nucleus	Vertigo, nystagmus
Cerebellum	Ipsilateral clumsiness, ataxia, intention tremor

TABLE 11-4:
Medial Medullary Syndrome (Alternating Hypoglossal Hemiplegia)

Likely cause: infarct of penetrating branches of anterior spinal artery or basilar artery

Site of Lesion	Signs and Symptoms
Corticospinal tracts within medullary pyramids	Hemiparesis, flaccid hemiparalysis, Babinski sign, loss of superficial reflexes in contralateral body
Medial lemniscus	Loss of vibration, fine touch, proprioception from contralateral arm and leg
Hypoglossal nucleus and nerve	Tongue weakness and atrophy ipsilateral to lesion; tongue deviates toward lesion on protrusion

TABLE 11-5:
Basal Pontine Syndrome (Locked-in Syndrome When Bilateral)

Likely cause: infarct of penetrating branches of basilar artery

Site of Lesion	Signs and Symptoms
Pontine base containing corticospinal tracts and descending cortical control of brainstem upper motor neurons	Hemiparesis, spastic hemiparalysis, Babinski sign, loss of superficial reflexes in contralateral body. Illustrated lesion is bilateral, which causes bilateral paralysis. Tongue weakness (without atrophy) and deviation away from side of lesion. Illustrated lesion completely paralyzes tongue.
Abducens nerve	Paralyzed eye ipsilateral to lesion with loss of lateral gaze. Illustrated lesion paralyzes lateral gaze for both eyes.

TABLE 11-6:
Dorsal Pontine Syndrome

Likely cause: infarct of penetrating branches of basilar artery

Site of Lesion	Signs and Symptoms
Facial motor nucleus or nerve	Paralyzed ipsilateral face, upper and lower
Abducens nerve	Paralyzed eye ipsilateral to lesion with loss of lateral gaze
Lateral gaze center	Loss of conjugate gaze ipsilateral to lesion
Medial lemniscus, if lesion extends anteriorly	Loss of fine touch, vibration, and proprioception from contralateral body
Spinothalamic tract, if lesion extends anteriorly and laterally	Loss of pain and temperature from contralateral face and body
Main trigeminal nucleus, if lesion extends sufficiently rostrally	Loss of fine touch and vibration from ipsilateral face
Descending spinal trigeminal tract, if lesion extends sufficiently laterally	Loss of pain and temperature from ipsilateral face

TABLE 11-7:
Weber Syndrome (Alternating Oculomotor Hemiplegia)

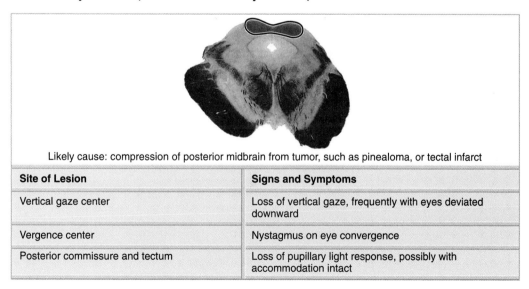

Likely cause: infarct of penetrating branches of posterior cerebral artery

Site of Lesion	Signs and Symptoms
Cerebral peduncles containing corticospinal tracts and descending cortical control of brainstem upper motor neurons	Hemiparesis, spastic hemiparalysis, Babinski sign, loss of superficial reflexes in contralateral body Hemiparesis or hemiparalysis in contralateral lower face Tongue weakness without atrophy and deviation away from side of lesion
Oculomotor nerve	Paralysis of eye ipsilateral to lesion with marked ptosis (eyelid droop), mydriasis (pupil dilation), lateral strabismus (with complete lesions, eye rolls down and out)

TABLE 11-8:
Parinaud Syndrome (Dorsal Midbrain Syndrome)

Likely cause: compression of posterior midbrain from tumor, such as pinealoma, or tectal infarct

Site of Lesion	Signs and Symptoms
Vertical gaze center	Loss of vertical gaze, frequently with eyes deviated downward
Vergence center	Nystagmus on eye convergence
Posterior commissure and tectum	Loss of pupillary light response, possibly with accommodation intact

TABLE 11-9:
Acoustic Neuroma (Vestibular Schwannoma)

Likely cause: schwannoma on vestibulocochlear nerve

Site of Lesion	Signs and Symptoms

Vestibulocochlear nerve
   Vestibular division
   Cochlear division
	
	Vertigo, nystagmus
	Tinnitus, hearing loss

Facial nerve	Facial weakness Loss of taste sensation, salivation, and tearing

Visual System

I. **Eye**
   A. **Layers** (Fig. 12-1)
      1. **Fibrous tunic**
         a. **Sclera:** surrounds eyeball
         b. **Cornea:** specialized, transparent sclera through which light enters eye
         c. **Meninges:** surround optic nerve and are continuous with sclera
      2. **Vascular tunic**
         a. **Choroid:** between sclera and retina
         b. **Ciliary body**
            (1) Continuous with choroid anteriorly
            (2) Supplies aqueous humor, which is similar to cerebrospinal fluid and fills anterior and posterior chambers
         c. **Scleral venous sinus** (Schlemm canal) drains aqueous humor to venous circulation.
         d. **Iris:** smooth muscle continuation of ciliary body
         e. **Lens** consists of protein and water.
      3. **Retina**
         a. **Central nervous system (CNS)** tissue derived as outpouching of diencephalon
         b. Consists of nuclear layers, which contain cell bodies, and plexiform layers, which contain synaptic processes
   B. **Blood supply**
      1. **Central retinal artery,** a branch of the ophthalmic artery, approaches retina within meningeal sheath containing optic nerve.

      > **Sudden painless loss of vision** in one eye indicates transient ischemic attack affecting the central retinal artery.

      2. **Choriocapillaries** run in subretinal space between retina and sclera.
      3. **Central retinal vein** exits through optic nerve sheath.

      > If intracranial pressure increases, the dural sheath surrounding optic nerve acts like a pressure cuff to restrict venous return, causing **papilledema** (swelling of retinal veins with edema of optic disc), which is seen on funduscopic exam.

   C. **Focusing**
      1. Cornea provides less than 40 diopters of focusing power.
      2. Lens adds 20 diopters and can thicken to increase focusing power.

Glaucoma: ↑ intraocular pressure caused by impaired circulation or reabsorption of aqueous humor

Cataracts: lens opacity caused by protein aggregates

Neovascularization in subretinal space: one cause of age-related macular degeneration

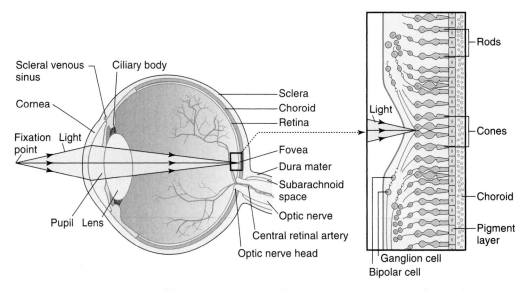

12-1: A, Anatomy of the eye. **B,** Major retinal cell types. Cones are concentrated at fovea; rods are concentrated toward periphery. Rods and cones communicate to bipolar neurons, which communicate to retinal ganglion cells. At fovea, cones communicate without convergence, and bipolar neurons and retinal ganglion cells are deflected away from light path. At periphery, rods communicate with much convergence.

3. Lens reverses image on retina, both top to bottom and right to left.
4. **Emmetropia** (normal vision): relaxed cornea–lens system focuses distant image on retina.
5. **Myopia** (nearsightedness): relaxed system focuses image in front of retina.
6. **Hyperopia** (farsightedness): relaxed system focuses image behind retina.
7. **Presbyopia** ("old eyes"): lens stiffens and loses ability to thicken on near focus, **beginning at about 40 years of age.**

Presbyopia: lens stiffens with age and will not thicken for close focus

II. **Retina**
   A. **Retinal cell types**
      1. **Rods**
         a. Work in dim light for monochromatic vision and provide motion detection
         b. Sensitive to single photons and saturate with a few photons
         c. Concentrated away from fovea: peripheral vision is more sensitive than central vision in dim light
         d. **Poor spatial resolution:** paths converge to amplify dim signals.
         e. Photosensitive pigment: **rhodopsin** (11-*cis*-retinal + scotopsin)
      2. **Cones**
         a. Work in bright light for color vision and provide high visual acuity
         b. Concentrated at fovea
         c. **Good spatial resolution:** little or no convergence.
         d. Photosensitive pigment: **iodopsins** (11-*cis*-retinal + photopsins)

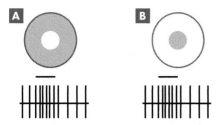

12-2: A, *On-center retinal ganglion cell response to illumination of center of receptive field.* **B,** *Off-center retinal ganglion cell response to illumination of surround of receptive field. Circles represent the receptive fields of individual retinal ganglion cells. Horizontal bars indicate the time of illumination. Vertical lines represent individual action potentials generated by each retinal ganglion cell in the dark and during the depicted pattern of illumination.*

3. **Bipolar cells**
   a. On—bipolar cells are excited by light (inhibited by glutamate from rods and cones).
   b. Off—bipolar cells are inhibited by light (excited by glutamate from rods and cones).
4. **Retinal ganglion cells (RGCs)**
   a. Excited by bipolar cells
   b. Provide for **contrast detection** (Fig. 12-2)
      (1) On-center RGCs are maximally excited when center of receptive field is illuminated relative to surround.
      (2) Off-center RGCs are maximally excited when surround of receptive field is illuminated relative to center.
   c. Project to lateral geniculate nucleus of thalamus
   d. Axons form the **optic nerves, optic chiasm, and optic tracts.**
5. **Interneurons**
   a. **Horizontal cells** modify and fine-tune synapses between rods or cones and bipolar neurons.
   b. **Amacrine cells** modify and fine-tune synapses between bipolar neurons and retinal ganglion. cells.

B. **Retinal layers**
   1. **Pigment epithelium** lines retina, absorbs stray light, and supports rods and cones.
   2. **Outer nuclear layer** contains rod and cone photoreceptors.
   3. **Outer plexiform layer** contains synapses between rods and cones, bipolar and horizontal cells.
   4. **Inner nuclear layer** contains bipolar, amacrine, and horizontal cells.
   5. **Inner plexiform layer** contains synapses between bipolar, amacrine, and retinal ganglion cells.
   6. **Ganglion cell layer** (innermost layer, closest to center of eyeball) contains retinal ganglion cells.

C. **Retinal anatomy**
   1. **Macula lutea:** central 5-mm region of retina
   2. **Fovea:** central 1.5 mm of macula

Multiple sclerosis: can cause blurred vision because CN II is part of the CNS

a. Point of focus; maximum visual acuity

b. Contains only cones

3. **Optic disc**

a. Point where retinal ganglion cell axons exit retina

b. Contains only axons, no photoreceptors

c. **Causes visual blind spot**

d. Blurring or bulging of optic disc (**papilledema**) is caused by increased intracranial pressure.

D. **Phototransduction**

1. **Phototransducer structure**

a. **Outer segment**

(1) Discs, formed as invaginations of cell membrane, contain photosensitive proteins called **opsins.**

(2) Discs form at base, migrate to cell tip and are phagocytosed by pigment epithelium.

b. **Inner segment**

(1) Connected to outer segment through **cilium,** contains nucleus and biosynthetic machinery

(2) **Synaptic terminal** releases glutamate onto retinal bipolar cells.

2. **Intracellular signaling: synaptic terminal release of glutamate when light is *not* present.**

a. Light hits opsin and 11-*cis* retinal in disc membrane.

b. **11-*cis*-retinal is converted to all-*trans*-retinal.**

c. All-*trans*-retinal activates a phosphodiesterase.

d. Phosphodiesterase decreases cyclic guanosine monophosphate (cGMP).

e. Decreased cGMP **decreases Na^+/Ca^{2+} current ("dark current")** (Fig. 12-3).

f. Photoreceptor hyperpolarizes, **decreasing glutamate release** onto bipolar cells.

III. **Nonvisual Retinal Outputs**

A. **Suprachiasmatic nucleus**

1. Projection through retinohypothalamic tract

2. **Function:** entrainment of circadian rhythms

B. **Midbrain pretectum**

1. Projection through brachium of superior colliculus

2. **Function:** pupillary light reflex (see section V, A)

C. **Superior colliculus**

1. Projection through brachium of superior colliculus

2. **Function:** orienting head to visual stimuli

IV. **Central Visual Pathways** (Fig. 12-4)

A. **Optic nerve**

1. Axons of retinal ganglion cells leaving retina

2. Damage causes **blindness in ipsilateral eye.**

Papilledema: sign of increased intracranial pressure

Retinal degeneration: disruption in migration and phagocytosis of photoreceptor discs

Olfactory groove meningioma: ipsilateral anosmia, blindness in ipsilateral eye, and papilledema in contralateral eye

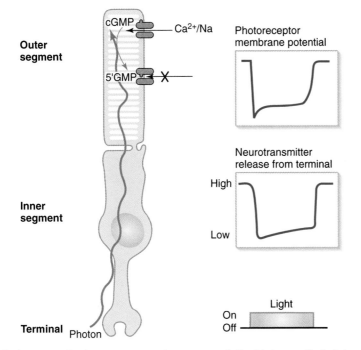

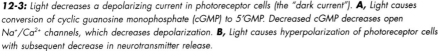

12-3: *Light decreases a depolarizing current in photoreceptor cells (the "dark current"). **A,** Light causes conversion of cyclic guanosine monophosphate (cGMP) to 5'GMP. Decreased cGMP decreases open Na⁺/Ca²⁺ channels, which decreases depolarization. **B,** Light causes hyperpolarization of photoreceptor cells with subsequent decrease in neurotransmitter release.*

B. **Optic chiasm**
  1. Retinal ganglion cell axons redistributing from left and right eye to carry left visual field of both eyes to right hemisphere and vice versa
  2. Damage to lateral chiasm (e.g., from aneurysm of distal internal carotid artery): ipsilateral **nasal field anopsia**
  3. Damage to central chiasm (e.g., from pituitary tumor or aneurysm of anterior communicating artery): **bitemporal hemianopsia** (sometimes described as "tunnel vision")

C. **Optic tract**
  1. Retinal ganglion cell axons carrying one visual field to contralateral thalamus (e.g., left optic tract carries right visual field of right eye and left eye to left thalamus).
  2. Damage to the optic tract causes **homonymous contralateral hemianopsia.**

D. **Lateral geniculate nucleus of thalamus**
  1. Receives input from contralateral visual field of both eyes
  2. Contains six layers: inputs from two eyes project to alternating layers.
    a. **Movement and contrast** are processed in layers 1 and 2.
    b. **Color and form** are processed in layers 3 to 6.

E. **Optic radiation**
  1. Massive fiber projection from thalamus to primary visual cortex

Aneurysm on internal carotid artery that compresses lateral optic chiasm: ipsilateral nasal hemianopsia

Damage to crossing fibers of the optic chiasm: bitemporal hemianopsia

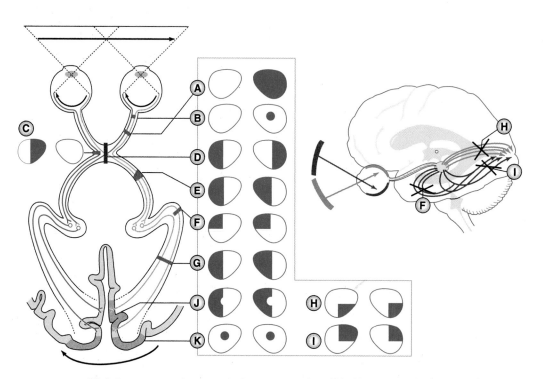

12-4: *Damage to visual pathways. A, Optic nerve: unilateral blindness; B, core of optic nerve: loss of central vision; C, lateral edge of optic chiasm: unilateral nasal hemianopsia; D, central chiasm: bitemporal hemianopsia; E, optic tract: homonymous hemianopsia; F, temporal lobe (Meyer loop): superior quadrant anopsia; G, optic radiation: homonymous hemianopsia; H, occipital lobe, superior to calcarine sulcus: inferior quadrant anopsia; I, occipital lobe, inferior to calcarine sulcus: superior quadrant anopsia; J, visual cortex: homonymous hemianopsia with macular sparing (tunnel vision); K, occipital pole: loss of central (macular vision).*

2. Damage to **complete radiation** in one hemisphere causes **homonymous hemianopsia.**
3. Damage to one fourth of a radiation in one hemisphere causes a **quadrantanopsia.**
   a. Projections that are most superior carry inferior visual field.
   b. Projections that are most inferior carry superior visual field, with some fibers sweeping forward around the inferior horn of the lateral ventricle **(Meyer loop).**

Damage to Meyer loop in the anterior temporal lobe: superior quadrant anopsia

> Damage to Meyer loop eliminates the **contralateral superior quadrant** of the visual field, causing a scotoma that is described as "pie in the sky."

F. **Primary visual cortex**
   1. Region of medial occipital lobe surrounding **calcarine sulcus**
   2. **Cuneate gyrus,** superior to calcarine sulcus, receives input from **contralateral inferior visual field.**

3. **Lingual gyrus,** inferior to calcarine sulcus, receives input from **contralateral superior visual field.**

4. Damage causes contralateral **homonymous hemianopsia with macular sparing** (macular vision) because macular retina is processed in a disproportionately large region occupying the posterior-most visual cortex.

5. **Damage to the occipital pole** causes **loss of macular vision.**

V. **Control of Pupil Size**

A. **Pupillary light response**

1. Light input is transmitted by optic nerve directly to pretectal region of posterior midbrain.

2. Pretectal midbrain projects to Edinger-Westphal nuclei (parasympathetic) bilaterally to activate direct and consensual responses.

   a. **Direct response:** constriction of ipsilateral pupil

   b. **Consensual response:** constriction of contralateral pupil.

3. **Damage affecting pupillary light reflex**

   a. **Optic nerve: afferent pupillary defect** (diminished or lost pupillary light reflex bilaterally)

      (1) Light directed to healthy eye: both pupils constrict.

      (2) Light directed to damaged eye: no direct or consensual pupillary constriction

      (3) Commonly seen in multiple sclerosis

   b. **Oculomotor nerve:** ipsilateral diminished or lost pupillary light reflex and ocular palsy.

      (1) Light directed to healthy eye: direct response intact, consensual response diminished or lost.

      (2) Light directed to damaged eye: direct response diminished or lost, consensual response intact.

   c. **Pretectal midbrain or posterior commissure:** loss of direct and consensual responses.

B. **Near reaction: response of eye on near focus**

1. **Vergent eye movement** mediated by midbrain vergence center and oculomotor nucleus

2. **Accommodation** (lens thickening) mediated by parasympathetic (Edinger-Westphal) component of oculomotor nerve

3. **Pupil constriction** mediated by parasympathetic component of oculomotor nerve

4. **Argyll-Robertson pupil**

   a. Pupil does *not* constrict to light (direct or consensual).

   b. Pupil *does* constrict with accommodation.

   c. Sign in **tabes dorsalis** (i.e., tertiary syphilis)

5. **Adie syndrome**

   a. Pupil may show greater constriction in near reaction than in response to light.

   b. Damage is loss of postganglionic parasympathetic innervation of pupillary constrictor muscles.

6. **Diabetes mellitus** may also cause loss of light response.

Afferent pupillary defect: bilateral loss of pupillary constriction after CN II damage

VI. **Eye Movements that Acquire a Target**
   A. **Saccades** (Table 12-1)
      1. Rapid conjugate movements to put target on fovea
      2. Can be generated in response to many stimuli (e.g., visual, auditory, tactile, memory)
      3. Frontal eye fields in frontal lobe generate voluntary saccades to contralateral visual space.
      4. Adversely affected by drugs, alcohol, fatigue, inattention
   B. **Smooth Pursuit**
      1. Slower tracking movements to keep image on fovea in response to moving visual stimulus
      2. Multiple regions of occipital, parietal, and frontal cortex generate smooth pursuits to ipsilateral visual space.
      3. Adversely affected by drugs, alcohol, fatigue, inattention
   C. **Vergence**
      1. Disconjugate movement: eyes move in opposite directions.
      2. Allows tracking of objects as they approach or recede

VII. **Eye Movements that Stabilize Eye during Head Movements**
   A. **Vestibulo-ocular reflex**
      1. Stabilizes image on fovea during **rapid** head movement
      2. Driven by vestibular system and does not require visual processing
      3. Requires only brainstem (i.e., not cortex)

   > **Doll's eye reflex** tests the vestibulo-ocular reflex in a comatose patient who has no injury to the cervical spine. If the reflex is incomplete or absent, the brainstem or vestibular system is damaged (see Fig. 13-7).

   B. **Optokinetic reflex**
      1. Stabilizes image on fovea during slow head movement
      2. Requires cortical involvement, including visual processing

VIII. **Brainstem Control of Eye Movement**
   A. **Vertical gaze center**
      1. Located in midbrain, near nerves necessary for vertical gaze
      2. Damage paralyzes vertical eye movement.
      3. Midbrain damage or barbiturate overdose can cause **vertical nystagmus.**

   > Damage to posterior midbrain **(Parinaud syndrome)** may occur due to pineal tumor or local infarcts in adults or ependymoma in children. Signs include loss of upward gaze with **downward deviation of eyes** ("sundowning"), **loss of convergence,** and **loss of pupillary light reflex. Hydrocephalus,** with expansion of third ventricle, may develop if the cerebral aqueduct is compressed by space-occupying mass.

TABLE 12-1:
Lesions Affecting Voluntary Eye Movement

SITE OF LESION	SIGNS	"LOOK RIGHT"
	Normal	
Left frontal eye field	Acute lesion causes left gaze preference, because activity of right frontal eye fields is unopposed. Eyes can move right as part of a tracking maneuver (smooth pursuit) or as a reflexive response. Large lesion paralyzes upper right body.	
Right abducens nerve	Loss of abduction in right eye. If lesion occurs as nerve passes apex of petrous temporal bone, trigeminal involvement is likely. If lesion occurs within cavernous sinus, oculomotor, trochlear, and trigeminal nerve damage is likely, in which case the right eye will be completely paralyzed.	
Right dorsomedial pons	Both abducens nucleus and horizontal gaze center are involved. Neither eye saccades right. Both eyes may deviate left. Complete paralysis of right side of face accompanies gaze paralysis.	
Left medial longitudinal fasciculus	**Internuclear ophthalmoplegia** Right eye abducts. Left eye will not adduct and remains in midline.	
Left oculomotor nerve or nucleus	Left eye deviated down and out, ptosis, pupil dilated. Paralysis of body contralateral to ocular paralysis suggests lesion to anterior midbrain.	

B. **Horizontal gaze center**
   1. Contiguous with abducens nucleus in pons
   2. Drives ipsilateral horizontal (lateral) gaze
C. **Medial longitudinal fasciculus**
   1. Extends through posterior medial brainstem and is continuous, caudally, with medial vestibulospinal tract
   2. Coordinates eye movements by supporting communication between vestibular, abducens, trochlear, oculomotor nuclei and cerebellum
      • On right lateral gaze, right lateral gaze center directs right eye to abduct (lateral rectus, innervated by abducens nerve) and, through left medial longitudinal fasciculus, directs left eye to adduct (medial rectus, innervated by oculomotor nerve).

Multiple sclerosis: most frequent cause of internuclear ophthalmoplegia

   3. Damage causes **internuclear ophthalmoplegia (INO)**
      a. On lateral gaze, abducting eye abducts (with possible nystagmus) while adducting eye reaches only midline position.
      b. In adults: associated with multiple sclerosis and with small brainstem infarcts.
      c. In children: may indicate a brainstem glioma

> **One-and-a-half syndrome:** rarely, stroke damages a portion of the posterior pons, including one horizontal gaze center and the ipsilateral medial longitudinal fasciculus. The result is paralysis of lateral gaze ipsilateral to the lesion and INO on gaze to the contralateral side.

Auditory and Vestibular Systems

I. **Anatomy of the Ear**

   A. **Outer ear** (Fig. 13-1)

     1. **Pinna** serves as a funnel to capture pressure (sound) waves.

     2. **External acoustic meatus** (ear canal) leads to tympanic membrane.

   B. **Middle ear**

     1. **Tympanic membrane** vibrates in response to pressure waves.

     2. **Ossicles** (malleus, incus, and stapes) transmit vibration to inner ear.

     3. **Auditory (eustachian) tube** connects middle ear to atmospheric pressure.

> When both sides of the tympanic membrane are exposed to atmospheric pressure, changes in pressure (e.g., in an airplane) do not affect the ability of the membrane to respond to rapid pressure waves. Blockage of the auditory tube causes changes in atmospheric pressure to be transmitted to the tympanic membrane, causing pain and decreased sound transmission.

   C. **Inner ear**

     1. **Bony labyrinth**

       a. Located in the petrous part of temporal bone

       b. Filled with **perilymph,** which is similar to cerebrospinal fluid and is in communication with subarachnoid space

     2. **Membranous labyrinth**

       a. Lines bony labyrinth and contains transduction apparatus.

       b. Filled with **endolymph,** which is similar to intracellular fluid (e.g., high in K^+)

         (1) Cilia of auditory and vestibular hair cells are exposed to endolymph.

         (2) Ionic differences between perilymph and endolymph establish potential differences similar to intracellular–extracellular potential differences.

     3. **Cochlea** (Figs. 13-2 and 13-3)

       a. **Oval window** transmits vibration of middle ear ossicles to fluid chambers of inner ear.

       b. **Scala vestibule** extends from oval window to helicotrema.

       c. **Helicotrema** is the small passage that connects scala vestibule to scala tympani

       d. **Scala tympani** extends to round window.

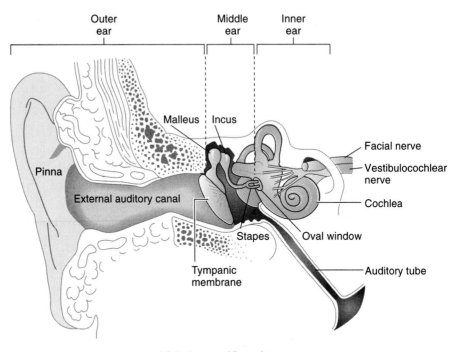

13-1: *Outer, middle, and inner ear.*

    e. **Round window** deflects in response to pressure waves within cochlea, preventing pressure waves from being damped.

    f. **Scala media** separates scala vestibuli and scala tympani along most of each structure's length.

      (1) **Vestibular membrane** (Reissner membrane) lies between scala media and scala vestibule.

      (2) **Basilar membrane with spiral** (Corti) **organ** lies between scala media and scala tympani and contains hair cells.

  4. Vestibular labyrinth

    a. **Static labyrinth:** macula of saccule and macula of utricle

    b. **Kinetic labyrinth:** three mutually perpendicular pairs of semicircular canals

II. Transduction

A. Hair cells

1. Convert mechanical energy into chemical signals
2. Constantly leak glutamate onto terminals of vestibulocochlear nerve, causing nerve to be tonically active
3. Cilia are arranged from short to tall, with linkages between adjacent cilia.
4. Deflection of cilia toward tallest (**kinocilium**) increases transmitter release; deflection away decreases transmitter release.

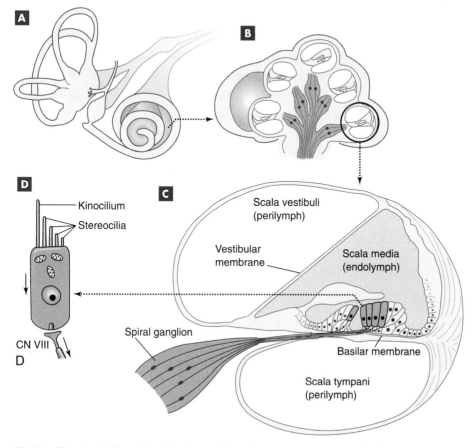

13-2: *Cochlea.* **A,** *Cochlea and semicircular canals share the inner ear compartment.* **B,** *Cross-section. Note cochlea wraps almost three times around its axis. Cell bodies of auditory branch of vestibulocochlear nerve distribute in spiral ganglion.* **C,** *Scala vestibuli, scala tympani, and scala media are separated by the vestibular and basilar membranes. Hair cells are innervated by the auditory branch of the vestibulocochlear nerve.* **D,** *Each hair cell is invested with a series of cilia that are surrounded by endolymph and innervated by one or more nerve endings.*

B. **Auditory system**
1. Detects frequency, amplitude, and location of sound
2. **Sound:** pressure wave transduced into an electrical signal by hair cells, which detect movement of the basilar membrane.
3. **Frequency coding**
   a. **Determines pitch**
      (1) The human ear detects frequencies between 20 and 20,000 Hz; the ability to hear higher frequencies diminishes with age.
      (2) Spoken language is typically in the 4,000- to 8,000-Hz range.
   b. Tonotopic representation of sound, relying on mechanical and electrical resonance, begins in inner ear.

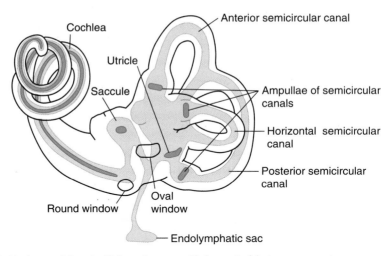

13-3: *Membranous labyrinth of left ear. Six regions (dark green) of the inner ear contain sensory apparatus with hair cells extending into endolymph region (light green).*

   c. **Mechanical resonance**
     (1) Entire basilar membrane vibrates, with location of maximum amplitude of wave determined by frequency.
     (2) Base of membrane near oval window is short (100 μm) and stiff; vibrates best at **high frequency**
     (3) Apex of membrane near helicotrema is wide (500 μm) and floppy; vibrates best at **low frequency**
   d. **Electrical resonance**
     (1) Hair cells are electrically tuned to operate efficiently at particular frequencies.
     (2) Hair cells near oval window are electrically predisposed to respond to higher frequencies.
  4. **Amplitude coding**
   a. **Loudness** (sound intensity) is detected at **inner ear** (Table 13-1).

> A jump to a 10-fold greater pressure is a jump of 20 dB; 0 dB is threshold (barely audible), and 140 dB hurts!

   b. Increases are coded by combination of more action potentials per fiber, and more fibers recruited.
  5. **Location coding**
   a. **Intensity** comparison: sounds are louder in ear ipsilateral to source of sound.
   b. **Timing** comparison: sounds arrive first at ear ipsilateral to source of sound first.
 C. **Vestibular system**
  1. Detects **position** and **movement of head**

dB	Sound
0	Threshold of hearing
10	Pin dropping at 30 feet
30	Whispered speech in quiet room
60	Normal speech
70	Auto traffic on busy street
100	Chainsaw
120	Threshold of discomfort; 747 jet taking off on runway
140	Threshold of pain
150	Military rifle firing 3 inches away; bones in ear may break
160	Instant perforation of eardrum

TABLE 13-1: Decibel Levels of Familiar Sounds Relative to Normal Hearing

2. **Static labyrinth** detects **linear acceleration,** including gravity.
   a. **Utricle** detects **horizontal** acceleration.
   b. **Saccule** detects **vertical** acceleration.
3. **Kinetic labyrinth** detects **angular acceleration** (spin).
   a. Consists of three mutually perpendicular pairs of **semicircular canals**
   b. For any direction of spin, one of each pair is excited as the other is inhibited.

III. **Auditory System**
   A. **Hair cells of cochlea** (Fig. 13-4)
      1. Located in **basilar membrane**
      2. **Inner hair cells** (~3,500 per cochlea) are the source of 90% of cochlear fibers.
         a. Each sensory axon innervates a single hair cell.
         b. Each hair cell is innervated by about 10 sensory axons.

Cochlear damage: produces pure tonal loss

> Because most axons innervate only one hair cell, most axons respond best to one **characteristic frequency.**

      3. **Outer hair cells** (~15,000 per cochlea) are the source of 10% of cochlear fibers.
         a. Each sensory axon innervates many hair cells.
         b. Cells are contractile and may enhance selective frequency response found along basilar membrane.
         c. **Otoacoustic emissions** (sound emanating from the ear after incoming sound) reflect outer hair cell response.

> Repeated **high-intensity noise, ototoxic drugs** (e.g., aspirin, salicylates, caffeine, and antibiotics), **presbycusis,** or **infection** (e.g., streptococcus or influenza) damages the cochlear hair cells, causing **pure tone loss.**

   B. **Vestibulocochlear nerve, auditory component**
      1. Bipolar neurons with cell bodies in **spiral ganglion** of cochlea.

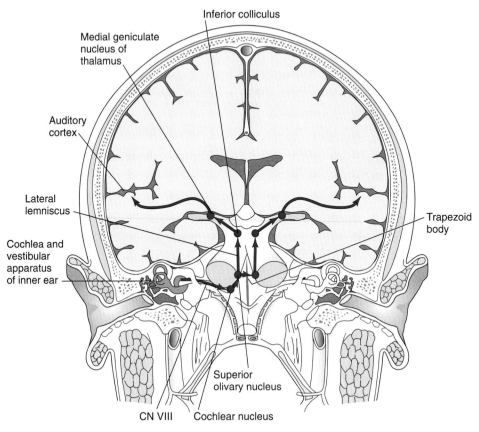

13-4: *Auditory pathway from cochlea to primary auditory cortex (arrows).*

2. Central projection courses through **internal auditory (acoustic) meatus,** enters the brainstem at the pontomedullary junction, and terminates on **cochlear nucleus.**
3. **Damage commonly results in high-frequency hearing loss and difficulty understanding speech.**

C. **Cochlear nucleus**
   1. Located at the **medullary-pontine junction** within field of anterior inferior cerebellar artery
   2. Each primary afferent sends branches to dorsal and ventral nuclei.
   3. Tonotopically organized: medial receives high frequencies; lateral receives low frequencies.
   4. Sends **bilateral outputs**
      a. To ipsilateral and, through trapezoid body, to contralateral superior olivary nucleus
      b. To inferior colliculus through **lateral lemniscus**

D. **Superior olivary nucleus**
   1. Receives input from each cochlear nucleus

2. **Localizes sounds particularly from contralateral space**
   a. Medial portion compares **time of arrival** of signal at each ear.
   b. Lateral portion compares sound **intensities.**
E. **Inferior colliculus**
   1. Receives input from cochlear nuclei bilaterally through lateral lemniscus and projects through brachium of inferior colliculus to medial geniculate nucleus of thalamus
   2. Responsible for **reflex orienting to auditory stimuli**
F. **Medial geniculate nucleus**
   1. Thalamic relay nucleus
   2. Projects through **auditory radiations** to ipsilateral primary auditory cortex
G. **Auditory cortex**
   1. Located in the **superior** (transverse) **temporal gyrus**
   2. Receives binaural input
   3. Sound is somewhat localized (e.g., right brain localizes sounds in left space).
   4. Tonotopic organization with higher frequencies more medial

> **Damage to auditory cortex** may cause tinnitus but does not yield deafness due to bilateral nature of auditory projections. Large lesions may affect **sound localization.**

Large lesion of auditory cortex: affects sound localization to contralateral side

H. **Additional innervation of ear**
   1. Stapedius muscle, innervated by **facial nerve** (CN VII), contracts in response to loud noise to limit movement of stapes and to **dampen sound.**

> Hyperacusis, seen in Bell palsy, reflects loss of stapedial reflex.

Damage to CN VII with intact CN VIII causes hyperacusis.

   2. **Tympanic membrane** receives sensory innervation
   a. **Trigeminal nerve** (CN V) (auriculotemporal branch): external membrane and external meatus
   b. **Vagus nerve** (CN X): inferior inner membrane and meatus

> Stimulating the tympanic membrane triggers the **vomiting reflex** through the vagus nerve.

   c. **Glossopharyngeal nerve** (CN IX): internal membrane

IV. **Tests of Auditory System**
   A. **Tuning fork tests** (using 256- or 512-Hz fork)
   1. **Basis of tests to differentiate conductive versus sensorineural hearing loss** (using 256- or 512-Hz fork)
      a. **Normal hearing:** Mechanical transduction apparatus amplifies sound, so vibration conducted through air is louder than vibration applied directly to bone.
      b. **Conductive hearing loss:** Mechanical transduction is inadequate, so vibration applied directly to bone is louder than vibration conducted through air.

2. **Weber test:** Place vibrating tuning fork on vertex of skull or forehead to transmit bone vibration to inner ears.
   a. **Conductive hearing loss:** sound is louder in affected ear.
   b. **Sensorineural hearing loss:** sound is diminished in affected ear.
      • Weber test can be approximated by mimicking conductive loss with a finger placed in the ear and imitating a tuning fork by humming. The humming seems louder in the plugged ear.
3. **Rinne test:** Place the vibrating tuning fork against the mastoid process and then near external acoustic meatus
   a. Place the vibrating tuning fork against the mastoid process. If sound is detected, neural pathways are intact.
   b. **Conductive hearing loss:** sound is louder when vibration is presented to mastoid process than to external ear (bone conduction is greater than air conduction).
   c. When sound disappears, move tuning fork near outer ear. If no sound is detected, suspect conductive loss.

B. **Audiometric tests**
1. **Stapedial reflex** (acoustic reflex)
   a. Loud noise in either ear elicits contraction of stapedius muscle through facial nerve (CN VII).
   b. Detected by tympanometry
2. **Otoacoustic emissions**
   a. Some hair cells contract in response to movement of the basilar membrane after a noise.
   b. Contraction of the outer hair cells in response to sound received moves the tympanic membrane and can be detected as sound generated by the ear.
   c. Emission implies auditory pathway is intact up to, and including, hair cells.
   d. **Used to screen hearing in infants** and to differentiate sensory versus neural source of sensorineural hearing loss.
3. **Brainstem auditory evoked responses**
   a. Evoked responses are recorded by surface electrodes on the head.
   b. Multiple waves are generated, each reflecting a different part of the auditory pathway from the peripheral portion of the vestibulo-cochlear nerve to the medial geniculate nucleus of the thalamus.
   c. Used to screen infants to detect deafness
   d. Monitor brainstem patency during surgery

Brainstem auditory evoked potentials responses: detect the 0.1% of infants that are born deaf

V. **Hearing Loss**
A. **Conductive hearing loss**
1. **Cause**
   a. **Outer ear obstruction** (e.g., earwax [cerumen], small objects)
   b. **Ear trauma** leading to **tympanic membrane perforation** and/or middle ear **ossicle disruption:** acute hearing loss, tinnitus, and vertigo

  c. **Otitis media** (middle ear infection affecting more than 75% of children younger than 3 years): decreased hearing and earache

  d. **Otosclerosis** (bone disease affecting the stapedial footplate): progressive hearing loss and tinnitus beginning as early as the third decade

Otosclerosis: causes progressive hearing loss

  e. Age: more common before 40 years of age

 2. **Signs and symptoms**

  a. Tinnitus

  b. Deafness in ipsilateral ear

  c. **Soft speech** because speaker's voice sounds loud to speaker

  d. Weber test: sound louder in ear with hearing loss

  e. Negative Rinne test

B. **Sensorineural hearing loss**

 1. **Causes**

  a. **Degeneration of hair cells**

  b. Damage to the vestibulocochlear cochlear nerve (e.g., acoustic neuroma) (Fig. 13-5)

  c. Damage to the brainstem, or supratentorial brain (e.g., stroke or tumor)

  d. Age: more common after 60 years of age

 2. **Signs and symptoms**

  a. Tinnitus

  b. Deafness in ipsilateral ear

  c. Dizziness, reflecting contribution of vestibular nerve component

  d. **Loud speech** because speaker's voice cannot be easily heard by speaker

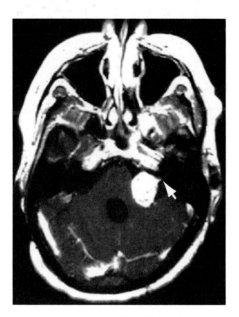

13-5: *Acoustic neuroma (vestibular schwannoma) on left vestibulocochlear nerve (arrow), Magnetic resonance imaging, horizontal view.*

Deafness for high
frequencies: interferes
with speech
comprehension and
affects one third of
people older than 65
years of age

   e. Difficulty with speech comprehension is **more pronounced in noisy environments.**

   f. Positive Rinne test

   g. **Presbycusis** (increased hearing loss with increasing age) presents initially with high-frequency hearing loss, affecting 20,000 to 4,000 Hz.

   h. **Central hearing loss** (i.e., due to central nervous system damage) findings vary with location of damage but **do not include unilateral deafness.**

VI. **Vestibular System**
  A. **Hair cells of vestibular organs** (see Figs. 13-1 and 13-3)
    1. Static labyrinth hair cells are located in **maculae of utricle and saccule**
    2. Kinetic labyrinth hair cells are located with **ampullary crests of three semicircular canals.**
  B. **Vestibulocochlear nerve, vestibular component**
    1. Bipolar neurons with cell bodies in **vestibular ganglion** (Scarpa ganglion) in temporal bone near inner ear.
    2. Central projection courses through **internal auditory meatus** and enters the brainstem at the pontomedullary junction.
    3. Most axons terminate in the **vestibular nucleus.**
    4. Some axons project directly to flocculonodular lobe of cerebellum.

> Because the **facial nerve** (CN VII) courses through the internal auditory meatus along with the **vestibulocochlear nerve,** tumors in this region **(acoustic neuromas)** produce facial weakness in addition to hearing loss and vertigo.

  C. **Vestibular nucleus**
    1. Extends through dorsolateral pons and medulla
    2. Projects to
      a. **Ocular motor nuclei** (oculomotor, trochlear, and abducens) through medial longitudinal fasciculus; important **for vestibulo-ocular reflex** (Fig. 13-6)
      b. **Cerebellum** through juxtarestiform body (primarily inferior cerebellar peduncle); important for **posture, balance, and equilibrium**
      c. **Spinal cord** (alpha and gamma motor neurons)
        (1) Through medial vestibulospinal tract; important for **reflexive positioning of head and neck**
        (2) Through lateral vestibulospinal tract; important for **reflexive extension of legs**

VII. **Tests of Vestibular System**
  A. **Vestibulo-ocular reflex (VOR)** (see Fig. 13-6)
    1. Serves to stabilize image on fovea during rapid head movements
    2. Hair cells in semicircular canals detect head turn and stimulate primary vestibular afferents.
    3. Primary afferents activate neurons in vestibular nuclei.

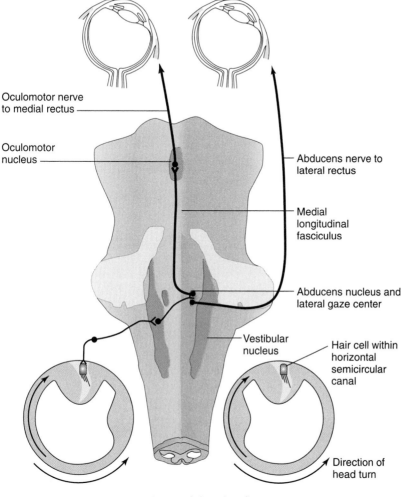

Oculomotor nerve to medial rectus

Oculomotor nucleus

Abducens nerve to lateral rectus

Medial longitudinal fasciculus

Abducens nucleus and lateral gaze center

Vestibular nucleus

Hair cell within horizontal semicircular canal

Direction of head turn

13-6: *Vestibulo-ocular reflex.*

    4. Vestibular nuclei direct ocular motor neurons (oculomotor, trochlear, and abducens) through interneurons with axons running in medial longitudinal fasciculus.

    5. If head moves sharply to right, VOR triggers compensatory movement of eyes to left

B. **Doll's eye (oculocephalic) reflex** (Fig. 13-7)

    1. Tests patency of vestibulo-ocular reflex

    2. Useful in unconscious individual with no damage to cervical region

    3. Less useful for alert individual who may override reflexive response

C. **Caloric test** (Fig. 13-8)

    1. Tests patency of vestibulo-ocular reflex (brainstem) and saccadic return of eyes to midposition (cortex)

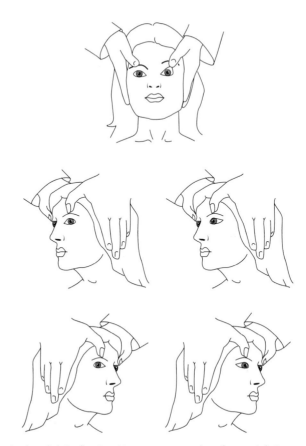

13-7: *Doll's eye (oculocephalic) reflex. Top, Unconscious patient lying face up. Left, Intact oculocephalic reflex indicates intact brainstem. Right, Absent oculocephalic reflex indicates loss of brainstem function.*

2. "Fools" the vestibular system into "thinking" that the head has turned.
   a. Cold water into right ear decreases vestibular nerve output from right labyrinth, which vestibular circuits interpret as head turns to the left.
   b. If brainstem circuits are intact, vestibulo-ocular reflex will elicit compensatory conjugate movement of both eyes to the right.
      • Slow eye movement toward "cold" ear is controlled in the brainstem (vestibulo-ocular reflex through the medial longitudinal fasciculus).
   c. If higher centers are also intact, the compensatory eye movement is followed by rapid saccade back to center (e.g., saccade left).
      • **Left beating nystagmus:** slow VOR movement of eyes to right followed by rapid saccade to left
   d. If higher centers are impaired, eyes deviate toward "cold" ear.
   e. If the brainstem is impaired, eyes do not fully move toward "cold" ear.
3. General predictors
   a. **Cold water** → nystagmus away → similar to destructive lesion of labyrinth

Cold opposite, warm same (COWS): direction of nystagmus in normal caloric test

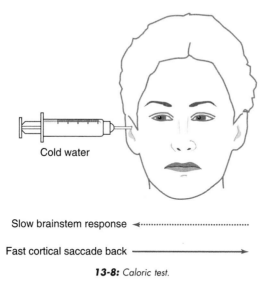

Cold water

Slow brainstem response ◄·······································

Fast cortical saccade back ─────────────►

13-8: *Caloric test.*

   b. **Warm water** → nystagmus toward → similar to irritative lesion of labyrinth

   c. Electro-oculogram can detect direction of nystagmus.

D. **Dix-Hallpike maneuver**
1. Distinguishes peripheral from central origin vertigo and nystagmus
2. Individual moved from the sitting to the supine position followed by head rotation
3. **Peripheral origin**
   a. Nystagmus begins after 3- to 10-second delay.
   b. Reduced effect with repeated tests (exhaustible)
4. **Central origin**
   a. Nystagmus begins immediately.
   b. No change with repeated tests (nonexhaustible)
   c. If vertical nystagmus is present, lesion is central (or caused by barbiturates).

VIII. **Vestibular System Damage and Vertigo**
  A. **Major signs of vestibular system damage**
    1. **Vertigo:** sensation that room or individual is spinning; frequently described as dizziness
    2. **Nystagmus:** involuntary, rhythmic, repetitive eye movements that can be vertical, horizontal, or rotary
  B. **Categories of vertigo**
    1. **Peripheral origin** (e.g., inner ear labyrinth or vestibular nerve) resulting in **unbalanced vestibular inputs**
    2. **Central origin** (e.g., brainstem, cerebellum, or cerebral cortex)
    3. **Systemic** (e.g., cardiovascular insufficiency or metabolic disorders)

C. **Peripheral origin vertigo**
   1. **General signs**
      a. Tinnitus or deafness due to auditory involvement
      b. Sensation can be reproduced with caloric test (see section VII, C).
      c. If caloric test is asymmetric, response is reduced on one side.
      d. Patient can fall toward side of lesion, away from nystagmus.
   2. **Acoustic (vestibular) neuroma** (see Fig. 13-5)
      a. **Schwannoma on the vestibulocochlear nerve** (CN VIII)
      b. **Auditory** signs: tinnitus and ipsilateral deafness
      c. **Vestibular** signs: vertigo, nausea, and nystagmus
      d. **Facial nerve** (CN VII) signs: ipsilateral facial paresis or paralysis, or loss of corneal reflex, taste (anterior two thirds of tongue), salivation, and tearing glands
         • **Hyperacusis,** which is a symptom of a facial nerve lesion, is not a feature of acoustic neuroma because the individual is deaf.
      e. Cerebellar signs possible if tumor in cerebellopontine angle
      f. Brainstem auditory evoked responses are a sensitive test.
   3. **Benign positional vertigo of peripheral origin** (episodic vertigo)
      a. **No hearing loss**
      b. Brief episodes of vertigo, possibly with nausea and vomiting (less frequent with central origin)
      c. Vertigo is fatigable (central origin is not fatigable)
      d. Caloric tests normal (lasting ~1 minute)
      e. Latency to nystagmus after new head position: 3 to 10 seconds (no latency with central origin)
      f. Vertical nystagmus is rare (vertical nystagmus is a central sign)
   4. **Ménière disease**
      a. Onset between 30 and 60 years of age
      b. **Disruption of endolymph circulation** increases pressure in labyrinth, causing auditory and vestibular symptoms.
      c. Signs and symptoms
         (1) Violent, sudden attack of nausea, vomiting, sweating, and decreased hearing
         (2) Sense of "stuffiness" or "fullness" in the affected ear may precede attack.
         (3) Nystagmus in either direction lasting 1 to 2 hours per attack
         (4) Recurrent attacks can cause residual tinnitus or hearing loss.
   5. **Middle ear disease with labyrinth involvement**
      • Recent ear infection, ototoxic drugs, or excess cerumen may cause middle ear disease.
   6. **Acute labyrinthitis secondary to bacterial or viral infection**

Ménière disease: disruption of endolymph circulation causing vertigo, tinnitus, and deafness

> Endolymph is produced in the cochlea and reabsorbed from the endolymph sac. Disruption in circulation of endolymph can result in increased pressure within the membranous labyrinth, with effects on both auditory and vestibular components (e.g., Ménière disease)

    7. **Post-traumatic vertigo**
       a. Likely due to blunt trauma to occipital or mastoid regions causing transverse fracture of temporal bone
       b. Damage extends to vestibular, cochlear, and possibly, facial nerves
       c. Blood pools behind tympanic membrane **(hemotympanum)**

D. **Central origin vertigo**
    1. **General signs**
       a. Disconjugate nystagmus (i.e., one eye moves more than the other)
       b. Direction of nystagmus can change, depending on direction of gaze.
       c. Oscillopsia (i.e., objects appear to move back and forth)
       d. Patient may fall toward lesion, toward nystagmus.
       e. Cerebellar ataxia, diplopia, papilledema, and dysarthria (in addition to vertigo and nystagmus) may be additional findings.
    2. **Posterior fossa tumors:** expect brainstem or cerebellar signs and elevated intracranial pressure (check fundi).
    3. **Vertebrobasilar insufficiency** (vascular disease): expect additional brainstem and/or cranial nerve signs and symptoms (e.g., diplopia, slurred speech, and difficulty with swallowing).
    4. **Lateral medullary** (Wallenberg) **syndrome**
       a. Vertigo, nausea, nystagmus, and oscillopsia
       b. Hoarseness and difficulty swallowing
       c. Loss of pain and temperature sensation in ipsilateral face
       d. Loss of pain and temperature sensation in contralateral body
       e. Ipsilateral Horner syndrome with miosis, ptosis, and anhidrosis
    5. Temporal lobe epilepsy
    6. Multiple sclerosis

Lateral medullary syndrome: may include vertigo and nystagmus

Homeostasis

I. **Autonomic Nervous System**
   A. **Function**
      1. **Effector limb** that communicates between hypothalamic and brainstem autonomic centers and peripheral targets
      2. Influences homeostatic functions by innervating muscles (smooth and cardiac) and glands (exocrine and endocrine)
      3. Primarily a motor system, but also carries and integrates sensory information from the viscera
   B. **Divisions**
      1. Sympathetic, parasympathetic, and enteric
      2. Control of one organ or tissue reflects dual innervation by sympathetic and parasympathetic divisions with opposing actions

      > In the iris, parasympathetic fibers control circular muscle, which produces pupil **constriction** (miosis), and sympathetic fibers innervate radial muscles, which produce **dilation** (mydriasis).

      3. Effects of sympathetic or parasympathetic divisions vary with target organ innervation (e.g., sympathetics both constrict arterioles in the skin and viscera and relax arterioles in heart and skeletal muscle).

Sympathetic neurons: preganglionic = short; postganglionic = long

II. **Sympathetic Division**
   A. **Preganglionic neurons** (Fig. 14-1)
      1. Cell bodies are located in intermediolateral cell column at **spinal levels T1 to L2.**
      2. **Myelinated axons** exit spinal cord through anterior roots to course in spinal nerve and leave spinal nerves through **white rami** to enter sympathetic trunk (Fig. 14-2).
         a. Some synapse with postganglionic neurons in **paravertebral ganglia.**
         b. Some ascend or descend one or more segments in the sympathetic trunk before synapsing with postganglionic neurons in paravertebral ganglia.
         c. Some exit sympathetic trunk as **splanchnic nerves** and synapse with postganglionic neurons in **prevertebral ganglia.**
   B. **Postganglionic neurons**
      1. Most cell bodies are in **paravertebral ganglia** (sympathetic chain ganglia)

SYMPATHETIC OUTFLOW

PARASYMPATHETIC OUTFLOW

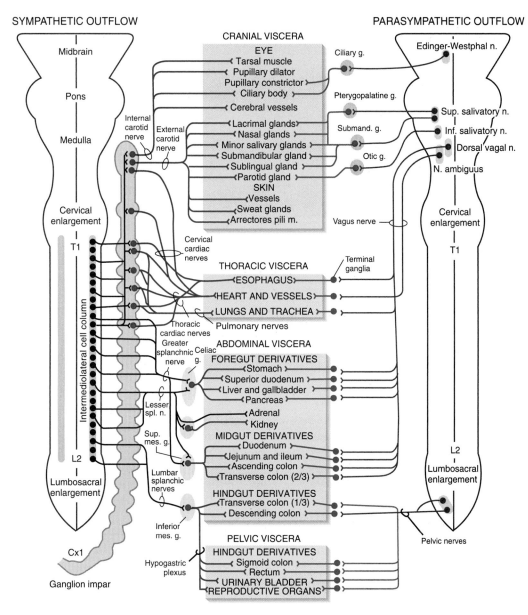

14-1: Sympathetic and parasympathetic innervation of major tissues and organs. Black, preganglionic neurons; green, postganglionic neurons.

    a. Cervical ganglia: superior, middle, and inferior

    b. First thoracic ganglion may fuse with inferior cervical ganglion to form stellate ganglion.

    c. **Unmyelinated axons** of postganglionic cell bodies in the paravertebral ganglia rejoin spinal nerves through **gray rami** to run to

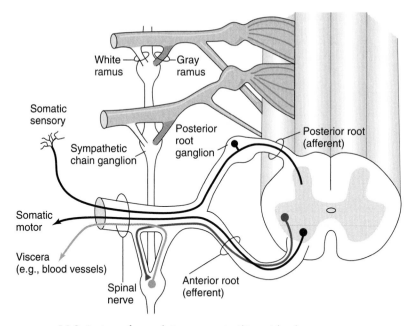

14-2: *Anatomy of sympathetic component within peripheral nervous system.*

target organs, (e.g. blood vessels, sweat glands, and arrector pili) (see Fig. 14-1).

2. Some cell bodies are in **prevertebral ganglia.**
   a. **Celiac ganglion** contains neurons that innervate liver, bile ducts, gallbladder, spleen, pancreas, stomach, small bowel, proximal colon, and kidney.
   b. **Aorticorenal ganglion** contains neurons that innervate kidney.
   c. **Superior mesenteric ganglion** contains neurons that innervate distal colon and rectum.
   d. **Inferior mesenteric ganglion** contains neurons that innervate anal sphincter, urinary bladder, internal urethral sphincter, genitalia, and uterus.
   e. **Terminal ganglia** contains neurons that innervate rectum and urinary bladder.
   f. **Adrenal medulla** is homologous to sympathetic ganglia; its neurons release **epinephrine** instead of norepinephrine.

Parasympathetic neurons:
preganglionic = long;
postganglionic = short

III. **Parasympathetic Division**
   A. **Preganglionic neurons** (see Fig. 14-1)
      1. Most cell bodies are located in **brainstem nuclei;** axons course in **cranial nerves.**
         a. **Edinger-Westphal nucleus** (oculomotor nerve): midbrain near oculomotor nucleus
         b. **Superior salivatory nucleus** (facial nerve): pons

    c. **Inferior salivatory nucleus** (glossopharyngeal nerve): medulla

    d. **Dorsal motor nucleus of the vagus** (vagus nerve): medulla

  2. Some cell bodies are located in intermediate gray in **S2 to S4;** axons course in **pelvic nerves.**

B. **Postganglionic neurons**

  1. Cell bodies of parasympathetic ganglia innervated by cranial nerves

    a. **Ciliary ganglion** (oculomotor nerve)

    b. **Pterygopalatine ganglion** (facial nerve)

    c. **Submandibular ganglion** (facial nerve)

    d. **Otic ganglion** (glossopharyngeal nerve)

    e. **Multiple thoracic and abdominal ganglia** to the level of the transverse colon (vagus nerve)

  2. Cell bodies of **parasympathetic ganglia** within the colon, rectum, and sphincters of lower gastrointestinal tract are innervated by pelvic splanchnic nerves.

IV. **Enteric Division**

A. **Components**

  1. **Intrinsic neurons** are located in and innervate the digestive systems.

  2. **Enteric plexus** contains neurons, glial-like cells and a blood–plexus barrier.

    a. **Myenteric** (Auerbach) plexus, between outer (longitudinal) and inner (circular) smooth muscle layers, controls **gut motility.**

    b. **Submucous** (Meissner) plexus, between inner smooth muscle layer and mucosa, regulates **secretory functions.**

B. **Function**

  1. Regulates peristalsis, gland secretion, water and ion transfer

  2. Operates independently of central nervous system, but can be influenced by sympathetic and parasympathetic divisions

> Absence of input from the central (autonomic) nervous system causes little or no change in intestinal activity.

C. **Clinical conditions**

  1. **Esophageal achalasia**

    a. Results from **denervation in the myenteric plexus** in the distal segment of esophagus

    b. Obstruction in terminal esophagus, with inability to relax lower esophageal sphincter, causes esophagus to fill and dilate with retained food.

  2. **Megacolon** (Hirschsprung disease)

    a. Congenital disorder in **which no ganglion cells are found in myenteric plexus**

    b. Affected intestinal tissue cannot relax in advance of normal peristaltic movement, causing lower gastrointestinal obstruction and severe abdominal distention.

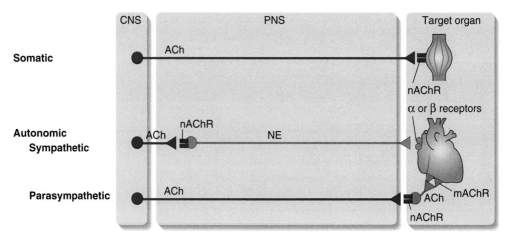

14-3: *Somatic efferent (dark green) fibers with cell bodies in the central nervous system (CNS) release acetylcholine (ACh) onto target skeletal muscles expressing nicotinic ACh receptors (nAChRs). Sympathetic preganglionic fibers (dark green) with cell bodies in the CNS release ACh onto target postganglionic neurons (gray) expressing nAChRs. Postganglionic axons release norepinephrine on target smooth and cardiac muscles expressing α- and β-adrenergic receptors. Parasympathetic preganglionic fibers (dark green) with cell bodies in the CNS release ACh onto target postganglionic neurons (light green) expressing nAChRs. Postganglionic axons release ACh onto target smooth and cardiac muscles expressing muscarinic acetylcholine receptors (mAChRs).*

V. **Neuropharmacology of Autonomic Nervous System**

A. **Cholinergic synapses** (Fig. 14-3 and Table 14-1)

Axillary sweat glands: Postganglionic sympathetic fibers are cholinergic.

1. **Acetylcholine** is the neurotransmitter used by sympathetic preganglionic, parasympathetic preganglionic, and parasympathetic postganglionic neurons.

2. **Receptors**

a. **Nicotinic** (neuronal subtype): on all autonomic postganglionic neurons, both sympathetic and parasympathetic

b. **Muscarinic (M_{1-3}):** on parasympathetic target organs

   • Muscarinic receptors are accessible by systemically administered drugs because they are outside the blood–brain barrier.

3. **Muscarinic cholinergic agonists**

a. **Carbachol** lowers intraocular pressure by causing constriction of iris and ciliary body and can be used to treat open-angle glaucoma.

b. **Bethanechol** has selectivity for gastrointestinal (GI) and urinary tract and can be used to manage ileus and urinary retention.

c. **Pilocarpine** stimulates gland secretion and can be used to induce sweating and to treat glaucoma.

4. **Muscarinic cholinergic antagonists**

Organophosphate poisoning: Atropine reverses effects of acetylcholinesterase inhibition.

a. **Atropine** prevents bradycardia and causes pupil dilation.

   • When the acetylcholinesterase inhibitor, edrophonium, is administered to diagnose **myasthenia gravis,** atropine is

TABLE 14-1:
Cholinergic
Receptor Location
and Pharmacology

Cholinergic Receptor Subtype	Important Locations (Effect of Activation)	Primary Agonists	Primary Antagonists
N—neuronal	Ganglia (stimulation) Adrenal medulla (secretion)	Epibatidine Nicotine Carbachol	Trimethaphan
M	Ganglia (stimulation) Bronchi (dilation)	Methacholine Pilocarpine Oxotremorine Carbachol	Atropine Pirenzepine
M-2	Sinoatrial node (bradycardia) Atrioventricular node (decreased conduction) Ventricle (decreased contractile force)		Atropine Tripitramine
M-3	Smooth muscle (contraction) Salivary glands (secretion) Pupil (constriction)		Atropine Darifenacin

frequently administered to counter the effects of increased acetylcholine at parasympathetic targets (e.g., cardiac arrhythmias, diarrhea).

b. **Scopolamine,** used to treat motion sickness, also blocks constriction of iris and gland secretion and causes side effects such as blurred vision and dry mouth.

B. **Adrenergic** (Table 14-2)

1. **Norepinephrine** is the neurotransmitter used by sympathetic postganglionic neurons.

> The adrenal medulla is innervated by sympathetic preganglionic fibers and serves a role equivalent to a postganglionic neuron pool, but with endocrine function. All catecholamines (epinephrine, norepinephrine, and dopamine) are released by the adrenal medulla.

2. **Receptors**
   a. **α Receptors** (α_{1-2})—primarily excitatory
   b. **β Receptors** (β_{1-3})—primarily inhibitory, except for heart rate and metabolism

3. **Adrenergic agonists**
   a. **Phenylephrine** (α_1 agonist) causes vasoconstriction and is used as a nasal decongestant.
   b. **Clonidine** (α_2 agonist) acts **centrally** to decrease sympathetic outflow and is used to treat hypertension; a transient increase in blood pressure on administration is mediated through receptors on vascular smooth muscle.

Ophthalmic application of phenylephrine: may produce rapid hypertension

TABLE 14-2: Adrenergic Receptor Location, Function, and Pharmacology

Adrenergic Receptor Subtype	Important Locations (Effect of Activation)	Primary Agonists	Primary Antagonists
α-1	Cardiac muscle (increased contractility) Vascular smooth muscle (constriction) Internal urinary sphincter (contraction) Smooth muscle of intestine (relaxation)	Epinephrine Isoproterenol Phenylephrine	Prazosin
α-2	Vascular smooth muscle (constriction) Pancreatic islet β-cells (decreased secretion of insulin)	Epinephrine Isoproterenol Clonidine	Yohimbine
β-1	Cardiac muscle (increased heart rate, contractility)	Isoproterenol Dobutamine	Metoprolol Atenolol
β-2	Vascular smooth muscle (relaxation) Bronchi (dilation) Detrusor muscle of urinary bladder (relaxation)	Isoproterenol Epinephrine Terbutaline	
β-3	Adipose tissue (lipolysis)	Isoproterenol Epinephrine	

      c. **Dobutamine** (β_1 agonist) increases cardiac output (heart rate and contractility).

      d. **Metaproterenol, albuterol, and terbutaline** (β_2 agonists) are used to treat bronchospasm.

    4. **Adrenergic antagonists**

      a. **Prazosin** (α_1 antagonist) is used to treat hypertension, pheochromocytoma, and pulmonary hypertension.

      b. **Yohimbine** (α_2 antagonist) is used to treat erectile dysfunction.
        • "Herbal Viagra" formations contain yohimbine

      c. **Atenolol** (β_1 antagonist) is used to treat hypertension.

      d. **Propranolol** (β antagonist) is used to treat hypertension and angina pectoris, and as prophylaxis for migraine headache.

VI. **Autonomic Control of Target Organs and Tissues** (Table 14-3; see also Fig. 14-1)

  A. **Arteries**

    1. **Sympathetic: vasoconstriction** of cutaneous arteries; **vasodilation** of skeletal muscle arteries

    2. **Parasympathetic: vasodilation** of arteries in brain, salivary glands, nasal mucosa, and genitals

  B. **Skin**

    1. **Sympathetic: secretion** (sweat glands) and **piloerection** (smooth muscles that erect the hairs)

    2. **Parasympathetic:** none

  C. **Eyes**

    1. **Sympathetic:** dilates pupil, increases palpebral fissure width

      a. Sympathetic fibers from superior cervical ganglion innervate ocular muscles, blood vessels, and glands of the head.

Organophosphate poisoning: blocks acetylcholinesterase and can cause miosis and cardiac slowing

TABLE 14-3:
Autonomic Receptor Location and Function

| Organ/Tissue | SYMPATHETIC | | | PARASYMPATHETIC | | |
	Response	Receptor Type	Ganglionic Blockade	Response	Receptor Type	Ganglionic Blockade
Adrenal medulla	Release of epinephrine	N*				
Arterioles			Vasodilates; ↑ blood flow; ↓ blood pressure			
Coronary	Dilates	β_2		Dilates	M	
	Constricts	$\alpha_1 > \alpha_2$				
Skin and mucosa	Constricts	$\alpha_1 > \alpha_2$				
Skeletal muscle	Constricts	$\alpha_1 > \alpha_2$		Dilates	M	
Lung	Dilate	β_2				
	Constricts	α_1				
Renal and mesenteric	Dilates	Dopamine, β_2		Dilates	M	
Splanchnic	Constricts	$\alpha_1 > \alpha_2$		Dilates	M	
Eye						
Iris						
Radial muscle	Contracts (pupil dilates = mydriasis)	α_1				
Sphincter muscle				Contracts (pupil constricts = miosis)	M_3	Pupil dilates
Ciliary muscle	Relaxes for far focus	β_2		Contracts for near focus	M_3	Loss of accommodation
Fat cells	Lipolysis	β_3				
GI tract						
Wall	Relaxes	α_2, β_2		Contracts	M	Constipation with ↓ tone and motility
Sphincters	Contracts	α_1		Relaxes	M	
Secretion	↓	α_2		↑	M	
Genitourinary system						
Penis, seminal vesicles	Ejaculation	α_2		Erection	M	
Urinary bladder	Relaxes	β_2		Contracts	M	
Detrusor trigone, sphincter	Contracts	α_1		Relaxes	M	Urine retention
Uterus, pregnant	Contracts	β_2				
	Relaxes	α_1				
Heart						
Sinoatrial node	↑ Heart rate	$\beta_1 > \beta_2$		↓ Heart rate	M_2	↑ Heart rate
Atrioventricular node	↑ Conduction velocity	$\beta_1 > \beta_2$		↓ Conduction velocity	M_2	
Contractility	↑	β_1		Slight ↓	M	
Kidney	↑ Renin secretion	β_1				
	↓ Renin secretion	α_1				

continued

TABLE 14-3:
Autonomic Receptor Location and Function—cont'd

Organ/Tissue	SYMPATHETIC			PARASYMPATHETIC		
	Response	Receptor Type	Ganglionic Blockade	Response	Receptor Type	Ganglionic Blockade
Lacrimal glands				Tearing	M	
Liver	Glycogenolysis, gluconeogenesis	α_1, β_2		Glycogen synthesis	M	
Lung, bronchial muscle	Relaxes	β_2		Contracts	M	
Pancreas, islets	↓ Insulin secretion ↑ Insulin secretion	α_2 β_2				
Pineal gland	Melatonin synthesis	β				
Salivary glands	K$^+$ and water secretion Amylase secretion	α β		K$^+$ and water secretion	M	Dry mouth

Skin
  Piloerection muscles
  Sweat glands
	
	Contracts
	Secretion
		
		α_1
		M
			
			No sweating			

Veins	Constricts Dilates	α_1 β_2	Dilates; pooling of blood; ↓ venous return			

* The adrenal medulla is equivalent to an autonomic ganglion. The preganglionic sympathetic terminals release acetylcholine onto nicotinic receptors at this gland.
M, muscarinic; N, nicotinic.

    b. **Horner syndrome** (pupil constriction and decreased palpebral fissure width in affected eye; decreased sweating on ipsilateral face) results from damage to sympathetic fibers (Fig. 14-4).
  2. **Parasympathetic:** constricts sphincter muscle of the pupil
    • **Argyll-Robertson pupil** (pupil constricts on near focus but not in response to light) results from damage to parasympathetic neurons or fibers.
 D. **Lacrimal glands**
  1. **Sympathetic:** vasoconstriction; decreased tearing
  2. **Parasympathetic:** secretion, tearing
 E. **Salivary glands**
  1. **Sympathetic:** vasoconstriction and production of **thick saliva rich in amylase**
  2. **Parasympathetic:** production of **watery saliva**
 F. **Heart**

Acute inflammatory demyelinating polyneuropathy (AIDP; Guillain-Barré syndrome) can cause acute autonomic failure with cardiac arrhythmias and swings in blood pressure.

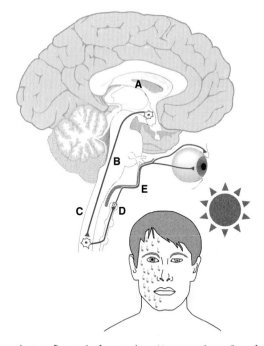

14-4: *Damage to sympathetic outflow to the face produces Horner syndrome (loss of sweating, pupil constriction, lid droop) ipsilateral to the lesion. A, Hypothalamic damage affects central control of autonomic outflow. B, Brainstem damage, including lateral medullary syndrome, may interrupt sympathetic outflow. C, Cervical spinal cord damage, including syringomyelia, interrupts descending control or directly affects sympathetic preganglionic cell bodies. D, Ascending sympathetic trunk damage, including apical lung tumors, and disruption of the superior cervical ganglion preganglionic axons. E, Postganglionic sympathetic fiber damage, including dissecting aneurysms of the carotid artery.*

    1. **Sympathetic: increases contractility and heart rate**
       a. Left cardiac sympathetic fibers increase cardiac contractility.
       b. Right cardiac sympathetic fibers increase heart rate.
    2. **Parasympathetic: slows heart rate** and rate of conduction

> Diabetes can cause parasympathetic loss with increased resting heart rate.

 G. **Respiratory system**
    1. **Sympathetic: dilation** of bronchi and bronchioles
    2. **Parasympathetic: constriction** and secretion
 H. **Esophagus**
    1. **Sympathetic:** increased tone in cardiac sphincter, decreased tone and motility in lower one third of the esophagus, and increased contraction in upper one third of esophagus
    2. **Parasympathetic:** increased tone and motility
  I. **Stomach and Intestines**
    1. **Sympathetic: inhibits peristaltic movement** and increases tone of sphincters

2. **Parasympathetic:** increases peristaltic movement and secretions, relaxes sphincters
   a. **Vagus** innervates the upper GI tract to the rostral two thirds of transverse colon.
   b. **Pelvic splanchnic nerves** innervate the lower gastrointestinal tract from distal one third of the transverse colon to rectum.
J. **Urinary bladder**
   1. **Sympathetic:** constricts internal urethral sphincter, relaxes detrusor muscle, allows filling of bladder
   2. **Parasympathetic:** relaxes internal urethral sphincter, stimulates contraction of detrusor muscle, empties bladder
K. **Prostate and testes**
   1. **Sympathetic:** vasoconstriction and contraction of smooth muscles of prostate, seminal vesicles, urethra, and vas deferens; emission of semen into urethra, **ejaculation**
   2. **Parasympathetic:** vasodilation and **erection**

Erectile dysfunction: most common autonomic neuropathy to accompany diabetes mellitus

VII. **Hypothalamus**
   A. **Overview**
      1. Connects with forebrain (particularly limbic areas), brainstem, and spinal cord
      2. With brainstem, contain suprasegmental integrating centers for autonomic, vegetative, emotional, and endocrine functions
   B. **Function of regions and nuclei**
      1. **Anterior region**
         a. **Anterior nucleus:** maintenance of body temperature
         b. **Lateral hypothalamic nucleus:** feeding center
         c. **Preoptic area (lateral and medial preoptic nuclei):** blood volume, temperature, and reproductive activity
         d. **Paraventricular and supraoptic nuclei:** release of oxytocin (for contraction of uterus and ejection of milk) and vasopressin (for water balance)
         e. **Suprachiasmatic nucleus:** circadian rhythms
      2. **Infundibular region**
         a. **Dorsomedial:** emotional behavior

Stimulating the dorsomedial infundibular region causes aggressive behavior (sham rage) in experimental models.

         b. **Ventromedial:** satiety center
         c. **Lateral hypothalamic nucleus:** feeding center
         d. **Tuberal nuclei (arcuate and infundibular** nuclei)
            (1) Produce **releasing factors** that regulate hormone release from anterior pituitary
            (2) Releasing factors are transmitted to anterior pituitary through the **hypophysial portal system**

(3) Clinically relevant releasing factors: **corticotropin releasing factor,** thyrotropin releasing factor, growth hormone releasing factors, prolactin releasing factor, gonadotropin releasing factor, and melanocyte stimulating hormone releasing factor

3. **Posterior region**
   a. **Mammillary nuclei:** limbic function

> **Korsakoff psychosis,** resulting from thiamine deficiency related to chronic alcoholism, is associated with anterograde and retrograde amnesia and with degeneration of the mammillary bodies and the dorsomedial nucleus of the thalamus.

Korsakoff psychosis: degeneration of the mammillary bodies and severe anterograde and retrograde amnesia

   b. **Lateral hypothalamic nucleus:** feeding center
   c. **Posterior nucleus:** blood pressure, emotional, maintenance of body temperature and analgesic functions

VIII. **Suprasegmental Control**
   A. **Cardiovascular centers** (Fig. 14-5)
      1. Input is from baroreceptors in carotid sinus (glossopharyngeal nerve) and aortic arch (vagus nerve) to the medulla.
      2. Elevated sinus pressure results in **decreased sympathetic discharge,** which decreases heart rate and contractility
      3. Reduced carotid sinus pressure results in **increased sympathetic outflow.**

> **Orthostatic hypotension** results from loss of the compensatory baroreceptor regulation of blood flow and pressure that normally occurs upon standing (see Fig. 14-5).

Sympathetic ganglionic blocking drugs may cause orthostatic hypotension.

   B. **Respiration centers**
      1. Input is from stretch receptors in lung and chemoreceptors in carotid and aortic bodies.
      2. **Medullary center** produces inspiration and expiration.
      3. **Pontine apneustic center,** if uncontrolled, prolongs inspiration.
      4. **Pontine pneumotaxic center** stimulation increases rate of respiration.
      5. Neurogenic influences regulate the depth, rate, and pattern of inspiration.
         a. **Cheyne-Stokes respiration:** rapid inspiration (hyperpnea) with gradually increasing and then decreasing depth with intermittent apnea; seen in individuals with either hemispheric or internal capsule damage
         b. **Central reflex apnea** (neurogenic hyperventilation): continuous deep breathing; seen in comatose individuals after midbrain damage
         c. **Apneustic** breathing: inspiratory spasms of varying length; seen in individuals with damage to the **lower pons.**
         d. **Ataxic** respiration: gasping with highly irregular rate and depth; seen in individuals with damage to the **medulla**

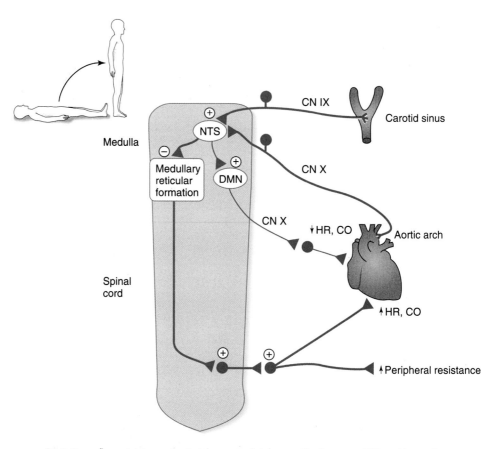

14-5: *Baroreflex maintains mean arterial pressure during postural adjustments. With rapid move from reclining to standing position, decreased blood pressure results in decreased activation of baroreceptors in carotid sinus and aortic arch. Decreased baroreceptor activity is conveyed by glossopharyngeal and vagus nerves to the caudal nucleus of the solitary tract (NTS). Decreased NTS activation results in decreased parasympathetic outflow from dorsal motor nucleus of vagus (DMN), which increases heart rate (HR). As heart rate increases, increased cardiac output (CO) causes increased blood pressure. In addition, decreased NTS output releases medullary reticular formation, acting through the reticulospinal tract, to stimulate sympathetic preganglionic neurons of thoracic spinal cord to increase cardiac output and peripheral resistance. Both factors increase blood pressure.*

C. **Vomiting (emetic) center**
1. Located in posterior lateral medulla
2. Receives input from
   a. Chemoreceptors located in **medullary chemoreceptor trigger zone (area postrema),** an area with no blood–brain barrier that can respond to chemicals (toxins) in the blood
   b. Gastrointestinal tract through afferents in vagus and splanchnic nerves
   c. Vestibular nuclei

d. Cerebral cortex

> The protective vomiting reflex involves rapid emptying of the stomach by contraction of abdominal muscles and relaxation of cardiac sphincter.

D. **Swallowing (deglutition) center**
  1. Located in the medullary reticular formation
  2. **Dysphagia** (difficulty in swallowing) characterizes motor neuron damage in the caudal brainstem.

E. **Feeding centers**
  1. Located in the infundibular region
  2. **Lateral hypothalamic nucleus:** feeding center.
     a. Stimulation: **induces urge to eat**
     b. Damage: **failure to eat** (neglect of eating—**aphagia**)
  3. **Ventromedial hypothalamic nucleus:** satiety center
     a. Stimulation: **inhibits urge to eat**
        • Activated by **increased glucose utilization** and increased afferent discharge from the gut.
     b. Damage: decreases physical activity and **increases appetite,** causing hyperphagia (excessive eating)

F. **Water and osmolar balance center**
  1. Located in **paraventricular and supraoptic** nuclei in **anterior hypothalamus**
  2. Releases vasopressin, which acts on kidney to increase water retention
     a. **Hyperosmotic blood** stimulates vasopressin release.
     b. **Hypotonic blood** inhibits vasopressin release.
  3. Bilateral damage to supraoptic nuclei causes diabetes insipidus, characterized by increased thirst (polydipsia) and pale, dilute urine.
  4. Damage to ventromedial and lateral hypothalamus results in **increased thirst.**

G. **Temperature centers**
  1. Located in **anterior and posterior hypothalamus**
  2. Contain thermal receptors that **monitor arterial blood (core body) temperature**
  3. Anterior hypothalamus stimulates **heat loss** (vasodilation).
     • Damage to the anterior hypothalamus causes **hyperthermia.**
  4. Posterior hypothalamus stimulates **heat conservation** (shivering, vasoconstriction, increased heart rate, elevated basal metabolic rate).
     a. Damage to the posterior hypothalamus destroys the heat conservation center as well as axons projecting from the anterior hypothalamic center, resulting in loss of thermoregulatory capacity (poikilothermia).
     b. In response to viral or bacterial infection, **endogenous fever-producing agents** (pyrogens, e.g., interleukin-1) act on thermal-sensitive neurons of the hypothalamus to raise the body temperature set-point, making the body a less hospitable host for the infecting pathogens.

Sympathomimetic amines (e.g., amphetamine) and cholecystokinin: suppress appetite

Leptin receptor suppresses appetite: Receptor mutations are associated with congenital obesity.

Postural hypotension: Administer vasopressin to increase blood volume.

Pyrogenic substances released by bacteria: stimulate hypothalamus to release vasopressin, which has antipyrogenic activity

H. **Circadian rhythms center**
   1. Located in the **suprachiasmatic nucleus**
   2. Biologic clock that maintains a near 24-hour cycle to influence
      a. Motor activity
      b. Sleep and wake cycles
      c. Eating and drinking
      d. Body temperature
      e. Release of neurotransmitters, pituitary hormones, and corticosterone
      f. Learning and memory retention
   3. Projections directly from the retina, through the retinohypothalamic tract, entrain internal clock to external environment.
      a. Absorption, distribution, metabolism, and elimination of drugs varies in a circadian fashion.
      b. **Chronotherapeutics** makes use of this knowledge to determine optimum timing of drug delivery (e.g., cancer chemotherapeutic, cisplatin, may be more effective when given in the evening rather than the morning).

> Asthma attacks: most common in the late night

I. **Sexual function**
   1. Psychic and somatic stimuli are integrated in the **limbic system** to influence outflow from **anterior and posterior hypothalamus** and **sacral spinal cord.**
   2. **Bilateral damage to amygdala** increases sexual behavior.
   3. Bilateral damage to sacral cord, pelvic nerves, or lower thoracic and upper lumbar sympathetic nerves decreases or abolishes both potency and emission.

> Depression: most frequent cause of impotence

> Retrograde ejaculation (orgasm without emission) may result from lesions to the pelvic nerves (e.g., in patients with diabetic neuropathy).

J. **Reproduction**
   1. **Paraventricular nucleus** (anterior hypothalamus) is the principal source of **oxytocin,** which causes expression of milk during breast-feeding and which stimulates uterine muscle during labor.
   2. **Oxytocin release** is increased by stimulation of the genital tract (distention of uterus and vagina) and suckling, increased osmolarity of the blood and acetylcholine (stimulates response to eject).

> Synthetic oxytocin is administered to induce labor or to increase the strength and duration of uterine contractions.

K. **Micturition** (Fig. 14-6)
   1. **Cerebral** cortical control **inhibits urinary bladder emptying by constricting external sphincter through pudendal nerve.**
   2. **Pontine micturition center** projects to sacral spinal cord and **allows voluntary bladder emptying.**
   3. **Sympathetic** control (T10–L2) through hypogastric nerve **allows bladder filling** by relaxing detrusor and contracting internal sphincter.

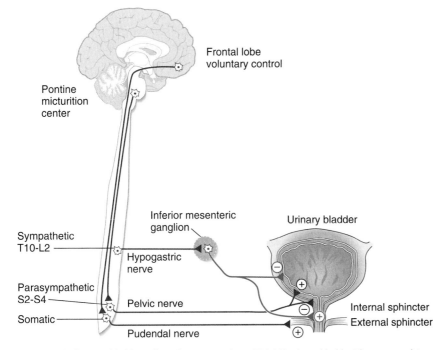

14-6: *Control of urinary bladder. Filling phase: sympathetic (T10–L2) relaxes bladder (detrusor muscle) and stimulates internal sphincter. Voiding phase: parasympathetic stimulates detrusor constriction and internal sphincter relaxation. Coordination of the spinal reflex is under control from the pontine micturition center. Voluntary constriction of the external urinary sphincter is controlled from the frontal lobe by way of lower motor neurons in the sacral spinal cord.*

4. **Parasympathetic** control (S2–S4) through pelvic nerve **activates bladder emptying** by constricting detrusor and relaxing internal sphincter.
5. **Micturition reflex,** initiated by stretch receptors in detrusor muscle, feeds back to spinal cord to inhibit sympathetic outflow and allow parasympathetic activation.
6. **Disorders of urinary bladder emptying**
   a. **Uninhibited bladder**
      (1) Loss of supraspinal control causing loss of voluntary inhibition with no loss of ability to perceive need to void
      (2) Leads to **urinary incontinence with urgency**
   b. **Automatic reflex bladder**
      (1) Follows loss of input from pontine micturition center (i.e., anywhere between pons and S2; start of parasympathetic output to bladder)
      (2) Leads to **urinary incontinence without urgency**
      (3) Bladder empties reflexively when full (1–4 hours) because spinal reflex arc is intact.

(4) Normal bladder in infants; in adults, lesion leads to frequent urination, incontinence, and urinary retention

(5) Occurs after initial recovery from spinal shock

> During spinal shock immediately after injury, acute atonic bladder (does not empty on its own) occurs, and urine must be drained through urethral catheter.

c. **Nonreflex (autonomous) bladder**

(1) Damage to sacral spinal cord or cauda equina (e.g., cauda equina trauma, myelomeningocele)

(2) Bladder is areflexic, and sphincters will not contract; bladder fills to maximum capacity, then dribbles (i.e., urinary retention and overflow incontinence).

d. **Paralytic bladder: sensory**

(1) Damage to sensory nerves (e.g. diabetes, lumbar disc herniation) or sensory tracts in spinal cord (e.g., tabes dorsalis)

(2) Loss of sensation leads to urinary retention and overflow incontinence

e. **Paralytic bladder: motor**

(1) Damage to motor nerves (e.g., acute inflammatory demyelinating polyneuropathy, poliomyelitis) or sensory tracts in spinal cord (e.g., tabes dorsalis)

(2) Loss of sensation leads to urinary retention and overflow incontinence

15 CHAPTER

States of Consciousness

I. **Consciousness**

A. **Overview** (Table 15-1)

1. State of mental function requiring both **arousal** and **awareness** of self and surroundings

2. Dependent on **cerebral cortex** and **ascending reticular activating system** (ARAS)

3. **Altered consciousness:** confusion and delirium

4. **Unconsciousness:** concussion, coma, persistent vegetative state, syncope and sleep

> Coma results from **bilateral cortical damage or from loss of ARAS** caused by diencephalic dysfunction or by discrete lesions of brainstem.

B. **Anatomy**

1. **Reticular formation**

a. Network of three columns of neurons extending from spinal cord continuously through the core of the brainstem to thalamus

(1) Median column: intermediate-sized neurons of raphe nuclei

(2) Medial column: large (magnocellular, gigantocellular) neurons

(3) Lateral column: small (parvicellular) neurons

b. Receives input from

(1) **Spinal cord:** spinoreticular, spinothalamic, medial lemniscus

(2) **Cranial nerves:** visual, auditory, vestibular

(3) **Diencephalon and subcortical regions:** thalamic, subthalamic, hypothalamic, basal ganglia

(4) **Cerebral cortex:** primary motor, primary sensory, limbic

2. From midpons rostrally, reticular system supplies cerebral cortex with **excitatory inputs necessary for arousal** and is the anatomic substrate for the ARAS.

3. From midpons caudally, reticular system provides drive to lower motor neurons of spinal cord through the medial and lateral reticulospinal tracts.

II. **Coma**

A. **Criteria**

1. Eyes are closed

2. No sleep–wake cycle

3. Unconscious as assessed by response to strong verbal and tactile (painful) stimuli

**TABLE 15-1:
Gradations in
Consciousness**

General Terms	Expected Behaviors and Responses to External Stimuli
Fully conscious	Fully awake, alert, oriented to environment Spontaneous (voluntary) speech at a normal rate Normal voluntary and reflex somatic motor activity Eyes open; normal oculomotor activity
Confusion, lethargy	Ability to respond to stimuli is intact, but *inattentive* Spontaneous sentences, spoken slowly Decreased speed of voluntary motor activity Eyes open; decreased oculomotor activity
Drowsiness	Spontaneous words, spoken infrequently Decreased speed and coordination of voluntary motor activity Eyes open or closed; decreased oculomotor activity Motor defenses are intact
Stupor	Vocalization only to stimuli that cause pain Markedly decreased spontaneous motor activity Eyes generally closed; some spontaneous eye movements Motor defenses still intact
Obtundation	No vocalization Appropriate defensive movements, generally flexor, to stimuli that cause pain Eyes generally closed
Semicoma (light coma)	No vocalization Only primitive mass movements to stimuli that cause pain Eyes closed; decreased spontaneous conjugate eye movements Abnormal body posturing
Coma	No vocalization Decerebrate posturing to stimuli that cause pain, or no response Eyes closed; spontaneous eye movements absent
Brain death	

4. **Glasgow coma scale:** standardized approach to rapidly assess neurologic function using a patient's verbal, gross motor, and eye movement responses (Table 15-2).

B. **Causes**

1. **Head trauma**

> **Diffuse axonal injury:** Head trauma causing rapid acceleration–deceleration or rotational movements of the head may cause damage through stretching and shearing of axons of the ARAS. Unconsciousness lasting less than 6 hours is termed concussion, whereas coma implies unconsciousness lasting at least 6 hours.

2. **Coma with focal signs**
   a. Tumor

> Unilateral structural intracranial masses may be sufficiently large to compress the contralateral hemisphere and disrupt contralateral cortical activity.

Motor vehicle crashes: leading cause of traumatic brain injury

Eyes Open

4 = Spontaneously
3 = To verbal command
2 = To pain
1 = Do not open

Best Verbal Response

5 = Oriented and converses
4 = Disoriented, confused, but converses
3 = Inappropriate words
2 = Incomprehensible sounds
1 = No response

Best Motor Response

6 = Obeys commands
5 = Purposeful movements localized to pain
4 = Withdrawal from pain
3 = Decorticate posturing
2 = Decerebrate posturing
1 = No response

**TABLE 15-2:
Glascow Coma
Scale**

Maximum score = 15
   15–13 = Mild head injury
    9–12 = Moderate head injury
    3–8 = Severe head injury, coma

    b. Stroke (hemorrhagic or ischemic)
    c. Infection (e.g., cerebral abscess)
  3. **Coma without head trauma and without focal signs**
    a. Stroke (e.g., hemorrhagic or ischemic; subarachnoid hemorrhage)
    b. Infection (e.g., meningitis, encephalitis)
    c. Metabolic disorders: respiratory (hypoxia, hypercapnia), cardiovascular (ischemia), hepatic, renal (uremia), pancreatic (hypoglycemia)
    d. Drug interactions or intoxication
    e. Seizure
  4. **Herniation syndromes**
    a. **Central herniation:** brain swelling or central mass lesions causing downward movement of diencephalon through the tentorial notch onto brainstem.
    b. **Lateral herniation:** expanding cerebral mass initially causing contralateral hemiparesis with eventual herniation of the medial temporal lobe through the tentorial notch, causing ipsilateral oculomotor palsy as the oculomotor nerve becomes stretched.
C. **Localizing signs** (Table 15-3)
  1. **Respiratory pattern** (Fig. 15-1)
    a. **Cheyne-Stokes:** hemispheres, upper brainstem, or metabolic encephalopathy

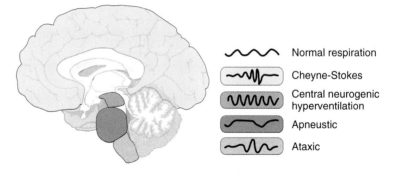

15-1: *Breathing patterns accompanying brain damage.*

TABLE 15-3:
Localizing Signs in Coma

Site of Lesion	Posture in Response to Painful Stimulus	Eyes	Respiratory Pattern
Hemispheres, bilaterally	Directed movement Withdrawal	PERLA Caloric yields nystagmus	Cheyne-Stokes
Diencephalon	Decorticate	PERLA Caloric: nystagmus	Cheyne-Stokes
Midbrain	Decorticate	Pupils do not constrict to light or accommodation. If CN III damaged, ipsilateral eye position "done and out"	Central reflex hyperpnea (central neurogenic hyperventilation)
Pons	Decerebrate	Pupils small If CN VI damage, loss of abduction in ipsilateral eye. If adjacent PPRF damaged, loss of conjugate horizontal eye movement to ipsilateral side	Cluster (Biot') or apneustic
Medulla	Flaccid paralysis	Pupils small	Ataxic

PERLA, *pupils equal, react to light and accommodation;* PPRF, *para pontine veticular formation.*

b. **Central neurogenic hyperventilation:** rostral midbrain

> Hyperventilation in coma patients may have causes other than damage to the rostral midbrain. Patients may hyperventilate as a response to hypoxia resulting from neurogenic pulmonary edema.

c. **Apneusis:** pons
d. **Cluster breathing** (Biot respiration): pons
e. **Ataxic breathing:** medulla

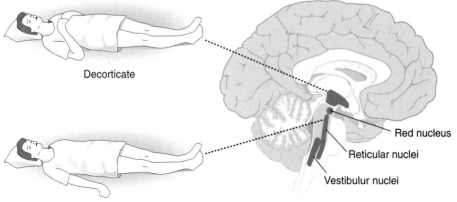

15-2: *Decorticate and decerebrate posturing.*

2. **Posturing** (Fig. 15-2)
   a. **Decorticate:** structural or metabolic damage to hemispheres or diencephalon
   b. **Decerebrate:** damage to midbrain or upper pons
3. **Pupils**
   a. **Reactive:** intact midbrain
   b. **Small, reactive:** metabolic encephalopathies
   c. **Bilateral pinpoint pupils:** narcotic overdose or pontine damage
   d. **Large, unreactive:** atropine, barbiturates, hypoxia
   e. **Fixed position and dilated:** midbrain lesion or atropine poisoning
   f. **Unilateral dilation** with no light reflex: oculomotor nerve compromise

   > **Unilateral dilated pupil** in the presence of signs of increased intracranial pressure suggests a tentorial temporal lobe (uncal) herniation and is a life-threatening emergency.

   g. **Small pupil as part of Horner syndrome** (miosis, ptosis, anhidrosis): diencephalon
4. **Eye position and movement**
   a. Both eyes deviate toward acute destructive cerebral lesions, driven by contralateral frontal eye fields.
   b. Both eyes deviate away from an irritative lesion or seizure (driven by overactive frontal eye fields).
   c. Both eyes deviate away from pontine lesion (driven by contralateral paramedian pontine reticular formation [PPRF], i.e., lateral gaze center).
   d. Eyelids closed means pons (facial nerve) is intact.
5. **Vestibulo-ocular reflex**
   a. No oculocephalic (**doll's eye**) reflex: brainstem function is compromised.
   b. Reactive pupils with no oculocephalic reflex can occur in response to **hypoglycemia or barbiturates.**

Decorticate posturing suggests CNS compromise above level of midbrain.

Decerebrate posturing suggests CNS compromise that includes midbrain but not lower brainstem.

TABLE 15-4: Comparison of Delirium and Dementia

Delirium	Dementia
Acute onset	Slow, insidious onset
Fluctuating	Progressive
Alterations in consciousness	Consciousness unimpaired until very late stages
Frequently due to treatable condition (e.g., systemic infection, drug intoxication) and reversible if underlying cause is treated.	Frequently due to a neurodegenerative process and irreversible

       c. No response to calorics: brainstem damage
         (1) Full nystagmus requires cortical function
         (2) Eyes partially or fully deviated toward "cold" ear: some brainstem function exists.
    D. **Noncoma causes of loss of consciousness**
       1. **Stupor** can be disrupted by strong stimuli.
       2. **Sleep** is readily reversible and has a cyclic variation in behavior and underlying electroencephalogram (EEG).
       3. **Syncope** (fainting) is transient.
       4. **Persistent vegetative state,** which occurs after coma of at least 2 weeks duration, includes sleep–wake cycle and spontaneous movements, including eye openings but no evidence of awareness or responsiveness to environment.
       5. **Locked-in syndrome:** patient appears unconsciousness but is **awake and aware.**
         a. Brainstem lesion damage, which destroys pontine base but spares all ascending sensory tracts and ascending reticular activating system, leaves patient fully paralyzed except for limited eye and eyelid movement.
         b. Causes: **infarct and central pontine myelinolysis** (loss of myelin from the base of the pons) due to **rapid correction of hyponatremia** that could have resulted from chronic alcoholism, often accompanied by malnutrition.

III. **Delirium**
    A. **Overview** (Table 15-4)
       1. **Syndrome** with **acute onset** (hours to days)
       2. **Fluctuating mental status** with alterations in level of consciousness, inattention, disorganized thought
       3. Changes in EEG, with slowing that accompanies periods of inattention
       4. Disrupted sleep–wake cycle
       5. Memory impairment
    B. **Causes**
       1. Central nervous system (CNS) damage resulting from stroke, head trauma, infection

2. An underlying systemic medical condition, especially of metabolic, infectious (e.g., HIV), endocrine, or cardiovascular origin

> In **elderly patients, delirium** may be the first sign of a systemic illness, such as a urinary tract infection.

Urinary tract infections in the elderly: may first present with delirium

3. Substance abuse or intoxication
4. Reaction to medication or interaction between medications

> Elderly individuals are particularly susceptible to delirium related to medications.

IV. **Dementia**
   A. **Overview** (see Table 15-4)
      1. **Set of syndromes** that produce sufficient cognitive impairments to **cause inability to maintain normal activities of daily living,** including normal social interactions
      2. Memory loss is most common initial finding
      3. Loss of judgment and planning ability
      4. Impairment in performance of complex motor activities (e.g., **apraxia**)
   B. **Permanent causes**
      1. Alzheimer, Parkinson, or Huntington disease
      2. Supranuclear palsy
      3. Multi-infarct (cerebrovascular) dementia
   C. **Reversible causes**
      1. Normal pressure hydrocephalus
      2. Thiamine (vitamin B_1) deficiency (beriberi, Korsakoff psychosis)
      3. Vitamin B_{12} deficiency

V. **Seizure**
   A. **Partial (focal) seizures**
      1. Begin in a limited region of one hemisphere.
      2. **Simple**
         a. **Do not impair consciousness**
         b. May cause sensory, motor, psychic, or autonomic signs and symptoms
         c. May be followed by **transient** (1–2 days) **sensory or motor deficit** (Todd paralysis)
      3. **Complex**
         a. Most frequently **originate from temporal lobe** and involve limbic structures (hippocampus, amygdala, parahippocampal gyrus)
         b. Cause **alterations in consciousness**
         c. Followed by **period of confusion during recovery**
         d. **Temporal lobe epilepsy** ("uncinate fits"): seizures that originate in or near **olfactory cortex** and produce an aura that includes **olfactory hallucinations**
   B. **Generalized seizure**
      1. Begin spontaneously in both hemispheres (primary) or begin as partial and spread to involve large portions of both hemispheres (secondarily generalized).

2. **Absence seizure**
    a. Formerly known as **petit mal**
    b. Characterized by **3 spikes/second EEG** pattern bilaterally
    c. Last only seconds, but may occur 100 or more times per day
    d. Start and end abruptly, with **no postictal confusion**
    e. Produce little or no abnormal motor activity
    f. May be misdiagnosed as daydreaming or inattention

3. **Myoclonic seizure**
    a. Brief muscle contractions affecting any muscle group
    b. May be unilateral or bilateral, synchronous or asynchronous
    c. Most frequent during **sleep–wake transitions**

4. **Tonic seizure**
    a. Sustained contraction of the limb muscles (flexion of the arms and flexion or extension of the legs)
    b. Lasts 1 minute or less
    c. Most frequent during drowsy period or rapid eye movement (REM) sleep and may occur many times per day
    d. Most often seen in children with generalized epilepsy

5. **Tonic–clonic seizure**
    a. Formerly known as grand mal
    b. **Most common type of seizure**
    c. **Tonic phase** occurs abruptly and includes limb extension bilaterally.
       • Air ejected forcefully against tightened vocal cords is responsible for the "epileptic cry" associated with a tonic–clonic seizure.
    d. **Clonic phase** follows as synchronous muscle contractions.
    e. Total seizure may last 1 to 2 minutes, but is followed by a postictal period of confusion lasting up to 30 minutes or longer.

6. **Atonic seizure**
    a. Known as **"drop attacks"**
    b. Characterized by partial or complete loss of muscle tone; seizure may only effect head and neck muscles ("head drop")
    c. Most frequently seen with diffuse encephalopathies

C. **Status epilepticus**
    1. Single seizure, or series of seizures without complete recovery interictally, that continues for at least 30 minutes
    2. **Medical emergency:** although incidence is low, mortality rate is high
    3. **Cause:** acute damage to CNS, especially cerebrovascular disease (adult) and fever and infection (children)
    4. Can be partial or generalized
    5. Can be convulsive (frequently tonic–clonic) or nonconvulsive (e.g., absence or complex partial)
       a. Convulsive generate multiple systemic and metabolic effects (e.g., hypoxia, elevated body temperature, loss of control of blood pressure, hypokalemia, hyponatremia, hypoglycemia)
       b. Nonconvulsive must be distinguished through EEG

D. **Psychogenic seizures**
    1. Represent between 15% and 30% of seizures diagnosed

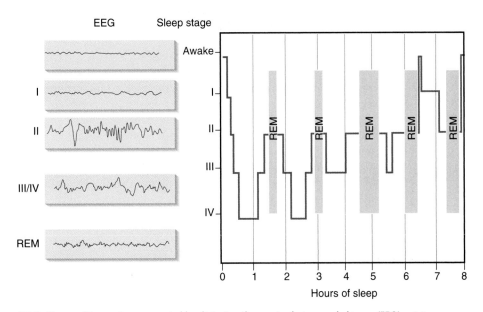

15-3: *Sleep architecture is accompanied by distinctive changes in electroencephalogram (EEG) activity. REM, rapid eye movement.*

2. May occur in individual who also experiences physiologic seizures
3. Occur without accompanying changes in EEG pattern
4. Postictal confusion may be absent (many physiologic seizures are followed by a period of confusion)
5. Evidence of loss of motor control during seizure (e.g., tongue bitten, urinary incontinence, injury) rare

VI. Sleep
A. Stages (Fig. 15-3)
1. Determined by **polysomnogram**
   a. EEG measures activity in the cerebral cortex.
   b. Electrooculogram (EOG) measures eye movement.
   c. Electromyogram (EMG) measures muscle activity.
2. **Awake, active mental state:** EEG shows high-frequency, low-amplitude beta waves (15–40 Hz).
3. **Relaxed, waking state:** EEG shows high-frequency, low-amplitude alpha waves (8–13 Hz).
4. **Non–rapid eye movement (NREM) stage 1 (drowsiness to light sleep):**
   a. EEG shows high-frequency, low-amplitude theta waves (3–7 Hz).
   b. Hypnic myoclonic contractions possible
5. **NREM stage 2 (light sleep)**
   a. EEG contains sleep spindles (12–14 Hz).
   b. Limited eye and body movement
6. **NREM stage 3 + 4 (deep sleep, slow-wave sleep)**
   a. EEG shows low-frequency, high-amplitude delta waves (2 Hz).

b. Stage 3 has up to 50%, and stage 4 has more than 50% delta waves.
c. Difficult to wake spontaneously
d. No eye movement and limited body movement
e. Parasympathetic control dominates, with slowed heart rate
f. Influenced by prior wakefulness: sleep deprivation causes increased stage 4 sleep.
g. **Night terrors** and somnambulism (**sleepwalking**) possible
h. Stage 4 is **suppressed by benzodiazepines**

Benzodiazepines control night terrors: suppress stage IV sleep

7. **REM sleep**
   a. Also called desynchronized, activated, or **paradoxical** sleep
   b. **EEG** shows high-frequency, low-voltage pattern that is very **similar to waking** beta-wave EEG.
   c. **Atonia due to paralysis of muscles,** excluding middle ear and eye and respiratory muscles, controlled from brainstem
   d. Dominates prenatally
   e. Sympathetic activity dominates.
   f. Penile erection
   g. Thermoregulatory control decreased
   h. Not influenced by prior wakefulness
   i. Vivid visual dreaming
      (1) Paralysis prevents acting out dreams
      (2) **REM sleep disorder:** loss of REM paralysis allows individual to act out dreams.
   j. **Suppressed by alcohol, barbiturates, and tricyclic antidepressants**

   Individuals are most likely to wake spontaneously from REM sleep, even though REM is the deepest sleep.

B. **Sleep architecture** (see Fig. 15-3)
   1. Normal: 90-minute cycle beginning with stage 1 - 2 - 3 - 4 - 3 - 2—REM
   2. First REM sleep is normally entered about 90 minutes into sleep.

   Individuals with REM sleep disorder or depression have early-onset REM sleep.

C. **EEG**
   1. Frequency varies with different stages of sleep
   2. **Beta** (13–30 Hz) awake, active ("desynchronized")
   3. **Alpha** (8–13 Hz) awake, relaxed
   4. **Theta** (4–7 Hz) sleep stages 1 and 2
   5. **Delta** (0.5–4 Hz) sleep stages 3 and 4 ("synchronized")

D. **Disorders**
   1. **Insomnia**
      a. **Definition**
         (1) Inability to achieve sufficient sleep
         (2) Subjective sense of insufficient sleep
         (3) Difficulty in falling asleep (30 minutes or more)
         (4) Symptom, not a disorder

  b. **Causes**
     (1) Anxiety, depression, stress, pain
     (2) Side effect of drugs, alcohol, poor sleep habits
     (3) Disruption of circadian rhythms
     (4) Increasing age
  c. **Effects**
     (1) Problems with memory and concentration
     (2) Potential link with cardiovascular disease
     (3) Four-fold increase in likelihood of depression
     (4) Impaired performance
  d. **Fatal familial insomnia** is a rare prion-mediated disorder that affects numerous brain regions, including thalamus.
2. **Sleep apnea**
  a. Consists of **brief periods of interrupted breathing** during sleep
  b. Diagnosed using polysomnogram and multiple sleep latency test: normal sleep latency is 10 to 20 minutes; sleep-deprived is less than 5 minutes
  c. **Obstructive sleep apnea**
     (1) **Major cause of daytime sleepiness**
     (2) Waking up to 500 times per night
     (3) Often accompanies heavy snoring
     (4) More common in **overweight individuals**
  d. **Treatment:** weight loss and continuous positive airway pressure
3. **Narcolepsy**
  a. Characterized by **sudden irresistible sleep attacks;** often 15 minutes of sleep refreshes
  b. **Second leading cause of daytime sleepiness;** affects about one in 2000 people, men and women of any age
  c. **Symptoms**
     (1) **Excessive daytime sleepiness**
     (2) Sleep latency is decreased on multiple sleep latency tests.
     (3) **Sleep-onset REM** (REM normally occurs after 90 minutes of sleep)
     (4) **Cataplexy**
        (a) Sudden loss of muscle tone ranging from slight weakness (head droop, facial sagging, jaw drop, slurred speech, buckling of knees) to total collapse
        (b) Triggered by intense emotion (laughter, anger, surprise, fear) or strenuous athletic activity
     (5) Paralysis at sleep onset and offset
     (6) Hypnagogic hallucinations

> Patients with hypnagogic hallucinations report vivid and often frightening dreams and sounds when falling asleep.

  d. **Cause:** associated with **lack of hypocretin** (orexin)

Narcolepsy tetrad: excessive daytime sleepiness, hypnagogic hallucinations, sleep onset paralysis and cataplexy

4. **Restless legs syndrome**
   a. Characterized by uncomfortable (not painful) sensation in legs, sometimes described as creeping or crawling
      (1) Most common in the evening or at night
      (2) Individual will have "restless" or "fidgeting" feet and legs when sitting down or lying down in the evening or at night.
   b. May be relieved by walking or stretching and may be exacerbated by rest
   c. **Epidemiology**
      (1) Affects about 5% of population
      (2) Affects up to 15% of pregnant women
      (3) Up to 80% of sufferers also have periodic limb movement of sleep (PLMS)
   d. **Cause**
      (1) Unknown, but apparent genetic component
      (2) Exacerbated by caffeine
5. **Periodic limb movements during sleep**
   a. Brief muscle twitches (2 or 3 times a minute)
   b. On and off during the night
   c. Usually legs
   d. Frequently seen in one third of individuals older than 65 years
6. **Nocturnal sleep-related eating disorder**
   a. Individuals eat food during the night while they appear to be asleep.
   b. Cannot remember nighttime eating
   c. One study indicates that more than two thirds of sufferers are women.
   d. Can occur during sleepwalking
   e. Causes
      (1) Medications (e.g., for depression or insomnia)
      (2) Sleep disorders that cause awakenings and trigger sleep-eating (e.g., sleep apnea, restless leg syndrome)
7. **Circadian related** (work-shift, jet lag)

16

Cortical Function

I. **Cortical Structure** (see Fig. 1-12)
   A. **Overview**
      1. Contains about 100 billion neurons
      2. Highly convoluted with sulci (grooves) and gyri (ridges) that increase surface area
   B. **Lobes**
      1. **Frontal:** anterior to central sulcus and superior to lateral sulcus
      2. **Parietal:** posterior to central sulcus and superior to lateral sulcus
      3. **Temporal:** inferior to the lateral sulcus
      4. **Occipital:** posterior to parietal and temporal lobes, from which it is separated on medial surface by parieto-occipital sulcus
   C. **Major cell types** (Fig. 16-1)
      1. **Pyramidal cells**
         a. Primary **excitatory** cell type in cortex (neurotransmitter: glutamate)
         b. Small (~10 μm) and medium pyramidal cells (~20 μm) project to areas of ipsilateral cortex
         c. Large (~50 μm) and giant pyramidal cells (~100 μm) project to ipsilateral and contralateral cortex and to subcortical areas, brainstem and spinal cord

> Pyramidal cells: source of corticobulbar and corticospinal tracts

      2. **Multipolar stellate cells** (interneurons): inhibitory (γ-aminobutyric acid [GABA])
      3. **Fusiform cells,** in the deepest layer of the cortex, are modified pyramidal cells with local projections.
   D. **Cortical layers** (see Fig. 16-1)
      1. **Layer I (molecular layer):** outermost, primarily an integrating layer, receives input from thalamus and brainstem and contains apical dendrites of deep pyramidal cells
      2. **Layer II (external granular layer):** primarily an input layer, contains small pyramidal cells whose axons project to ipsilateral cortex
      3. **Layer III (external pyramidal layer):** primarily an output layer, contains **medium pyramidal cells** whose axons project to ipsilateral cortex
      4. **Layer IV (internal granular layer):** the major **input** layer, receives input from thalamus
      5. **Layer V (internal pyramidal layer):** the major **output** layer, contains **medium, large, and giant pyramidal cells** whose axons project as association fibers to ipsilateral cortex, as commissural fibers to contralateral cortex, and as projection fibers to brainstem and spinal cord

	Golgi stain	Nissl stain	Weigert stain

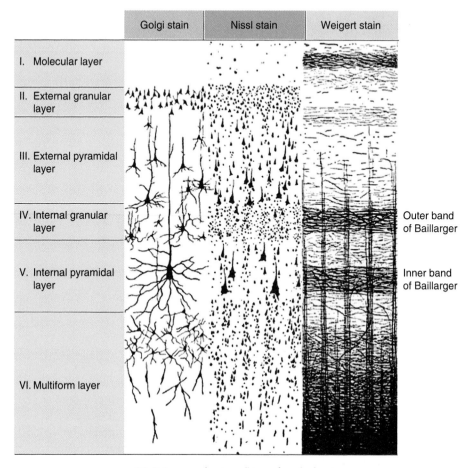

I. Molecular layer

II. External granular layer

III. External pyramidal layer

IV. Internal granular layer — Outer band of Baillarger

V. Internal pyramidal layer — Inner band of Baillarger

VI. Multiform layer

16-1: Layers and major cell type of cerebral cortex.

6. **Layer VI (multiform layer):** contains **fusiform cells** whose axons project as short association fibers to ipsilateral cortex
7. **Homogenetic cortex** contains all six layers.
   a. **Homotypical** cortex has all six layers well represented.
   b. **Heterotypical granular** cortex is sensory cortex with expanded input layer IV.
   c. **Heterotypical agranular** cortex is motor cortex with expanded output layer V.
8. **Heterogenetic cortex** is phylogenetically older cortex (e.g., piriform, entorhinal, and hippocampal) containing three to five layers.

E. **Vertical columns**
1. Each contains about 200 neurons.
2. Form functional units for input–output processing with extensive interconnections among cortical layers but only minor connections to neurons outside column.
3. Activation of one column tends to inhibit activity in adjacent columns.

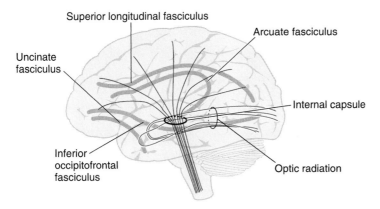

16-2: *Major fiber systems of cerebral cortex.*

II. **Fiber Systems** (Fig. 16-2)
   A. **Association fibers**
      1. **Short association fibers** (e.g., arcuate fibers) connect adjacent gyri within one hemisphere.
      2. **Long association fibers** (e.g., uncinate fasciculus, superior longitudinal fasciculus, cingulum bundle, inferior longitudinal fasciculus, and inferior frontal occipital fasciculus) connect different cortical regions within one hemisphere
         • **Arcuate fasciculus** connects receptive language centers of the temporal lobe with expressive motor speech centers of the frontal lobe, supporting repetition of spoken language.
   B. **Commissural fibers**
      1. Connect the two hemispheres
      2. **Anterior commissure** connects olfactory system, amygdala, and temporal lobe.
      3. **Hippocampal commissure** connects the two hippocampi.
      4. **Corpus callosum** connects homologous regions of the two hemispheres.
         a. Rostral and genu portions connect the frontal lobes.
         b. Body connects parietal and temporal lobes.
         c. Splenium and posterior portion connect auditory and occipital cortex
         d. Not all cortical regions are connected (e.g., there are no known connections between right and left primary visual cortex).
      5. **Posterior commissure** connects the pretectal areas and Edinger-Westphal nuclei and includes fibers that support consensual light response.
   C. **Projections fibers**
      1. Connect cerebral cortex with subcortical, brainstem, and spinal cord regions.
         a. **Corticofugal** (output) fibers (e.g., corticospinals and corticobulbars)
         b. **Corticopetal** (input) fibers (e.g., thalamocorticals, including sensory and optic radiations)

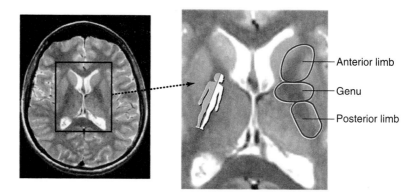

16-3: *Major fiber pathways coursing through the internal capsule. Anterior limb, corticopontine; genu, corticobulbar (upper motor neuron axons to cranial nerve nuclei) and thalamocortical (sensory information from the contralateral side of the head); posterior limb, corticospinal (upper motor neurons controlling muscles in the contralateral body) and thalamocortical (sensory information from the contralateral side of the body).*

2. Enter and leave cortex through the **internal capsule** (Fig. 16-3)
   a. **Anterior limb** of the internal capsule carries corticopontine fibers to the pontine nuclei.
   b. **Genu** (apex) of the internal capsule carries corticobulbar fibers to cranial nerve motor nuclei.
   c. **Posterior limb** of the internal capsule carries (primarily) corticospinal tract to spinal cord and thalamocortical fibers to cortex.

III. **Functional Regions**
   A. Divided into about 50 different regions (Brodmann areas)
   B. **Primary sensory cortex**
      1. **Primary somatosensory area** (general sensory)
         a. **Location:** lateral and medial surface of the postcentral gyrus (parietal lobe)
         b. **Function:** general sensation; receives general sensory information (touch, pain, and temperature) and conscious proprioceptive information (position sense, vibratory sense, and two-point discrimination) from the contralateral body
         c. **Sensory homunculus** (from lateral sulcus, extending over lateral convexity to medial surface of postcentral gyrus, ending superior to cingulate gyrus, medially): pharynx, tongue, jaw, face, hand, arm, trunk, thigh, leg, foot, and genitals
         d. **Stimulation:** contralateral **numbness and tingling** (paresthesia)
         e. **Damage: contralateral loss** of all **sensation** and astereognosis
      2. **Primary visual cortex**
         a. **Location:** calcarine gyrus (medial occipital lobe)
         b. **Function:** primary vision; receives primary visual information from contralateral visual field
         c. Foveal fibers terminate in the posterior portion of the gyrus (**macular region**).

        d. **Stimulation:** crude sensations of bright flashes of light

        e. **Damage:** loss of vision in the contralateral visual field

   3. **Primary auditory cortex**

        a. **Location:** superior temporal gyrus

        b. **Function:** hearing; receives primary auditory information from both ears

        c. **Stimulation:** tinnitus (buzzing, humming, or ringing)

        d. **Damage:** slight contralateral hearing loss

   4. **Primary vestibular cortex**

        a. **Location:** face region of primary sensory cortex (parietal lobe)

        b. **Function:** appreciation of spacial orientation

        c. **Stimulation:** hallucinations of body movement (vertigo)

   5. **Primary olfactory cortex**

        a. **Location:** inferior temporal lobe

        b. **Function:** smell; only sensory system that does *not* synapse in thalamus

        c. **Stimulation:** hallucinations of disagreeable smells

   6. **Primary gustatory cortex**

        a. **Location:** parietal operculum, ventral to primary sensory cortex

        b. **Function:** taste; receives input from tongue and pharynx

        c. **Damage:** loss of taste on contralateral side

C. **Unimodal association cortex**

   1. **Somatosensory association cortex**

        a. **Location:** posterior parietal lobe

        b. **Function:** early sensory processing, goal-directed voluntary movement, and object manipulation

   2. **Visual association cortex**

        a. **Location:** occipital lobe adjacent to primary visual cortex

        b. **Function**

           (1) **Conjugate eye movements,** through connections to frontal eye fields, superior colliculi, and motor nuclei of extraocular muscles

           (2) Transfer of **monocular learned behavior** to the opposite hemisphere

        c. **Stimulation:** hallucinations of formed images

        d. **Damage:** visual agnosia (individual can see objects but cannot to recognize them)

   3. **Auditory association cortex (Wernicke area** in dominant hemisphere)

        a. **Location:** superior temporal gyrus

        b. **Function:** comprehension of spoken word

        c. **Stimulation:** tinnitus

        d. **Damage:** receptive (Wernicke) aphasia, a syndrome of pure word deafness. (Individual can hear sounds and words, but is unable to relate them to previous experiences; individual has difficulty with speech, speaks words that sound like nonsense.)

D. Multimodal association cortex

   1. Anterior association area

        a. **Location:** anterior to premotor areas, that is, prefrontal cortex

        b. **Function:** affective behavior and judgment, motor planning, planning for the future, language production, "holding" or working memory

---

Tumors within visual cortex: patient may report seeing bright flashes of light

Posterior cerebral artery occlusion: contralateral vision loss with macular sparing

Uncinate fits: Seizures originating in temporal lobe may be preceded by hallucinations of disagreeable smell.

    c. **Damage:** changes in mood, behavior, and personality: individual neglects appearance, laughs or cries inappropriately, and demonstrates no appreciation of social norms.

2. **Posterior association area**

    a. **Location:** parietotemporal region, and includes supramarginal and angular gyri

    b. **Function:** complex multisensory perception, including visuospatial localization, language processing, attention

    c. **Damage to dominant hemisphere (Gerstmann syndrome)**

      (1) **Expressive aphasia:** nonfluent speech

      (2) **Agraphia:** inability to write

      (3) **Alexia:** inability to read

      (4) **Agnosia:** inability to synthesize, correlate, or recognize multisensory perceptions

      (5) **Finger agnosia:** inability to recognize different fingers

      (6) **Acalculia:** inability to calculate or use numbers

      (7) **Left–right confusion:** inability to recognize left from right side of body

    d. **Damage to nondominant hemisphere**

      (1) **Hemineglect syndrome,** contralateral neglect, extinction

      (2) **Constructional apraxia:** inability to copy simple drawings

      (3) Disturbances in awareness of body image

E. **Motor association cortex**

1. **Supplementary motor cortex**

    a. **Location:** anterior to medial extension of primary motor cortex in frontal lobe

    b. **Function:** complex movements (e.g., raising the contralateral arm)

2. **Premotor cortex**

    a. **Location:** frontal lobe, anterior to primary motor cortex

    b. **Function:** movements initiated by primary motor cortex; gross movements that require coordination among muscles (e.g., walking)

3. **Premotor cortex: frontal eye fields**

    a. **Location:** middle frontal gyrus

    b. **Function:** direct voluntary conjugate eye movements to contralateral visual space

    c. **Stimulation:** conjugate deviation of both eyes to the contralateral side

    d. **Damage:** conjugate deviation of both eyes to the ipsilateral side

Conjugate deviation of both eyes to contralateral side: can be seen during epileptic seizures

4. **Premotor cortex: motor speech area (Broca area)**

    a. **Location:** inferior frontal gyrus, rostral to the primary motor cortex in dominant hemisphere

    b. **Function:** speech production and aspects of comprehension

    c. **Stimulation:** inhibition of speech or uttering of vowel sounds

> **Damage:** individual may comprehend language but cannot express language (**expressive aphasia**)

F. **Primary motor cortex**

1. **Location:** precentral gyrus

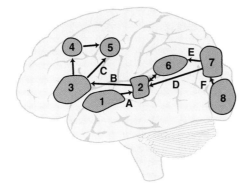

16-4: *Language disorders. 1, Primary auditory cortex; 2, Wernicke area; 3, Broca area; 4, supplementary motor area; 5, primary motor strip; 6, word recognition area; 7, visual association cortex; 8, primary visual cortex.*

2. **Function:** movement contralateral head and body
3. **Motor homunculus** (from lateral sulcus, extending over lateral convexity to medial surface of precentral gyrus, ending superior to cingulate gyrus, medially): pharynx, tongue, jaw, face, hand, arm, trunk, thigh, leg, foot, and genitals
4. **Stimulation:** discrete and isolated contralateral movement limited to a single joint or muscle
5. **Damage to motor cortices (primary cortex, precortex, and supplementary cortex):** upper motor neuron signs on the contralateral side of the body that vary with time (e.g., initial hypotonia, hyporeflexia, or flaccid paralysis and chronic hyperreflexia and spasticity. Babinski sign, if present, occurs from the outset).
6. **Damage restricted to primary motor cortex** may affect distal extremities, whereas **damage sparing primary motor cortex** may affect production of skilled and complex movements without causing noticeable decrease in muscle power.

IV. **Aphasias** (Fig. 16-4 and Table 16-1)
   A. **Definition**
      1. **Disorders of language function (comprehension, processing, or production)** caused by cortical or subcortical damage, as opposed to disorders of motor aspects of speech production (dysarthrias)
      2. Most often related to damage within the left hemisphere
   B. **Assessment**
      1. **Spontaneous speech:** is it fluent? (words per minute, words per phrase, word finding effort, agrammatic or telegraphic speech)
      2. Auditory **comprehension**
      3. **Repetition**
      4. Object **naming**

**TABLE 16-1:
Overview of
Language
Disorders***

Area Involved	Language Deficit	Clinical Disorder
Primary auditory area	Comprehension (spoken language) Repetition (spoken) Response to non-language sounds	Cortical deafness
Connection A	Comprehension (spoken) Repetition (spoken)	Pure word deafness
Auditory association area (Wernicke)	Comprehension (spoken and written language) Repetition (spoken language) Spontaneous speech Speech is fluent but impaired	Wernicke aphasia
Connection B	Repetition (spoken language) Spontaneous speech Speech is fluent but impaired	Conduction aphasia
Motor area (Broca)	Spontaneous speech Repetition (spoken language) Reading aloud Naming objects	Broca aphasia
Connection C	Spontaneous speech Repetition (spoken language) Reading aloud Naming objects	Aphemia
Supplementary motor area	Spontaneous speech	Transcortical motor aphasia
Connection D	Comprehension (written language) Reading aloud	Alexia without agraphia
Word recognition area	Comprehension (spoken and written language) Naming objects Spontaneous speech	Transcortical aphasia
Connection E	Naming objects	Aphasia without alexi
Connection F	Comprehension (written) Naming objects Reading aloud	Visual agnosia
Auditory association, motor area and connection B	Comprehension (spoken and written) Repetition Naming of objects Reading aloud	Global aphasia

* See Figure 16-3.

5. **Reading**
6. **Writing**

An individual with nonfluent aphasia may be able to communicate verbally, with difficulty, whereas an individual with fluent aphasia may easily produce volumes of words that make no sense to him or to the listener.

C. **Broca aphasia**
1. Damage to inferior frontal lobe (**Broca area**)
2. Speech fluency decreased, with **word-finding difficulty, telegraphic speech,** and few (almost no) words produced; **repetition and naming are poor.**
3. Comprehension appears good, although careful exam may reveal deficits ("The bear was killed by the lion. Which animal is dead?")

D. **Wernicke aphasia**
1. Damage to posterior superior temporal gyrus (**Wernicke area**)
2. **Speech** fluency may be normal, with normal rate and phrasing; however, **content is nonsensical** and may include neologisms and **paraphasic** substitutions; **comprehension, repetition, and naming are poor.**

E. **Conduction aphasia**
1. Damage to arcuate fasciculus connecting Wernicke and Broca areas
2. **Repetition is poor**
3. Speech may be fluent and comprehension good

F. **Global (total) aphasia**
1. Damage includes the **area surrounding lateral sulcus,** probably due to infarction of left middle cerebral artery. (Look for right-sided weakness.)
2. **Speech is nonfluent; comprehension, repetition, and naming are poor; reading and writing are impaired.**

G. **Transcortical sensory aphasia**
1. Damage to **posterior parietal lobe,** sparing Wernicke area
2. **Speech is fluent, but paraphasic** with empty content; comprehension is poor.
3. Repetition is good.

H. **Transcortical motor aphasia**
1. Damage is to **anterior inferior frontal lobe,** sparing Broca area
2. **Speech is nonfluent with word-finding difficulty.**
3. Comprehension and repetition are good.

I. **Transcortical mixed (isolation) aphasia**
1. Damage is to both transcortical sensory and motor areas, likely due to a **watershed infarct** in the distribution of the internal carotid artery **(anterior and middle cerebral artery boundary zone).**
2. Speech is nonfluent; comprehension is poor.
3. Repetition is good.
4. Transcortical aphasias have in common preservation of repetition despite disruption to speech comprehension or production.

J. **Anomia**
1. Damage reflects transcortical lesions, likely involving angular gyrus.
2. Difficulty naming objects, with speech fluency, comprehension, and repetition intact

K. **Writing**
1. **Damage to angular gyrus** (parietotemporal lobe junction)
2. May produce **agraphia** (difficulty with writing)

V. **Cerebral Dominance**
   A. **Dominant hemisphere**
      1. **Psychomotor activities** (handedness, language and spatial relationships)
      2. Speech and written language comprehension

Left cerebral hemisphere: usually responsible for language dominance

> The term "dominant hemisphere" refers to language dominance. Most left-handed individuals with right hemisphere motor dominance are left hemisphere dominant for language.

   B. **Nondominant hemisphere**
      1. Appreciation of spatial dimensions, totality of a scene (including recognition of faces), and nonverbal symbolism
      2. Right temporal stores tone memories
      3. Right parieto-occipital stores perception and spatial relationships.
      4. **Damage to parietal lobe: hemi-neglect syndrome** (neglects contralateral half of body)

Parietal lobe damage in nondominant hemisphere: individual may deny that anything is wrong with an affected limb

> Subtle hemi-neglect may be revealed by extinction on simultaneous stimulation. Individual reports sensation when stimulus is applied to affected limb or visual field. However, individual denies visual and tactile sensation on affected side when stimuli are applied simultaneously, bilaterally.

   C. **Commissurotomy**
      1. Can be used to prevent the spread of seizures between hemispheres
      2. Produces **disconnection syndrome**
         • Individual can recognize and describe an unseen object placed in the right hand but cannot recognize or describe the same object when it is placed in left hand.

> **Cortical plasticity:** after damage to one hemisphere, the intact hemisphere may assume some of the lost functions. This is most evident when the damage occurs during early development and decreases with advancing age, although it is always a factor in recovery from damage.

VI. **Limbic System**
   A. **Major components**
      1. **Hippocampal formation** (dentate gyrus and hippocampus)

Surgery for intractable epilepsy: amygdala can be damaged

      a. **Location:** medial temporal lobe
         b. **Function:** acquisition of explicit (declarative) memories
         c. **Damage** (bilateral): anterograde amnesia (unilateral damage has no significant effect on memory)
      2. **Amygdala**

Occlusion of small-caliber anterior choroidal artery: can cause acute death of hippocampal neurons

      a. **Location:** anterior temporal lobe, at the level of the uncus, anterior and superior to hippocampus
         b. **Function**

(1) **Autonomic:** heart rate, respiration, blood pressure, and gastric motility

> "Fight or flight" response: increased respiration with increased or decreased blood pressure and pulse.

(2) **Mood and emotion:** interpret and recall emotional content (especially fear and stress) of visual inputs and events

3. **Septum**
   a. **Location:** medial wall of anterior horn of the lateral ventricle
   b. **Function:** related to endogenous reward circuits

B. **Major connections**
   1. **Medial forebrain bundle:** complex longitudinal fiber system that connects the limbic forebrain–hypothalamus–limbic midbrain
   2. **Stria medullaris** (from the septal region to the habenula) and **fasciculus retroflexus** (from the habenula to the interpeduncular nucleus) connect to brainstem **autonomic nuclei.**
   3. **Fornix:** connects hippocampus to mammillary bodies

C. **Disorders**
   1. **Amnestic confabulatory syndrome** (Korsakoff psychosis)
      a. Associated with **chronic alcoholism** resulting in malnutrition (thiamine/vitamin B_1 deficiency)
      b. Damage to thalamus, mammillary bodies, and periaqueductal gray

      > Individuals experience anterograde amnesia (inability to remember recent events), tendency to confuse and fabricate, and a decrease in spontaneity and initiative

   2. **Temporal lobe epilepsy**
      a. Olfactory hallucinations often precede seizure
      b. Most common form: **complex partial seizures** (psychomotor) with unconscious actions (e.g., lip smacking)
   3. **Kluver-Bucy syndrome**
      a. Originally described in primates with anterior temporal lobectomies (amygdala)
      b. **Signs and symptoms:** loss of fear and aggression, **hyperorality** (excessive attention to stimuli with oral tendencies), **hypersexuality, visual agnosia** (inability to recognize familiar objects)

CHAPTER 17

Neurologic Exam

I. **History and Physical Exam**
   A. **Time course and duration of symptoms**
      1. **Rapid** onset (minutes to hours) suggests **stroke.**
      2. Changes that occur over a period of **weeks to months** may indicate **tumor or infection.**
      3. Processes that have been ongoing for **years** suggest **neurodegenerative** processes.
      4. Headache with no previous history or **headache that changes** in position and increases over time may be significant; severe headache that resembles previous headaches may not be significant.
   B. **Autonomic findings**
      1. **Blood pressure and heart rate: orthostatic hypotension** indicates autonomic dysfunction.
      2. **Respiration:** abnormal pattern helps locate level of brainstem damage.
      3. **Changes in heart rate and blood pressure** or **diaphoresis** (profuse sweating) may indicate pain in an otherwise unresponsive individual.

II. **Mental Status**
   A. **Arousal**
      1. Patients in **coma** cannot be aroused; patients who are **asleep** can be aroused; patients with **pontine lesions** can demonstrate arousal through directed eye movements.
      2. Requires participation of brainstem ascending reticular activating system (ARAS) and hemispheres; coma indicates loss of ARAS or bilateral hemispheric damage.
   B. **Awareness**
      1. Patients who are **awake** but unresponsive to a variety of stimuli are unaware.
      2. Patients in a **vegetative state** demonstrate arousal without awareness.
   C. **Attentiveness**
      1. Test a variety of stimuli: inattention to verbal stimuli could be due to hearing loss.
      2. Test both left and right sides: parietal lobe damage can reduce attention to contralateral space.
   D. **Orientation**
      1. **Place:** ask the patient, "Where are we now?"
      2. **Time:** ask the patient, "What day of the week is it? What day of the month? What season?"
      3. **Person:** ask the patient, "Do you know who I am?"

E. **Language**
   1. **Repetition:** ask the patient to repeat, "No ifs, ands, or buts."
   2. **Naming:** point to items such as button, pen, and stethoscope and ask patient to name each one.
   3. **Writing:** is the patient able to write a complete sentence?

   > Broca aphasia results in deficits in speech and writing. Loss of speech with retained writing ability, although rare, indicates a disorder resulting from a lesion to an area other than Broca area.

   4. **Aphasia** implies cortical dysfunction.
      a. **Receptive:** test speech comprehension, "The deer was killed by the wolf. Which animal is dead?"
      b. **Expressive:** is speech spontaneous and fluent with appropriate content?
   5. **Dysarthria** implies motor dysfunction: upper motor neuron (UMN), lower motor neuron (LMN) (glossopharyngeal nerve, CN IX; vagus nerve, CN X), or cerebellar involvement.

F. **Memory**
   1. **Immediate retention:** ask the patient to repeat three words, such as apple, wristwatch, pencil; then ask patient to repeat the three words after 3- to 5-minute delay
   2. Long-term retention: ask the patient about historic, general, and personal events.

G. **Right–left orientation and finger recognition**
   1. Instruct patient, "Touch your right ear with your left thumb."
   2. **Damage to dominant parietal lobe** is revealed by several findings, termed **Gerstmann syndrome.**
      a. Right–left confusion
      b. Finger agnosia
      c. Agraphia (difficulty writing)
      d. Acalculia (difficulty manipulating numbers)

H. **Double simultaneous stimulation**
   1. Patient, with eyes closed, identifies touches on one side of body, the other side, or both sides simultaneously.
   2. **Extinction** (simultagnosia) to double simultaneous stimulation suggests damage to posterior parietal lobe contralateral to overlooked touch, termed **hemi-neglect** or **contralateral neglect**
      a. More commonly involves **non-dominant hemisphere**
      b. Constructional tests (e.g., drawing a clock face, bisecting a line, copying a simple drawing) may reveal more activity in right visual space.

III. **Cranial Nerves**
   A. **Findings observable during general physical examination**
      1. **Eyelid droop** (ptosis): oculomotor nerve (CN III) or sympathetic (Horner syndrome)

2. Complaints of **double vision:** CN III, trochlear nerve (CN IV), or abducens nerve (CN VI), or brainstem (medial longitudinal fasciculus)
3. **Asymmetry in facial expression:** facial nerve (CN VII)
4. **Pupil asymmetry:** CN III or sympathetic (Horner syndrome due to lateral medullary damage)
5. **Hoarseness** (dysarthria) or difficulty swallowing (dysphagia): CN IX and CN X

B. **Olfactory nerve** (CN I)
1. Test using weak, familiar odors (e.g., vanilla, coffee, tobacco). Strong odors (e.g., ammonia) act as irritants and are detected by trigeminal (CN V).
2. **Loss of sense of smell** common with colds, aging; if accompanied by visual disturbance, may be an indication of a tumor
   • **Olfactory groove meningioma** (Kennedy-Foster syndrome) compresses one olfactory bulb (unilateral anosmia) and ipsilateral optic nerve (visual loss in that eye) and produces contralateral papilledema.
3. **Olfactory hallucinations:** an aura may precede **temporal lobe seizure** ("uncinate fits").

C. **Optic nerve** (CN II)
1. **Visual acuity**
2. **Confrontational visual fields**
   a. **Blindness in one eye:** damage to eye or optic nerve
   b. **Bitemporal hemianopsia:** medial damage at chiasm
      • Causes include pituitary tumor or aneurysm of anterior communicating artery.
   c. **Unilateral loss of nasal visual field:** lateral damage at chiasm
      • Causes include internal carotid aneurysm
   d. **Homonymous hemianopsia:** damage central to chiasm and contralateral to visual loss
      • Causes include damage to optic tract approaching lateral geniculate nucleus (LGN), damage to LGN, damage to optic radiation or damage to visual cortex.
   e. **Superior quadrant anopsia:** temporal lobe damage (Meyer loop)
      • Causes include stroke involving the portion of the middle cerebral artery supplying lateral optic radiation and Meyer loop.
   f. **Inferior quadrant anopsia:** parietal lobe damage
   g. Visual loss with **macular sparing:** primary visual cortex
      (1) **Superior quadrant anopsia:** *below* calcarine sulcus
      (2) **Inferior quadrant anopsia:** *above* calcarine sulcus
      (3) Possible cause: posterior cerebral artery occlusion
3. **Funduscopic** examination: **papilledema** indicates increased intracranial pressure.
4. **Pupils**
   a. **PERRLA:** *p*upils *e*qual, *r*ound, *r*eactive to *l*ight and *a*ccommodation
   b. **Anisocoria:** pupils of **unequal** size
      (1) Congenital likely benign (e.g., Adie pupil)

(2) Acute appearance could be **medical emergency.**
  (a) Dissecting carotid aneurysm producing Horner syndrome
  (b) Medial temporal lobe herniation producing dilated ("blown") pupil

c. **Pupillary light reflex:** shine light in one eye
  (1) **Normal response**
    (a) Pupil of stimulated eye constricts (direct response).
    (b) Pupil of other eye constricts (consensual response).
  (2) **Afferent pupillary defect:** optic nerve damage
    (a) Light in healthy eye: both pupils constrict
    (b) Light in damaged eye: no pupillary constriction, either direct or consensual
  (3) **Unilateral large, unreactive ("blown") pupil:** CN III damage
    (a) Light in healthy eye: healthy eye constricts, damaged eye does not constrict
    (b) Light in damaged eye: healthy eye constricts, damaged eye does not constrict
  (4) **Neither eye responds to light:** midbrain involvement

d. **Near reflex triad**
  (1) Patient alternately focuses on close and distant objects
    (a) **Convergence:** medial rectus (CN III) bilaterally
    (b) **Accommodation:** lens thickens
    (c) **Miosis:** pupillary constriction (increases depth of focus)
  (2) Pupil does *not* constrict as response to light but *does* constrict with accommodation: Argyll-Robertson pupil or Adie syndrome, a benign condition.

e. **Pupils unreactive**
  (1) Fixed, dilated pupils: midbrain damage
  (2) Pinpoint pupils: pontine damage or narcotic overdose

D. **Oculomotor, trochlear, abducens nerves** (CN III, IV, VI)
 1. Test eye movement in lateral and vertical directions.
 2. Observed nystagmus may indicate damage to vestibulocochlear (CN VIII), brainstem, or cerebellum.
 3. **Oculomotor nerve damage: eye moves downward and outward,** pupil dilates, eyelid droops
 4. **Trochlear nerve damage: inability to direct gaze downward and inward,** diplopia when walking down stairs
 5. **Abducens nerve damage:** inability to abduct, diplopia on lateral gaze

E. **Trigeminal nerve** (CN V)
 1. Test sensation using light cotton and pinprick on forehead, cornea (V_1), cheek, nose, upper teeth (V_2), for jaw, chin, lower teeth, front of tongue (V_3)
 2. **Test motor strength** (V_3)
  a. Push jaw laterally against resistance (pterygoid muscles)
  b. Resist opening of jaw (masseter and temporalis muscles)
  c. **Bite weakness**

(1) **LMN lesion:** unilateral weakness of bite

(2) **UMN lesion:** produces minimal effect due to bilateral cortical control

d. **Jaw-jerk reflex** tests V_3 (sensory and motor)

e. **Corneal reflex** tests V_1 (sensory) and CN VII (motor)

F. **Facial nerve** (CN VII)

1. **Tests:** wrinkle forehead, wrinkle nose, close eyes, purse lips, whistle

2. **Paralysis of upper and lower face** with possible ipsilateral hyperacusis, loss of salivation, tearing and taste from front of tongue: **ipsilateral** LMN or peripheral nerve lesion (e.g. **Bell palsy**)

   a. Facial weakness with loss of hearing and balance indicates peripheral lesion at internal acoustic meatus.

   b. Facial weakness with paralysis of ipsilateral lateral gaze indicates dorsomedial pontine lesion.

3. **Paralysis of *lower* part of the face,** with retained ability to wrinkle forehead: **contralateral** UMN lesion.

G. **Vestibulocochlear nerve** (CN VIII)

1. **Vestibular branch**

   a. Spontaneous nystagmus occurs away from destructive lesion or toward irritating lesion.

   b. Caloric testing investigates function of vestibular pathways.

2. **Auditory branch**

   a. Test hearing in each ear by speaking softly or by rubbing fingers together near each ear.

   b. Loss of hearing in one ear: conductive or sensorineural hearing loss are identified with tuning fork tests (Rinne and Weber)

H. **Glossopharyngeal nerve** (CN IX) and **vagus nerve** (CN X)

1. Test visceral function with pulse, respiration, and heart and carotid reflexes

2. Test motor function by elevation of palate with speaking, swallowing, and vocal cord function

   a. Ask patient to say "ah": look for symmetric elevation of palate

   b. Damage: difficulty with swallowing and speech

3. **Gag reflex** tests: CN IX (sensory) and CN X (motor)

I. **Spinal accessory nerve** (CN XI)

1. Test by turning head (sternocleidomastoid) and lifting of the shoulder (trapezius) against pressure

2. Damage: difficulty turning head to contralateral side plus ipsilateral shoulder droop

J. **Hypoglossal nerve** (CN XII)

1. Examine tongue for atrophy or fasciculations.

2. Test function by protrusion of the tongue.

   a. **LMN lesion:** tongue deviates to weak side (i.e., toward lesion)

   b. **UMN lesion:** tongue deviates to weak side (i.e., away from lesion)

IV. **Motor Systems**
   A. **Strength**
   - 0 = total paralysis; 1 = contraction visible or felt on palpation; 2 = movement in absence of gravity; 3 = movement against gravity; 4 = full range, but decreased strength; 5 = normal strength

   B. **Tone**
   1. **Flaccid** muscle tone indicates an LMN or acute UMN lesion.
   2. Increased tone that fades at end of movement **(clasp-knife rigidity)** indicates a UMN lesion.
   3. Increased tone throughout range of movement **(lead-pipe or plastic rigidity)** indicates basal ganglia disease.

   > **Cog-wheel rigidity** produces ratchet-like catches and releases and accompanies parkinsonism.

   4. **Decreased tone** (hypotonia) with **pendular reflexes** indicates cerebellar damage.

   C. **Appearance**
   1. **Severe muscle wasting** (atrophy) indicates denervated muscle of end-stage LMN lesion.
   2. **Fasciculations** (visible twitches of individual motor units) indicate damage to LMN cell bodies or motor nerve roots.
   3. **Fibrillations** (twitches of individual muscle fibers) are **not visible;** are measured by electromyogram (EMG) and indicate muscle disease or denervated muscle.

   D. **Involuntary movements**
   1. **Resting tremor** is a sign of contralateral basal ganglia damage.
   2. **Intention tremor,** most apparent at the end of a goal-directed movement, is a sign of ipsilateral cerebellar damage.
   3. **Athetosis or choreiform movements** indicate basal ganglia dysfunction.
   4. **Ballismus** indicates contralateral basal ganglia (subthalamic nucleus) damage.

   E. **UMN damage**
   1. Caused by damage involving corticospinal tract and indirect pathways (rubrospinal, vestibulospinal, reticulospinal) or cortical control of these pathways
   2. **Signs:** distal extremity weakness and loss of fine control, hyperreflexia, spastic paralysis, clasp-knife rigidity, ankle clonus, and Babinski
   3. Damage to spinal cord: ipsilateral body affected
   4. Damage to brain: contralateral body affected

   F. **LMN damage**
   1. Caused by damage to motor neuron innervating muscle
   2. **Signs:** weakness or flaccid paralysis, hyporeflexia or areflexia, severe muscle wasting, and fasciculations
   3. Damage is ipsilateral to affected side of the body.

   G. **Test: arm extension with eyes closed**
   1. Drift down with pronation of the hand and flexion of the arm: UMN damage with hypertonia

    2. Drift down without pronation: cerebellar damage with hypotonia

    3. Drifts up: sensory damage (lack of proprioceptive information)

V. **Gait, Coordination, Balance, and Equilibrium**

  A. **Gait**

    1. Walking on heels, toes, and both tests cerebellar function.

    2. Wide-based (ataxic) gait suggests cerebellar damage.

    3. Festinating gait, short-stepped and accelerating, suggests Parkinson disease.

    4. **Movement:** problems with initiating or slowing of movement are usually due to damage to UMNs or the basal ganglia.

  B. **Coordination**

    1. Lack of coordination (ataxia) is frequently due to ipsilateral cerebellar damage.

    2. **Rapid alternating movements:** tapping alternating fingers, slapping palm and back of hand alternately against thigh

    3. **Goal-directed movements:** finger to nose, heel to shin

  C. **Romberg test**

    1. Patient stands with feet close together and closes eyes.

    2. Instability indicates **decreased proprioceptive sense** and is a positive test.

    3. Inability to stand with feet together and **eyes open** indicates cerebellar damage.

VI. **Reflexes**

  A. **Deep tendon reflexes**

    1. Designed to test sensory limb, motor limb, and UMN modulation of muscle stretch reflex

    2. 0 = absent; 1+, ++ = hypoactive; 2+, ++ = normal; 3+, +++ = hyperactive; 4+, ++++ = clonus present

    3. Biceps (C5, C6); triceps (C6, C7, C8); knee (L2, L3, L4); ankle (L5, S1, S2)

  B. **Superficial reflexes**

    1. Plantar (S1) (Fig. 17-1): appearance of Babinski sign indicates corticospinal tract damage.

    2. Abdominal (T8–T12), cremasteric (L1, L2): absent reflex indicates damaged reflex loop or corticospinal tract damage.

VII. **Sensory Systems**

  A. **Tests**

    1. Spinothalamic tract: pain (sharp object) and temperature (warm and cold stimuli)

    2. Posterior column–medial lemniscal system: light touch (cotton), vibration (128-Hz tuning fork), proprioception

  B. **Signs of peripheral damage**

    1. Dermatomal loss indicates peripheral, segmental damage.

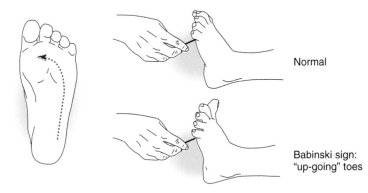

Normal

Babinski sign:
"up-going" toes

17-1: *Babinski sign. Normal response to stroking of plantar surface of foot is plantar flexion. Abnormal response, fanning of toes with extension of great toe, called Babinski sign or Babinski reflex, or, simply, "up-going toes," indicates damage to corticospinal tract.*

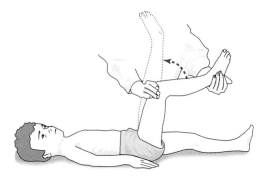

17-2: *Kernig sign. Thigh is flexed to 90 degrees from body (sitting or supine). Attempt is then made to straighten leg. Inability to straighten, due to severe stiffness of hamstrings, is termed Kernig sign. In meningitis, hamstring stiffness stems from muscles spasms due to inflammation in region of lumbar spinal roots.*

    2. "Stocking-and-glove" distribution of loss suggests metabolic peripheral neuropathy.

C. **Signs of cortical (parietal) damage**

    1. **Tactile atopognosis:** inability to locate point of stimulus with eyes closed

    2. **Astereognosis:** inability to identify common items (e.g., paper clip, coin, key) by touch and manipulation

    3. **Decreased two-point discrimination**

VIII. **Other Tests**

A. **Kernig** sign (Fig. 17-2): meningitis or subarachnoid hemorrhage

B. **Brudzinski** sign (Fig. 17-3): meningitis or subarachnoid hemorrhage

C. **F wave:** nerve velocity conduction test that reveals anterior spinal root damage (e.g., Guillain-Barré syndrome)

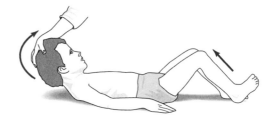

17-3: Brudzinski sign. With patient supine, passively flex neck, bringing chin to chest. Involuntary flexion at hips is termed Brudzinski sign. Seen in meningitis, it results from inflammation and exudates near lumbar roots.

    D. **H reflex:** nerve velocity conduction test that slows with many peripheral neuropathies

    E. **Brainstem evoked auditory responses** test peripheral and central auditory pathways and may reveal peripheral CN VIII damage (e.g., vestibular neuroma) (acoustic schwannoma).

    F. **Visual evoked responses** test central visual pathways and may reveal damage from multiple sclerosis.

Common Laboratory Values

Test	Conventional Units	SI Units
Blood, Plasma, Serum		
Alanine aminotransferase (ALT, GPT at 30°C)	8–20 U/L	8–20 U/L
Amylase, serum	25–125 U/L	25–125 U/L
Aspartate aminotransferase (AST, GOT at 30°C)	8–20 U/L	8–20 U/L
Bilirubin, serum (adult): total; direct	0.1–1.0 mg/dL; 0.0–0.3 mg/dL	2–17 µmol/L; 0–5 µmol/L
Calcium, serum (Ca^{2+})	8.4–10.2 mg/dL	2.1–2.8 mmol/L
Cholesterol, serum	Rec: <200 mg/dL	<5.2 mmol/L
Cortisol, serum	8:00 AM: 6–23 µg/dL; 4:00 PM: 3–15 µg/dL 8:00 PM: ≤50% of 8:00 AM	170–630 nmol/L; 80–410 nmol/L Fraction of 8:00 AM: ≤0.50
Creatine kinase, serum	Male: 25–90 U/L Female: 10–70 U/L	25–90 U/L 10–70 U/L
Creatinine, serum	0.6–1.2 mg/dL	53–106 µmol/L
Electrolytes, serum		
Sodium (Na^+)	136–145 mEq/L	135–145 mmol/L
Chloride (Cl^-)	95–105 mEq/L	95–105 mmol/L
Potassium (K^+)	3.5–5.0 mEq/L	3.5–5.0 mmol/L
Bicarbonate (HCO_3^-)	22–28 mEq/L	22–28 mmol/L
Magnesium (Mg^{2+})	1.5–2.0 mEq/L	1.5–2.0 mmol/L
Estriol, total, serum (in pregnancy)		
24–28 wk; 32–36 wk	30–170 ng/mL; 60–280 ng/mL	104–590 nmol/L; 208–970 nmol/L
28–32 wk; 36–40 wk	40–220 ng/mL; 80–350 ng/mL	140–760 nmol/L; 280–1210 nmol/L
Ferritin, serum	Male: 15–200 ng/mL Female: 12–150 ng/mL	15–200 µg/L 12–150 µg/L
Follicle-stimulating hormone, serum/plasma (FSH)	Male: 4–25 mIU/mL Female:	4–25 U/L
Premenopause, 4–30 mIU/mL		4–30 U/L
Midcycle peak, 10–90 mIU/mL		10–90 U/L
Postmenopause, 40–250 mIU/mL		40–250 U/L
Gases, arterial blood (room air)		
pH	7.35–7.45	[H^+] 36–44 nmol/L
Pco_2	33–45 mmHg	4.4–5.9 kPa
Po_2	75–105 mmHg	10.0–14.0 kPa
Glucose, serum	Fasting: 70–110 mg/dL 2 hr postprandial: <120 mg/dL	3.8–6.1 mmol/L <6.6 mmol/L
Growth hormone–arginine stimulation	Fasting: <5 ng/mL Provocative stimuli: >7 ng/mL	<5 µg/L >7 µg/L

continued

Test	Conventional Units	SI Units
Blood, Plasma, Serum—cont'd		
Immunoglobulins, serum		
IgA	76–390 mg/dL	0.76–3.90 g/L
IgE	0–380 IU/mL	0–380 kIU/L
IgG	650–1500 mg/dL	6.5–15 g/L
IgM	40–345 mg/dL	0.4–3.45 g/L
Iron	50–170 µg/dL	9–30 µmol/L
Lactate dehydrogenase, serum	45–90 U/L	45–90 U/L
Luteinizing hormone, serum/ plasma (LH)	Male: 6–23 mIU/mL	6–23 U/L
	Female:	
	Follicular phase, 5–30 mIU/mL	5–30 U/L
	Midcycle, 75–150 mIU/mL	75–150 U/L
	Postmenopause, 30–200 mIU/mL	30–200 U/L
Osmolality, serum	275–295 mOsm/kg	275–295 mOsm/kg
Parathyroid hormone, serum, N-terminal	230–630 pg/mL	230–630 ng/L
Phosphatase (alkaline), serum (p-NPP at 30°C)	20–70 U/L	20–70 U/L
Phosphorus (inorganic), serum	3.0–4.5 mg/dL	1.0–1.5 mmol/L
Prolactin, serum (hPRL)	<20 ng/mL	<20 µg/L
Proteins, serum		
Total (recumbent)	6.0–8.0 g/dL	60–80 g/L
Albumin	3.5–5.5 g/dL	35–55 g/L
Globulin	2.3–3.5 g/dL	23–35 g/L
Thyroid-stimulating hormone, serum or plasma (TSH)	0.5–5.0 µU/mL	0.5–5.0 mU/L
Thyroidal iodine (^{123}I) uptake	8–30% of administered dose/24 hr	0.08–0.30/24 hr
Thyroxine (T_4), serum	4.5–12 µg/dL	58–154 nmol/L
Triglycerides, serum	35–160 mg/dL	0.4–1.81 mmol/L
Triiodothyronine (T_3), serum (RIA)	115–190 ng/dL	1.8–2.9 nmol/L
Triiodothyronine (T_3) resin uptake	25–38%	0.25–0.38
Urea nitrogen, serum (BUN)	7–18 mg/dL	1.2–3.0 mmol urea/L
Uric acid, serum	3.0–8.2 mg/dL	0.18–0.48 mmol/L
Cerebrospinal Fluid		
Cell count	0–5 cells/mm³	$0–5 \times 10^6$/L
Chloride	118–132 mEq/L	118–132 mmol/L
Gamma globulin	3–12% total proteins	0.03–0.12
Glucose	50–75 mg/dL	2.8–4.2 mmol/L
Pressure	70–180 mm H_2O	70–180 mm H_2O
Proteins, total	<40 mg/dL	<0.40 g/L
Hematology		
Bleeding time (template)	2–7 min	2–7 min
Erythrocyte count	Male: 4.3–5.9 million/mm³	$4.3–5.9 \times 10^{12}$/L
	Female: 3.5–5.5 million/mm³	$3.5–5.5 \times 10^{12}$/L
Erythrocyte sedimentation rate (Westergren)	Male: 0–15 mm/hr	0–15 mm/hr
	Female: 0–20 mm/hr	0–20 mm/hr
Hematocrit (Hct)	Male: 40–54%	0.40–0.54
	Female: 37–47%	0.37–0.47

Test	Conventional Units	SI Units
Hematology—cont'd		
Hemoglobin A$_{IC}$	≤6%	≤ 0.06%
Hemoglobin, blood (Hb)	Male: 13.5–17.5 g/dL	2.09–2.71 mmol/L
	Female: 12.0–16.0 g/dL	1.86–2.48 mmol/L
Hemoglobin, plasma	1–4 mg/dL	0.16–0.62 mmol/L
Leukocyte count and differential		
Leukocyte count	4500–11,000/mm^3	4.5–11.0 × 10^9/L
Segmented neutrophils	54–62%	0.54–0.62
Bands	3–5%	0.03–0.05
Eosinophils	1–3%	0.01–0.03
Basophils	0–0.75%	0–0.0075
Lymphocytes	25–33%	0.25–0.33
Monocytes	3–7%	0.03–0.07
Mean corpuscular hemoglobin (MCH)	25.4–34.6 pg/cell	0.39–0.54 fmol/cell
Mean corpuscular hemoglobin concentration (MCHC)	31–37% Hb/cell	4.81–5.74 mmol Hb/L
Mean corpuscular volume (MCV)	80–100 μm^3	80–100 fl
Partial thromboplastin time (activated) (aPTT)	25–40 sec	25–40 sec
Platelet count	150,000–400,000/mm^3	150–400 × 10^9/L
Prothrombin time (PT)	12–14 sec	12–14 sec
Reticulocyte count	0.5–1.5% of red cells	0.005–0.015
Thrombin time	<2 sec deviation from control	<2 sec deviation from control
Volume		
Plasma	Male: 25–43 mL/kg	0.025–0.043 L/kg
	Female: 28–45 mL/kg	0.028–0.045 L/kg
Red cell	Male: 20–36 mL/kg	0.020–0.036 L/kg
	Female: 19–31 mL/kg	0.019–0.031 L/kg
Sweat		
Chloride	0–35 mmol/L	0–35 mmol/L
Urine		
Calcium	100–300 mg/24 hr	2.5–7.5 mmol/24 hr
Creatinine clearance	Male: 97–137 mL/min	
	Female: 88–128 mL/min	
Estriol, total (in pregnancy)		
30 wk	6–18 mg/24 hr	21–62 μmol/24 hr
35 wk	9–28 mg/24 hr	31–97 μmol/24 hr
40 wk	13–42 mg/24 hr	45–146 μmol/24 hr
17-Hydroxycorticosteroids	Male: 3.0–9.0 mg/24 hr	8.2–25.0 μmol/24 hr
	Female: 2.0–8.0 mg/24 hr	5.5–22.0 μmol/24 hr
17-Ketosteroids, total	Male: 8–22 mg/24 hr	28–76 μmol/24 hr
	Female: 6–15 mg/24 hr	21–52 μmol/24 hr
Osmolality	50–1400 mOsm/kg	
Oxalate	8–40 μg/mL	90–445 μmol/L
Proteins, total	<150 mg/24 hr	<0.15 g/24 hr

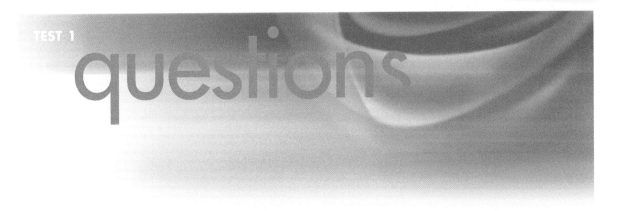

questions

DIRECTIONS: Each numbered item or incomplete statement is followed by options arranged in alphabetical or logical order. Select the best answer to each question. Some options may be partially correct, but there is only **ONE BEST** answer.

1. A 32-year-old woman has a progressive loss of pain and temperature sensation across both hands and arms. Vibration and proprioceptive sense are intact. She begins to have weakness and fasciculations in both hands and lower arms. Further testing reveals hyperactive patellar and Achilles tendon reflexes in the right leg. Sensation is normal in both legs. Which of the following is the most likely cause of her symptoms?

A. Bilateral damage to the posterior horn and adjacent white matter of lateral spinal cord (C5–T1)

B. Bilateral damage to the anterior horn and adjacent white matter of anterolateral spinal cord (C5–T1)

C. Damage to the central spinal cord extending bilaterally into anterior horn and white matter of lateral spinal cord (C5–T1)

D. Bilateral damage to white matter of posterior and lateral spinal cord (C1–C3)

E. Bilateral damage to white matter of anterior and lateral spinal cord (C1–C3)

2. A 67-year-old man experiences weakness in his right face. He cannot wrinkle his forehead symmetrically or close his right eye against resistance. His smile is lopsided, with the right side being noticeably weak. His right eye cannot abduct, and he has double vision on right lateral gaze. Motor exam of arms and legs is normal. Damage to which of the following is the most likely cause of his signs and symptoms?

A. Oculomotor and trigeminal nerves as they run through the cavernous sinus

B. Trigeminal and abducens nerves as they run through the cavernous sinus

C. Abducens and facial nerves in the posterior pons

D. Abducens and facial nerves in the anterior pons

E. Abducens and facial nerves in the internal acoustic meatus

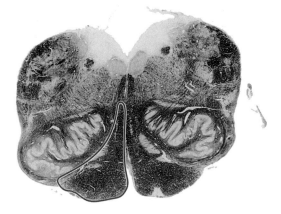

3. A 53-year-old woman experiences an ischemic stroke as a result of occlusion of penetrating branches of the anterior spinal artery, affecting the region outlined in the accompanying section. Which of the following is most likely as a result of this vascular lesion?

A. Ipsilateral Babinski sign with a loss of joint position sense from the contralateral body
B. Ipsilateral Babinski sign with a loss of pain sensation from the contralateral body
C. Ipsilateral Babinski sign with deviation of the tongue to the contralateral side on protrusion
D. Contralateral Babinski sign with a loss of joint position sense from the ipsilateral body
E. Contralateral Babinski sign with a loss of pain sensation from the ipsilateral body
F. Contralateral Babinski sign with deviation of the tongue to the ipsilateral side on protrusion

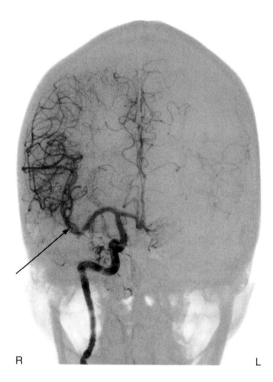

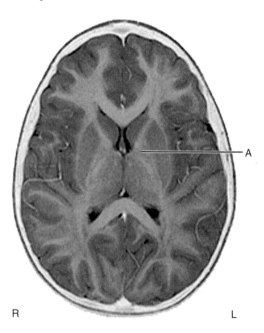

4. A 63-year-old man suffers stroke damage to the brain region indicated by the "A" in the accompanying normal MRI. Which of the following is most likely with damage to this structure?
A. Deviation of the tongue to the right on protrusion
B. Deviation of the tongue to the left on protrusion
C. Decreased bite strength on the right
D. Decreased bite strength on the left
E. Decreased strength in the right leg
F. Decreased strength in the left leg

5. A 56-year-old woman is seen in the emergency department for an acute, intense headache that was brought on while straining at the stool. Arterial angiogram revealed a leaking aneurysm, causing arterial vasospasm in the area indicated by the arrow. Right (R) and left (L) are as indicated. Which of the following deficits is most likely to occur?
A. Expressive aphasia
B. Loss of vision in the right eye
C. Weakness in the left arm
D. Loss of sensation in the right arm
E. Complete paralysis of the left lower leg
F. Loss of sensation in the right lower leg

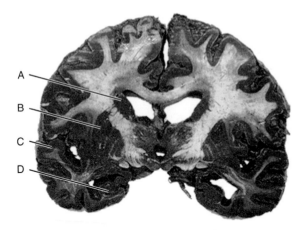

7. A 42-year-old woman is seen in the emergency department for numbness in the left arm. Examination reveals a loss of fine touch and vibration sensation from the right face and left body. Which of the following is the most likely level of the lesion in the accompanying MRI?
   A. A
   B. B
   C. C
   D. D

8. A 22-year-old woman is seen in the emergency department for double vision. She can track an object moving to left of center. On attempted right lateral gaze, her right eye abducts, but her left eye does not move beyond a midline position. Which of the following structures is most likely damaged?
   A. Left medial longitudinal fasciculus
   B. Right medial longitudinal fasciculus
   C. Left lateral gaze center
   D. Right lateral gaze center
   E. Left superior colliculus
   F. Right superior colliculus

6. A 64-year-old man experiences an extended episode of decreased cerebral perfusion during which he exhibits profound anterograde amnesia, with loss of ability to form new explicit memories. Which of the labeled areas in the figure (above) would result in memory loss following a bilateral ischemic event?
   A. A
   B. B
   C. C
   D. D

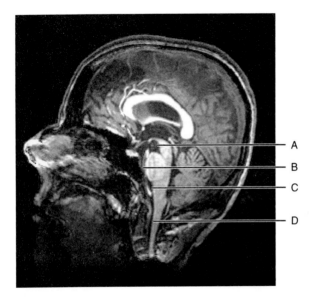

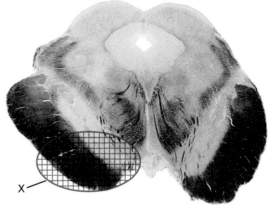

9. A 66-year-old man has an ischemic episode that results in damage to the indicated region ("X"). Which of the following is most likely?
   A. Eyelid droop and pupil constriction ipsilateral to the lesion

B. Paralysis of abduction in the ipsilateral eye
C. Weakness of the tongue contralateral to the lesion
D. Paralysis of the lower face ipsilateral to the lesion

10. A 35-year-old man is seen in the emergency department for a headache that appears to be localized in the front of the head. Confrontational visual testing reveals a loss of peripheral visual fields. He sees little that is presented to his right eye to the right of center and little to the left of center with his left eye. Which of the following is the most likely cause of the visual deficit?
A. Pituitary tumor
B. Pineal tumor
C. Olfactory groove meningioma
D. Schwannoma

11. Drug A induces seizure activity in neurons. At rest, the membrane potential of these neurons is −68 mV. Application of drug A causes these neurons to depolarize to −55 mV. The Nernst (equilibrium) potentials of the ions to which this cell can become permeable are

E_{Na^+}	+60 mV
E_{K^+}	−90 mV
E_{Cl^-}	−70 mV
$E_{Ca^{2+}}$	+120 mV

Which of the following is the most likely mechanism of action of this drug?
A. Open Cl^- channels
B. Block Ca^{2+} channels
C. Block K^+ channels
D. Block Na^+ channels

12. A 46-year-old man is on heart–lung bypass during surgery. An intravenous line is inadvertently flushed with KCl rather than with normal saline, causing K^+ ion concentration $[K^+]$ to increase in the extracellular space. Which of the following is most likely to occur to the resting membrane potential of neurons as a result of increased extracellular $[K^+]$?

A. Remains the same
B. Becomes hyperpolarized
C. Becomes depolarized
D. Oscillates between slightly depolarized and hyperpolarized

13. A 28-year-old man is brought to the emergency department for shortness of breath, headache, dizziness, and vomiting. He was spraying crops with an insecticide 2 hours earlier. The diagnosis is acute organophosphate poisoning. Which of the following is the most likely finding?
A. Increase in acetylcholine release from nerve endings
B. Blockade of acetylcholine receptors due to steric hindrance
C. Increase in the frequency of miniature end-plate potentials at the motor end plate
D. Hyperactivity followed by paralysis as acetylcholine receptors desensitize
E. Hypoactivity followed by paralysis as acetylcholine receptors desensitize

14. A 23-year-old student is brought to the emergency department complaining of headache and fever that began the previous evening. Examination reveals stiff neck (nuchal rigidity) and a bending of the knees in response to passive flexing of the chin to the chest (Brudzinski sign). Cerebrospinal fluid findings following lumbar puncture reveal cloudy CSF with increased numbers of polymorphonuclear leukocytes (5000/µL), decreased glucose (30 mg/dL), increased protein (1100 mg/dL), and an increased opening pressure (20 mmHg). Gram stain is positive. Which of the following would most likely explain these findings?
A. Tuberculous meningitis
B. Bacterial meningitis
C. Viral encephalitis
D. Viral meningitis

15. A 22-year-old woman presents at the emergency department with a red and tearing right eye, the result of a corneal abrasion. She reports that her right eye feels numb when she inserts her contact lens. Which of the following is most likely responsible for the loss of sensation from the cornea?

A. Optic nerve
B. Oculomotor nerve
C. Trigeminal nerve
D. Facial nerve
E. Ciliary body

16. A 29-year-old man has a 4-year history of headache. The history indicates that most of his headaches have a lancinating pain behind one eye with ipsilateral nasal congestion and tearing. The headaches occur at the same time every afternoon, last less than 1 hour, and are so severe that they wake him from sleep. The neurologic exam is otherwise normal. Which of the following is the most likely cause of these findings?

A. Temporal arteritis
B. Classic migraine headache
C. Common migraine headache
D. Cluster headache
E. Slow-growing tumor in the frontal lobe

17. A 47-year-old man has a 14-year history of alcohol abuse. Examination reveals gait instability and a widened base. Heel-to-shin test demonstrates profound ataxia in the legs. Which of the following is the most likely cause of the movement disorder?

A. Demyelination of the posterior columns
B. Bilateral degeneration of the caudate and putamen
C. Meningioma compressing one cerebellar hemisphere
D. Degeneration of the superior cerebellar vermis
E. Degeneration of the mammillary bodies

18. A 65-year-old man presents with tremor in his right hand at rest. Examination reveals that he has difficulty performing rapid alternating movements in that they are both slowed and decreased in amplitude. When asked to walk, he hesitates and then takes small steps, which become faster as he proceeds. MRI reveals a loss

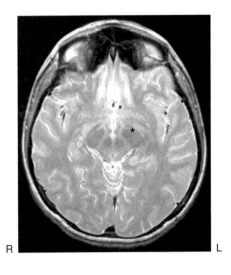

R   L

of cells bodies in the area indicated by the asterisk in the accompanying normal MRI. Which of the following would most likely cause the symptoms described?

A. Decreased dopamine release into the putamen
B. Decreased dopamine release into the substantia nigra
C. Decreased glutamate release into the caudate
D. Decreased glutamate release into the right cerebellar hemisphere
E. Normal changes seen with aging

19. A 73-year-old man has increasing difficulty with daily activities like dressing and brushing his teeth. Examination reveals a tremor in both hands at rest, a ratcheting resistance to passive movement, and bradykinesia. He receives L-dopa to alleviate these symptoms. Which of the following is the most likely basis for this treatment?

A. Block cholinergic receptors in the central nervous system
B. Increase the concentration of dopamine in the basal ganglia
C. Increase the activity of peripheral adrenergic neurons
D. Act directly on skeletal muscle
E. Decrease brain serotonin levels

20. Passive flexion of the right arm of a 69-year-old man is met with excessive resistance that is uniform through the range of movement. Degeneration of which of the following is the most likely cause of these findings?
A. Cell bodies in the left motor cortex
B. Axons in the left medullary pyramids
C. Axons in lateral funiculus in the right spinal cord
D. Neurons in the midbrain substantia nigra
E. Purkinje cells in the right cerebellar hemisphere

21. A 62-year-old woman is brought to the emergency department because of difficulty walking. She has decreased muscle tone in the right leg. Deep tendon reflex testing reveals pendular reflexes on the right side. Muscle tone and reflexes on the left are normal. Which of the following structures would most likely be damaged?
A. Left caudate nucleus
B. Right caudate nucleus
C. Left internal capsule
D. Right internal capsule
E. Left cerebellar hemisphere
F. Right cerebellar hemisphere

22. A 57-year-old woman is brought to the emergency department because of recurring episodes of dizziness and difficulty maintaining her balance. She always feels nauseous and frequently vomits during an attack. Examination reveals a left-beating nystagmus. She has tinnitus and mild hearing loss in both ears. Which of the following is the most likely cause of her symptoms?
A. Vestibular neuroma in the left cerebellopontine angle
B. Otosclerosis affecting both ears
C. Hemorrhage into the flocculonodular lobe of the cerebellum
D. Bilateral increase in endolymph pressure
E. Infarct in the left lateral vestibular nucleus

23. A 49-year-old woman experiences sudden onset of headache with nausea and vertigo. She has difficulty keeping her balance and finds that she falls to the left. On examination, she has decreased muscle tone in her left arm and leg, although muscle mass is normal. The patellar tendon reflex is normal on the right and pendular on the left. There is some intention tremor associated with movements of the left arm. Which of the following arteries is most likely involved?
A. Left posterior inferior cerebellar artery
B. Left anterior inferior cerebellar artery
C. Left posterior cerebral artery
D. Right posterior inferior cerebellar artery
E. Right anterior inferior cerebellar artery
F. Right posterior cerebral artery

24. A 56-year-old woman is brought to the emergency department because of sudden and repeated violent and uncontrolled flinging movements of her left arm and leg. History reveals that the movements are worse when she becomes anxious. Examination reveals weakness on the left side. Which of the following structures is most likely damaged?
A. Left subthalamic nucleus
B. Right subthalamic nucleus
C. Left dentate nucleus
D. Right dentate nucleus
E. Left red nucleus
F. Right red nucleus

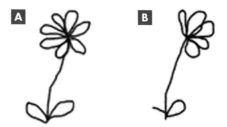

25. A 62-year-old man is seen because of weakness on the left half of his body. He also has a dense left hemianopsia. He is asked to copy Figure A and produces a sketch resembling Figure B.

Which of the following is the most likely cause for his symptoms?
A. Occlusion of distal posterior cerebral artery branches supplying the right calcarine sulcus
B. Lacunar infarct involving the genu and posterior limb of the right internal capsule
C. Tumor in the right temporal lobe involving Meyer loop causing a midline shift and compression of the left cerebral peduncle against the tentorium
D. Ischemic stroke involving most of the territory of the right middle cerebral artery

26. A 19-year-old man is seen because of fever and headache. The previous day he felt listless and unenergetic. He has chills, a stiff neck, and a headache that has increased in intensity throughout the day. Examination reveals a Kernig sign. Which of the following is the most likely cause of his symptoms?
A. Meningitis
B. Subarachnoid hemorrhage
C. Tension headache
D. Cluster headache

27. A 65-year-old man with Alzheimer disease and associated paranoid delusions has been treated with haloperidol for 6 months. Which of the following is most likely to be an effect of chronic antipsychotic treatment?
A. Tremor
B. Rigidity
C. Bradykinesia
D. Tardive dyskinesia
E. Ballism

28. A 58-year-old man is seen because he has difficulty reading. Confrontational visual fields testing reveals a scotoma (visual deficit) in the inferior portion of the left half of his visual fields, bilaterally. Which of the following is most likely damaged?
A. Axons running in the optic radiation of the left temporal lobe
B. Axons running in the optic radiation of the right temporal lobe

C. Axons terminating in the left cuneate gyrus
D. Axons terminating in the right cuneate gyrus

29. A 59-year-old man with an 8-month history of dull headache is seen in the emergency department. He is obtunded, and his left pupil is dilated and unreactive. His wife reports that his headache has become more severe in the past 2 weeks. Which of the following is the most likely cause of his symptoms?
A. Supratentorial tumor
B. Cluster headache
C. Subarachnoid hemorrhage
D. Classic migraine

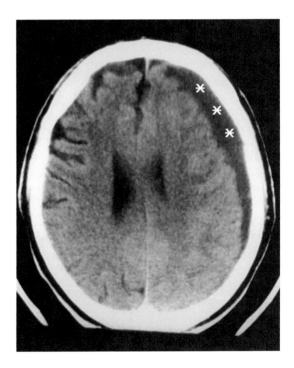

30. A 34-year-old woman is seen in the emergency department after a low-speed motor vehicle crash during which her head struck the windshield. A CT scan (above) reveals an accumulation of blood (indicated by several asterisks) consistent with a subdural hematoma and no evidence of skull fracture. Which of the following is the most likely source of this blood?

A. Arterial blood resulting from the rupture of the anterior cerebral artery

B. Arterial blood resulting from the rupture of the middle meningeal artery

C. Arterial blood resulting from the rupture of an aneurysm

D. Venous blood resulting from the rupture of the superior sagittal sinus

E. Venous blood resulting from the rupture of bridging vessels

31. A 58-year-old man is seen because of increasing difficulty in performing activities of daily living, such as eating, dressing, and brushing his teeth. Examination reveals a "pill-rolling" tremor in both hands with a frequency of 7 Hz, rigidity (lead-pipe) with increased resistance to flexion and extension of the arm at the elbow, bradykinesia, and postural instability. Which of the following would most likely be found in the cerebrospinal fluid?

A. Decreased homovanillic acid

B. Decreased vanillylmandelic acid

C. Increased 3-methoxy-4-hydroxyphenylglycol

D. Increased 5-hydroxyindole acetic acid

32. A 68-year-old man is seen in the emergency department because of weakness on his right side. His wife reports that he fell and fractured his hip 3 months earlier. Examination reveals paresis of the right body and a left hemianopic scotoma. CT reveals a mass on the lateral and ventral surface of the brain on the right side with a right-to-left midline shift. Which of the following is most likely damaged?

A. Right optic nerve

B. Right optic tract

C. Left optic nerve

D. Left optic tract

E. Optic chiasm

33. A 71-year-old man presents with sudden onset of paralysis of the left side of his body. Examination reveals flaccid paralysis of the left arm and leg, deviation of the tongue to the right side on protrusion, and markedly reduced touch and vibration sensation on his left side. Occlusion of

penetrating branches from which of the following is most likely to result in these findings?

A. Anterior cerebral artery

B. Posterior inferior cerebellar artery

C. Anterior inferior cerebellar artery

D. Anterior spinal artery

E. Posterior spinal artery

34. A 15-year-old girl is brought to the emergency department disoriented, confused, and unable to follow simple commands. The history reveals that she was fine when she came home from a skating outing, but within half an hour began to get drowsy and confused. Examination reveals a badly bruised right forehead and elbow. Further examination reveals a dilated and poorly reactive right pupil. The left pupil is normal. Which of the following is the most likely cause for her findings?

A. Subarachnoid hemorrhage

B. Horner syndrome

C. Complex partial seizures

D. Epidural hematoma

35. A 45-year-old man is seen in the emergency department because of sudden weakness on the left side of his face and body. Examination reveals a flaccid paralysis involving the lower face and arm on the left side and paralysis of voluntary eye movement to the left with a right gaze preference. Which of the following is most likely damaged?

A. Right supratentorial brain

B. Right midbrain

C. Right pons

D. Left spinal cord

36. A 24-year-old woman with excessive daytime sleepiness is admitted to a sleep clinic for observation. Which of the following findings would give the most support to a diagnosis of narcolepsy?

A. Abnormally long period of time spent initially in stage 1 sleep

B. Rapid transition from wakefulness to stage 2 sleep

C. Direct transition from wakefulness to delta sleep
D. Rapid transition from wakefulness to REM sleep
E. Delay (90 minute) between sleep onset and the first episode of REM sleep

37. A 19-year-old man is subject to uncontrollable sleep attacks lasting up to 30 minutes and occurring several times per day. He reports that he tosses and turns at night and awakens at least once most nights. On occasion, he experiences dramatic and frightening hallucinations as he drifts off to sleep. Most disturbing to him is that he feels completely paralyzed at these times. Which of the following additional findings is he most likely to experience?
A. Difficulty in falling asleep
B. No REM sleep on an average night
C. Overwhelming weakness when he is emotional
D. Snoring
E. Frequent limb flailing during REM sleep

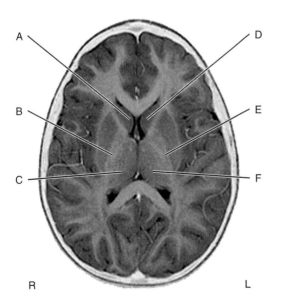

38. Three months ago a 55-year-old man suffered a stroke that resulted in a loss of all sensation from the left body and face. He is now experiencing episodes of spontaneous, excruciating pain on left side of his face and body. Damage to which of the labeled regions in the above normal MRI is most likely to give rise to these findings?
A. A
B. B
C. C
D. D
E. E
F. F

39. An 18-year-old man is administered the acetylcholinesterase inhibitor, edrophonium, during a diagnostic procedure for myasthenia gravis. He experiences cardiac arrhythmia and is immediately administered atropine to counter the autonomic effects of the edrophonium. Which of the following is most likely if he is administered excess atropine?
A. Tachycardia
B. Weakness of respiratory muscles
C. Constricted pupils
D. Transient Horner syndrome

40. A 43-year-old man is seen because of shaking in both hands. He reports that the shaking is worse when he is stressed and better after he consumes a glass or two of beer. Examination reveals tremor in both hands with a frequency of 10 Hz. The tremor increases when his arms are outstretched and decreases during movement. His father has a similar tremor. Which of the following is the most likely cause for his symptoms?
A. Parkinson disease
B. Alcoholic cerebellar degeneration
C. Benign essential tremor
D. Dystonic tremor

41. A 48-year-old man is seen in the emergency department following a blunt injury to his left index finger. He has no feeling or mobility in the finger. Further examination reveals that the nerve was crushed in the distal one third of the finger. Which of the following is most likely?

A. Within a day, Schwann cells will begin to break down myelin of the axon distal to the lesion.

B. Axons distal to the lesion will degenerate owing to the loss of retrogradely transported trophic factors.

C. Axon regrowth will occur, dependent on the fast axonal transport of tubulin and actin.

D. Microglia will be recruited to the area to remove debris.

42. A 58-year-old man is unable to move both eyes (conjugately) to the right. Eye movements to the left are normal. When the corner of his left cornea is touched with a cotton wisp, his left eye blinks, but his right eye does not. Which of the following is most likely to explain these findings?

A. Schwannoma in the left cerebellopontine angle

B. Schwannoma in the right cerebellopontine angle

C. Small infarct in the left pons

D. Small infarct in the right pons

43. A 17-year-old high school student is brought to the emergency department following an automobile accident. He is initially unconscious but eventually makes a partial recovery. Four years later, he is paraplegic with hyperreflexia and Babinski sign in the legs bilaterally, no voluntary motor control, and no sensation below the umbilicus. He has full use of both arms with normal biceps and triceps reflexes. Which of the following is the most likely additional finding?

A. His bladder is atonic and does not empty reflexively.

B. His bladder partially empties reflexively when full, with urine retention.

C. His bladder fills and empties completely and frequently, but without voluntary control.

D. Control of the external urinary sphincter is intact.

44. A 42-year-old man experiences numbness and tingling in both legs. Examination reveals diminished vibratory sensation in lower legs and feet, bilaterally. Deep tendon reflexes (ankle and patellar) are diminished in both legs. Nerve conduction tests reveal a normal F response. A Romberg sign is elicited. Which of the following is the most likely cause of these findings?

A. Entrapment neuropathy

B. Sensory neuropathy of metabolic origin

C. Radicular neuropathy affecting the anterior lumbar roots

D. Damage to the posterior columns

45. An MRI taken of an 18-year-old woman reveals a hypothalamic tumor located superior to the optic chiasm and inferior to the anterior commissure. Which of the following is most likely if she spends several hours sunbathing on a very hot day?

A. An increase in basal metabolism

B. Hyperthermia

C. Cutaneous vasodilation

D. Cutaneous vasoconstriction

E. Uncontrolled shivering

46. A 63-year-old woman has a slow-growing tumor located near the tip of the arrow in the accompanying normal MRI. Which of the following is most likely as the tumor continues to expand?

A. Bitemporal hemianopsia ("tunnel vision")

B. Difficulty directing gaze while going down stairs

C. Internuclear ophthalmoplegia

D. One or both eyes deviated down and out with eyelid droop

E. Loss of corneal blink reflex

47. A 56-year-old man has a 10-year history of numbness in his legs and feet. When asked, he reports that he feels like he is walking on cotton. Examination reveals decreased proprioceptive and vibratory sensation. He sways from side to side and attempts to compensate with a

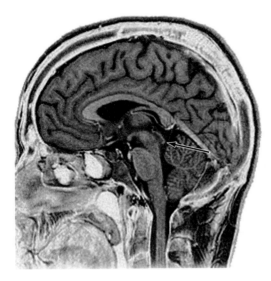

A. Right ventrolateral nucleus of the thalamus
B. Left frontal cortex
C. Right cerebellar hemisphere
D. Left substantia nigra
E. Right vestibular nucleus

49. A 32-year-old man lost sight in both eyes as a result of damage from an explosion. His circadian rhythms are disrupted, and he now sleeps at intervals that no longer correspond to the day–night cycle. Which of the following is most likely damaged?
A. Supraoptic–hypophyseal tract
B. Retinohypothalamic tract
C. Tuberohypophyseal tract
D. Retinogeniculate tract
E. Retinocollicular tract

broad-based stance. His pupils do not react to light but do constrict on near focus. CSF reveals a mild mononuclear pleocytosis and elevated protein. Which of the following is most likely damaged?
A. Ventral posterolateral nuclei of the thalamus
B. Dorsal reticular nuclei of the thalamus
C. Cerebellum
D. Posterior column/medial lemniscal system
E. Posterior limb of the internal capsule

48. A 50-year-old man is brought to the emergency department because of difficulty with balance and walking. Examination reveals hypotonia, dysmetria, decomposition of movement, and pendular reflexes on the right side. When asked to walk, he deviates to the right side. Which of the following is most likely damaged?

50. A 55-year-old woman is seen in the emergency department because of burning pain over the right shoulder and upper part of the right arm. The pain intensifies when she moves her neck or coughs. Examination reveals weakness and fasciculations in the right shoulder and upper arm muscles. There is also a reduction in somatic sensation (fine touch, vibration, proprioception, pain, temperature, crude touch) along the right shoulder and the lateral aspect of the arm. There is atrophy in the right upper arm. Which of the following is the most likely damaged?
A. Posterior and anterior roots
B. Posterior limb of the internal capsule
C. Ipsilateral side of the spinal cord
D. Contralateral side of the spinal cord
E. Ventrolateral medulla

answers

1. C (damage to the central spinal cord extending bilaterally into anterior horn and white matter of lateral spinal cord [C5–T1]) is correct. Damage to the anterior white commissure of the spinal cord disrupts pain transmission axons serving the arm as they cross to join the contralateral spinothalamic tract, causing loss of pain and temperature from both arms, but sparing pain ascending from the lower body. As the lesion extends to the anterior horn, lower motor neurons innervating the arms begin to die, causing early (weakness and fasciculations) and then later (paralysis and atrophy) signs of lower motor neuron damage. Involvement of the lateral funiculus causes upper motor neuron signs, including hyperreflexia.

A (bilateral damage to the posterior horn and adjacent white matter of lateral spinal cord [C5–T1]) is incorrect. That would cause complete loss of all sensation from both arms, including vibration and proprioception. It would not explain the fasciculations in the hands.

B (bilateral damage to the anterior horn and adjacent white matter of anterolateral spinal cord [C5–T1]) is incorrect. That would cause bilateral loss of pain and temperature from both legs. It would not explain the hyperreflexia in the legs.

D (bilateral damage to white matter of posterior and lateral spinal cord [C1–C3]) is incorrect. That would cause loss of vibration and proprioception for the whole body, while sparing pain and temperature. It would not explain the fasciculations in the hands.

E (bilateral damage to white matter of the anterior and lateral spinal cord [C1–C3]) is incorrect. That would cause bilateral loss of pain and temperature from the both arms and legs. It would not explain the fasciculations in the hands.

2. C (abducens and facial nerves in the posterior pons) is correct. The facial motor nucleus axons wrap around the abducens nucleus in the pons, so it would be easy to involve both in one lesion. This lesion would likely affect the right abducens nucleus, in which case, neither eye would perform well on attempted right lateral gaze.

A (oculomotor and trigeminal nerves as they run through the cavernous sinus) is incorrect. The oculomotor nerve is not involved in abduction. Damage to this nerve causes the eye to rotate down and out. The trigeminal nerve carries most facial sensation, but the only motor control it exerts relates to muscles of mastication. If it is damaged, bite strength is weak, but muscles of facial expression are unaffected.

B (trigeminal and abducens nerves as they run through the cavernous sinus) is incorrect. Although abducens nerve damage explains the diplopia, trigeminal nerve damage does not explain the facial weakness. The trigeminal nerve carries most facial sensation, but the only motor control it exerts relates to muscles of mastication. If it is damaged, bite strength is weak, but muscles of facial expression are unaffected.

D (abducens and facial nerves in the anterior pons) is incorrect. Although abducens nerve damage explains the diplopia and facial nerve damage explains the facial weakness, to damage both of those in the anterior pons requires a large lesion that would certainly also damage upper motor neuron tracts, causing upper motor neuron signs in the contralateral body.

E (abducens and facial nerves in the internal acoustic meatus) is incorrect. The abducens nerve and superior orbital fissure runs through the cavernous sinus.

3. **F** (contralateral Babinski sign with deviation of the tongue to the ipsilateral side on protrusion) is correct. Damage to the corticospinal tracts in the medullary pyramids causes a contralateral Babinski sign. Damage to the hypoglossal nerve weakens the ipsilateral tongue, and the tongue deviates to the weak side.

A (an ipsilateral Babinski sign with a loss of joint position sense from the contralateral body) is incorrect. Damage to the corticospinal tracts in the medullary pyramids causes a contralateral, not an ipsilateral, Babinski sign.

B (an ipsilateral Babinski sign with a loss of pain sensation from the contralateral body) is incorrect. Damage to the corticospinal tracts in the medullary pyramids causes a contralateral, not an ipsilateral, Babinski sign. Damage to the medial lemniscus causes loss of joint position sense, not pain sensation.

C (an ipsilateral Babinski sign with deviation of the tongue to the contralateral side on protrusion) is incorrect. Damage to the corticospinal tracts in the medullary pyramids causes a contralateral, not an ipsilateral, Babinski sign. Damage to the hypoglossal nerve weakens the ipsilateral tongue, and the tongue deviates to the weak side.

D (a contralateral Babinski sign with a loss of joint position sense from the ipsilateral body) is incorrect. Damage to the medial lemniscus causes loss of joint position sense from the contralateral, not the ipsilateral, body.

E (a contralateral Babinski sign with a loss of pain sensation from the ipsilateral body) is incorrect. Damage to the medial lemniscus causes loss of joint position sense, not pain sensation.

4. **A** (deviation of the tongue to the right on protrusion) is correct. The internal capsule contains axons of upper motor neurons. Those axons located close to the genu innervate lower motor neurons controlling muscles of the contralateral head and neck. Loss of upper motor neuron innervation to the right hypoglossal nucleus leaves the right side of the tongue weak. The tongue deviates to the weak side on protrusion.

B (deviation of the tongue to the left on protrusion) is incorrect. The tongue will deviate to the left when the left side is weak. Loss of upper motor neuron control of the left hypoglossal nucleus could cause such weakness. Upper motor neuron axons innervating the left hypoglossal nucleus pass through the genu of the right, not the left, internal capsule.

C (decreased bite strength on the right) is incorrect. Muscles of mastication on the right are innervated by lower motor neurons of the right trigeminal motor (masticator) nucleus. These lower motor neurons are innervated bilaterally from the cortex. Although axons of the genu of the left internal capsule are lost, those of the right internal capsule are still intact.

D (decreased bite strength on the left) is incorrect. Muscles of mastication on the left are innervated by lower motor neurons of the left trigeminal motor (masticator) nucleus. These lower motor neurons are innervated bilaterally from the cortex. Although axons of the genu of the left internal capsule are lost, those of the right internal capsule are still intact.

E (decreased strength in the right leg) is incorrect. The internal capsule contains axons of upper motor neurons. Those axons innervating lower motor neurons controlling muscles of the leg are located in the posterior limb. Those axons located close to the genu innervate lower motor neurons controlling muscles of the contralateral head and neck.

F (decreased strength in the left leg) is incorrect. The internal capsule contains axons of upper motor neurons that innervate lower motor neurons of the contralateral leg. In addition, axons innervating lower motor neurons controlling muscles of the leg are located in the posterior limb. Those axons located close to the genu innervate lower motor neurons controlling muscles of the contralateral head and neck.

5. **C** (weakness in the left arm) is correct. The occluded artery is the right middle cerebral, which supplies the portion of the motor cortex that controls the contralateral arm.

A (an expressive aphasia) is incorrect. The occluded artery is the right middle cerebral. Because most individuals are left hemisphere dominant for language, aphasias generally arise from damage to language-related areas of the left, not the right, hemisphere.

B (loss of vision in the right eye) is incorrect. Loss of vision in the right eye results from damage to the right eye or the right optic nerve. Vascular insufficiency affecting the right eye is likely to involve the right ophthalmic artery. The occluded artery is the middle cerebral.

D (loss of sensation in the right arm) is incorrect. Sensation from the right body is processed within the left cerebral cortex. The occluded artery is the right middle cerebral, which supplies portions of the right cerebral cortex.

E (complete paralysis of the left lower leg) is incorrect. The lower leg is represented on the medial aspect of the motor cortex, in the field of the anterior cerebral, not the middle cerebral artery. Although axons from the motor cortex controlling the lower leg may pass though the field of the middle cerebral artery, this is unlikely to produce a complete paralysis.

F (loss of sensation in the right lower leg) is incorrect. Sensation from the right body is processed within the left cerebral cortex. The occluded artery is the right middle cerebral, which supplies portions of the right cerebral cortex.

6. **D** (D) is correct. This region, the hippocampus, is necessary for establishing new explicit (declarative) memories.

A (A) is incorrect. This region, the caudate nucleus, is a component of the basal ganglia. The basal ganglia are important to procedural learning, but not to storage of explicit memories.

B (B) is incorrect. This region, the putamen, is a component of the basal ganglia. The basal ganglia are important to procedural learning, but not to storage of explicit memories.

C (C) is incorrect. This region, the superior temporal gyrus, is the primary auditory cortex.

7. **B** (B) is correct. Damage at the level of the pons can affect the right pontine trigeminal nucleus, which relays fine touch and vibration from the right face, and can affect the right medial lemniscus, which carries fine touch and vibration sensation from the left body.

A (A) is incorrect. Damage at the level of the midbrain that causes loss of fine touch and vibration sensation will affect the medial lemniscus. Damage to the right medial lemniscus would cause loss of these sensations from the left face and body.

C (C) is incorrect. Damage at the level of the medulla can affect the right medial lemniscus, causing loss of fine touch and vibration from the left body. However, fine touch and vibration sensation from the face enter the brainstem at the pons and ascend from there. They do not descend to the medulla.

D (D) is incorrect. Damage to the spinal cord will not affect fine touch and vibration sensation from the face.

8. **A** (the left medial longitudinal fasciculus) is correct. This tract communicates between the right abducens nucleus in the pons and the left oculomotor nucleus. If it is damaged, right lateral gaze will be affected. The right abducens nucleus and nerve will cause the right eye to gaze right, but communication to the left oculomotor is disrupted, paralyzing the left eye on right gaze.

B (the right medial longitudinal fasciculus) is incorrect. This tract communicates between the left abducens nucleus in the pons and the right oculomotor nucleus. If it is damaged, the left lateral gaze will be affected.

C and **D** (left or right lateral gaze center) are incorrect. Damage to this region results in complete paralysis of both eyes on attempted left or right gaze, respectively.

E and **F** (left or right superior colliculi) are incorrect. The superior colliculi integrate sensory information (e.g., visual, auditory) that orient the head toward a stimulus. Damage to the superior colliculi results in the inability to reflexively turn the head to the opposite side.

9. **C** (weakness of the tongue contralateral to the lesion) is correct. Damage to the cerebral peduncle disrupts descending corticobulbar and corticospinal tract axons that control the contralateral face and body, including the contralateral tongue.

A (eyelid droop and pupil constriction ipsilateral to the lesion) is incorrect. This lesion will affect the oculomotor nerve, causing severe eyelid droop. However, it will also cause loss of parasympathetic control of the pupil. The unopposed sympathetic activity will result in pupil dilation.

B (paralysis of abduction in the ipsilateral eye) is incorrect. This lesion will affect the oculomotor nerve, causing severe paralysis of eye movement, including the ability to adduct. The abducens nerve (CN VI), in the pons, is responsible for abduction and is unaffected by this lesion.

D (paralysis of the lower face ipsilateral to the lesion) is incorrect. Damage to the cerebral peduncle disrupts descending corticobulbar and corticospinal tract axons that control the contralateral face and body, including the contralateral tongue. Only the lower portion of the contralateral face will be affected by this lesion because corticobulbar control of facial motor neurons innervating the upper face is bilateral.

10. **A** (pituitary tumor) is correct. The deficit is a bitemporal hemianopsia and results from damage at the optic chiasm. The pituitary gland is located centrally beneath the optic chiasm and a sufficiently large tumor will compress the chiasm.

B (pineal tumor) is incorrect. The pineal gland sits centrally, superior to the superior colliculi of the midbrain. A tumor of this gland may compress the dorsal midbrain but will not affect visual pathways.

C (olfactory groove meningioma) is incorrect. A tumor within the olfactory groove may compress a single optic nerve, resulting in loss of vision from one eye.

D (Schwannoma) is incorrect. A schwannoma, or Schwann cell tumor, affects axons of the peripheral nervous system (frequently CN VIII). The optic nerve is actually part of the central nervous system and, as such, is myelinated by oligodendrocytes, not Schwann cells. This makes it susceptible to multiple sclerosis, but not to schwannomas.

11. **C** (block K$^+$ channels) is correct. Because the equilibrium potential for K$^+$ is -90 mV, any increase in K$^+$ conductance serves to move the membrane potential from -68 mV to a value closer to -90 mV, and any decrease in K$^+$ conductance will move membrane potential in the other direction, that is, to a value more positive than -68 mV.

A (open Cl$^-$ channels) is incorrect. Opening Cl$^-$ channels moves the membrane potential from its current value (-68 mV) toward Cl$^-$ equilibrium potential (-70 mV).

B (Block Ca^{2+} channels) is incorrect. Opening Ca^{2+} channels moves the membrane potential from its current value (-68 mV) toward Ca^{2+} equilibrium potential ($+120$ mV). Blocking Ca^{2+} channels would be expected to move membrane potential in the other direction, that is, to a value more negative than -68 mV.

D (block Na$^+$ channels) is incorrect. Opening Na$^+$ channels moves the membrane potential from its current value (-68 mV) toward Na$^+$ equilibrium potential ($+55$ mV). Blocking Na$^+$ channels would be expected to move membrane potential in the other direction, that is, to a value more negative than -68 mV.

12. **C** (becomes depolarized) is correct. Increasing extracellular [K$^+$] decreases the concentration gradient driving K$^+$ out of neurons. The result is that the opposing electrical gradient for K$^+$ at equilibrium also decreases, that is, equilibrium potential for K$^+$ becomes less negative. The major determinate of membrane potential at rest is K$^+$ ion flux. As equilibrium potential for K$^+$ becomes more depolarized, resting membrane potential also becomes more depolarized.

A (remains the same), **B** (becomes hyperpolarized), and **D** (oscillates between slightly depolarized and hyperpolarized) are incorrect. Increasing extracellular [K$^+$] decreases the concentration gradient driving K$^+$ out of neurons. The result is that the opposing electrical gradient for K$^+$ at equilibrium also decreases, that is, equilibrium potential for K$^+$ becomes less negative (depolarized). The major determinate of membrane potential at rest is K$^+$ ion flux. As equilibrium potential for K$^+$ becomes more depolarized, resting membrane potential also becomes more depolarized.

13. **D** (hyperactivity followed by paralysis as acetylcholine receptors desensitize) is correct. Organophosphates inhibit acetylcholinesterase, blocking the degradation of acetylcholine (Ach) in the synapse. The prolonged presence of Ach in the synapse results in continued stimulation of both nicotinic and muscarinic Ach receptors. Atropine, a muscarinic antagonist, is used as the antidote for acute organophosphate poisoning.

A (increase in Ach release from nerve endings) is incorrect. Organophosphates increase ACh concentration in the synapse by preventing breakdown of released ACh through inhibition of acetylcholinesterase, but they do not directly affect release of ACh from terminals.

B (blockade of ACh receptors due to steric hindrance) is incorrect. Blockade of receptors by steric hindrance is accomplished by receptor antagonists. Acetylcholinesterase inhibitors, such as the organophosphates, do not bind ACh receptors.

C (increase in the frequency of miniature end-plate potentials at the motor end plate) is incorrect. Acetylcholinesterase inhibitors, such as the organophosphates, prolong the action of ACh in the synapse but do not increase the rate of spontaneous vesicle release from nerve terminals.

E (hypoactivity followed by paralysis as ACh receptors desensitize) is incorrect. The acute effect of prolonged survival of ACh in the synapse is hyperactivity, not hypoactivity. However, prolonged exposure to ACh does cause receptor desensitization, resulting in paralysis.

14. B (bacterial meningitis) is correct. *Neisseria meningitides* (most often responsible for sporadic outbreaks on college campuses) is the probable causative organism. Fever, chills, headache, nausea, vomiting, stiff neck, exhaustion, irritability, and confusion and CSF findings (increased opening pressure, pleocytosis, decreased glucose and increased protein) are common findings in bacterial meningitis. Acute onset and a positive Gram stain are pathognomic for bacterial infection.

A (tuberculous meningitis) is incorrect. CSF findings do include increased opening pressure, increased protein, decreased glucose, but the increased white cell count will be due to mononuclear leukocytes. Subacute onset with headache, fever, vomiting, irritability, nocturnal wakefulness, anorexia, and abdominal pain are common in tuberculous meningitis.

C (viral encephalitis) is incorrect. CSF findings would show at most a mild increase in protein with normal glucose. In addition, encephalitis will present with more findings related to direct CNS involvement, including focal neurologic signs. Acute illness with fever, convulsions, confusion, stupor or coma, aphasia, hemiparesis with asymmetry of tendon reflexes and Babinski sign, involuntary movements, and ataxia could all accompany encephalitis.

D (viral meningitis) is incorrect. CSF findings would show at most a mild increase in protein with normal glucose. An elevated white cell count would be due to mononuclear leukocytes. Viral meningitis presents as acute illness with symptoms similar to the flu. Most cases are associated with enteroviruses, although other viruses (e.g., herpes, HIV) can cause meningitis.

15. C (trigeminal nerve) is correct. The trigeminal nerve carries all forms of somatic sensation, including fine touch, vibration, pain, and temperature from the face, including the cornea and the front two thirds of the tongue.

A (optic nerve) is incorrect. The optic nerve is formed from the axons of retinal ganglion cells and carries information related to light impinging on the retina to be used for vision, in pupillary light reflexes, and to entrain circadian rhythms. It is not related to touch sensation.

B (oculomotor nerve) is incorrect. This motor nerve controls most aspects of eye movement, pupillary constriction, and elevation of the upper eyelid. It has no sensory components.

D (facial nerve) is incorrect. The facial nerve controls muscles of facial expression, including orbicularis oculi, which is responsible for closing the eye (winking and blinking). The facial nerve has a minor somatic sensory component (near ear) and a special sensory component (taste for front two thirds of tongue), but does not carry any sensation from the eye.

E (ciliary ganglion) is incorrect. This parasympathetic ganglion relays input from the Edinger-Westphal nucleus and mediates pupil constriction and lens thickening. It has no sensory component.

16. D (cluster headache) is correct. The pain of cluster headache is commonly centered behind one eye and is so severe as to increase the risk for suicide. An autonomic component (nasal congestion and tearing) is another feature of many cluster headaches. They are named for their timing: they appear in clusters, with a headache occurring at the same time of day for several days or weeks at a time, followed by a period without headache.

A (temporal arteritis) is incorrect. Temporal, or giant cell, arteritis most commonly occurs in elderly people. It is generally diagnosed as a new headache or as a new type of headache in an individual with a history of headache. The quality is generally throbbing and the radiation generalized rather than localized behind one eye. Scalp tenderness is common. Other signs and symptoms, including polymyalgia rheumatica, are common.

B (classic migraine headache) and **C** (common migraine headache) are incorrect. Migraine headaches, while generally unilateral, do not isolate to the orbit. Their quality is throbbing rather than stabbing or lancinating. They do not awaken the sufferer; rather, it is common for someone with migraine to rest quietly and attempt to sleep to relieve the headache.

E (slow-growing tumor in the frontal lobe) is incorrect. Tumor headache pain tends to be dull, with the pain worst upon first arising in the morning. Autonomic findings are unlikely. A critical finding related to a headache due to tumor might be a headache that changes or increases in intensity over a period of weeks or months.

17. **D** (degeneration of the superior cerebellar vermis) is correct. Gait ataxia (without limb ataxia) is a hallmark of alcohol-induced cerebellar damage. The anterior lobe of the cerebellum, which includes the superior vermis, is particularly susceptible to degeneration related to long-term alcohol abuse. This cerebellar region is responsible for coordination of gait and propulsive movements.

A (demyelination of the posterior columns) is incorrect. Damage to the posterior columns causes a sensory ataxia that, because of loss of proprioception, produces a stamping gait. Demyelination of the posterior columns may result from multiple sclerosis, tabes dorsalis, or Friedrich ataxia, but not from alcohol abuse.

B (bilateral degeneration of the caudate and putamen) is incorrect. Degeneration of the caudate and putamen (striatum) is consistent with Huntington disease. Choreoathetotic movements are a hallmark of HD.

C (meningioma compressing one cerebellar hemisphere) is incorrect. Unilateral cerebellar lesions would be expected to produce unilateral (ipsilateral) findings, not the bilateral ataxia described. In addition, damage to a cerebellar hemisphere is more likely to result in loss of coordination in the extremities. Intention tremor is more likely than gait ataxia. There may be difficulty with tasks such as rapidly alternating supination and pronation movements of the hand, termed *dysdiadochokinesia*). Finally, meningioma is not related to alcohol abuse.

E (degeneration of the mammillary bodies) is incorrect. Long-term alcohol abuse can result in Wernicke-Korsakoff syndrome. Korsakoff psychosis, or amnestic confabulatory syndrome, is associated with degeneration in the mammillary bodies, the thalamus, and the periaqueductal gray of the midbrain and results in severe anterograde and retrograde amnesia. Wernicke encephalopathy causes cerebellar damage and gait ataxia. Thus, long-term alcohol abuse may result in both gait ataxia and degeneration of the mammillary bodies, but the ataxia is not due to mammillary degeneration.

18. **A** (decreased dopamine release into the putamen) is correct. The description matches that of Parkinson disease, which is a result of degeneration of dopaminergic neurons in the substantia nigra of the midbrain, the region indicated by the asterisk. These dopaminergic neurons project to the caudate and putamen, where they release dopamine. The fact that the tremor is currently only in the right hand is consistent with the degeneration, which is currently limited to the left substantia nigra.

B (decreased dopamine release into the substantia nigra) is incorrect. The description matches that of Parkinson disease, which is a result of degeneration of dopaminergic neurons in the substantia nigra. However, these dopaminergic neurons project to the caudate and putamen, where they release dopamine.

C (decreased glutamate release into the caudate) is incorrect. The description matches that of Parkinson disease, which is a result of degeneration of neurons in the substantia nigra. These neurons project to the caudate and putamen, where they release dopamine, not glutamate.

D (decreased glutamate release into the right cerebellar hemisphere) is incorrect. The tremor typical of cerebellar damage is seen particularly at the end of targeted movements and is called intention or action tremor. A tremor seen at rest is called a resting tremor and is a common finding in Parkinson disease, which affects the basal ganglia. The remaining movement difficulties described and the brain region indicated by the asterisk are consistent with Parkinson disease. Initial degeneration in the left substantia nigra would affect the right body.

E (normal changes seen with aging) is incorrect. The description matches that of Parkinson disease, which is a result of degeneration of dopaminergic neurons in the substantia nigra. These dopaminergic neurons project to the caudate and putamen, where they release dopamine.

19. B (increase the concentration of dopamine in the basal ganglia) is correct. L-dopa is a precursor to dopamine, which, unlike dopamine itself, can cross the blood–brain barrier. The description includes three of the hallmark signs of Parkinson disease: resting tremor, rigidity (cog-wheel, in this case), and bradykinesia. Parkinson is the result of degeneration of dopaminergic neurons of the substantia nigra with subsequent loss of dopamine released into the caudate and putamen.

A (block cholinergic receptors in the central nervous system), C (increase the activity of peripheral adrenergic neurons), D (act directly on skeletal muscle), and E (decrease brain serotonin levels) are incorrect. L-dopa is a dopamine precursor that is given because it can cross the blood–brain barrier, unlike dopamine itself. It will not act on central or peripheral cholinergic receptors, nor will it affect the biogenic amine, serotonin.

20. D (neurons in the midbrain substantia nigra) is correct. Uniform increase in resistance to passive movement, sometimes called lead-pipe rigidity or plastic rigidity, is a hallmark of Parkinson disease resulting from degeneration of neurons of the substantia nigra.

A (cell bodies in the left motor cortex) and C (axons in lateral funiculus in the right spinal cord) are incorrect. These upper motor neuron lesions would likely produce an increase in resistance at the beginning of passive limb flexion or extension, but that resistance would then fade away rather than remaining uniform. This would be described as clasp-knife rigidity.

B (axons in the left medullary pyramids) is incorrect. Damage restricted to the medullary pyramids results in weakness and flaccid paralysis without rigidity.

E (Purkinje cells in the right cerebellar hemisphere) is incorrect. Cerebellar damage may produce hypotonia, but it is not associated with an increase in resistance.

21. F (right cerebellar hemisphere) is correct. Damage to a cerebellar hemisphere results in limb ataxia, reduced muscle tone, and pendular reflexes, plus additional motor changes, including decomposition of movement and loss of coordination on the ipsilateral side. Other findings may include headache, vomiting, and a change in consciousness. Pure cerebellar disorders are rare because vascular disorders usually affect both the cerebellum and brainstem.

A and **B** (left and right caudate nuclei) are incorrect. Damage to the caudate nuclei results in Huntington disease, an autosomally dominant disorder characterized by behavioral changes with irritability and depression, choreoathetotic movements, and dementia.

C and **D** (left and right internal capsule) are incorrect. Damage to the posterior limb of the internal capsule results in an upper motor neuron disorder on the contralateral side. In the acute stage, this would result in a flaccid paralysis; in the chronic stage, this would result in spastic paralysis with hyperreflexia and hypertonia.

E (left cerebellar hemisphere) is incorrect. Damage to a cerebellar hemisphere causes ipsilateral, not contralateral, findings.

22. **D** (bilateral increase in endolymph pressure) is correct. Increase in endolymph pressure (Ménière disease) results in vertigo, hearing loss, and tinnitus. Bilateral forms of the disease are usually related to either the presence of autoantibodies or a familial genetic predisposition.

A (vestibular neuroma at the left cerebellopontine angle) is incorrect. This would affect only hearing in the left ear. In general, vestibular (acoustic) neuromas can result in tinnitus, asymmetric (one-sided) sensorineural hearing loss, and vertigo.

B (otosclerosis affecting both ears) is incorrect. Otosclerosis is usually characterized by new bone formation in the stapes, reducing its ability to vibrate and resulting in conductive hearing loss, but it will have no vestibular effects.

C (hemorrhage into the flocculonodular lobe) is incorrect. Damage to the flocculonodular lobe usually results in unsteady gait with a wide-base stance to maintain balance. Nystagmus is typical. There is no hearing loss.

E (infarct in the left lateral vestibular nucleus) is incorrect. Damage to the lateral vestibular nucleus will not cause any auditory problems, although it results in dizziness, ataxia, and unsteady gait.

23. **A** (left posterior inferior cerebellar artery) is correct. Occlusion of the posterior inferior cerebellar artery (PICA) results in lateral medullary (Wallenberg) syndrome. Damaged structures include the spinothalamic tract (loss of pain and temperature on contralateral body), spinal trigeminal tract (loss of pain and temperature on ipsilateral face), and descending sympathetic fibers (ipsilateral Horner syndrome). Nausea, vertigo, and limb ataxia (ipsilateral side) result from damage to the cerebellum, inferior cerebellar peduncle, and vestibular nuclei.

B and **E** (left and right anterior inferior cerebellar artery) are incorrect. The anterior inferior cerebellar arteries supply the inner ear and cochlear nuclei. Occlusion results in monaural hearing loss. The facial nerves and pontine gaze center may also be affected.

C and **F** (left and right posterior cerebral artery) are incorrect. Damaged structures include occipital cortex resulting in a contralateral homonymous hemianopia with macular sparing. There are no cerebellar or vestibular signs.

D (right posterior inferior cerebellar artery) is incorrect. Signs and symptoms would be on the right side.

24. **B** (right subthalamic nucleus) is correct. Hemiballismus (violent, flinging movements in the arm and leg) usually results from a small stroke in the subthalamic nucleus. It appears that disinhibition of the ventrolateral thalamic nucleus results in paroxysmal surges of neuronal firing in the motor cortex, giving rise to the violent movements in the contralateral arm and leg.

A (left subthalamic nucleus) is incorrect. The left subthalamic nucleus is part of the left basal ganglia. These are in communication with the left cortex, through which they affect the contralateral body. Damage to the left subthalamic nucleus would result in hemiballistic movements of the right arm and leg.

C and **D** (left and right dentate nuclei) are incorrect. Dentate nuclei are the principal relay nuclei from the cerebellar hemispheres to cerebral cortex. Damage to one of these nuclei would result in signs such as decomposition of movement, intention tremor, and past-pointing on the ipsilateral side.

E and **F** (left and right red nuclei) are incorrect. Red nuclei are the origin of the rubrospinal tracts. There are no known clinical syndromes that follow damage to the red nuclei or the rubrospinal tracts.

25. **D** (ischemic stroke involving most of the territory of the right middle cerebral artery) is correct. The sketch suggests hemi-neglect, which results from damage to the posterior parietal lobe, more commonly in the nondominant hemisphere. The left body weakness further locates the damage to the right hemisphere surrounding the central sulcus. The left hemianopsia is consistent with a right hemisphere injury, damaging much of the optic radiation.

A (occlusion of distal posterior cerebral artery branches supplying the right calcarine sulcus) is incorrect. This would explain left hemianopsia but would not account for the hemi-neglect. Occlusion of proximal branches of PCA that supply the cerebral peduncle would produce left side weakness or paralysis, but occlusion of only distal branches would not.

B (lacunar infarct involving the genu and posterior limb of the right internal capsule) is incorrect. This would account for the left-sided weakness but would not cause hemi-neglect or a visual field loss.

C (tumor of the right temporal lobe involving Meyer loop causing a midline shift and compression of the left cerebral peduncle against the tentorium) is incorrect. Damage to portions of the optic radiation in the temporal lobe (Meyer loop) will cause a superior quadrant anopsia, not a full hemianopsia, because other portions of the optic radiation will still be intact. Compression of the left cerebral peduncle will affect the right, not the left body. Neither temporal lobe nor peduncle damage will produce hemi-neglect.

26. **A** (meningitis) is correct. Headache and stiff neck are hallmarks of meningitis. Although not always present, Kernig sign is consistent with meningeal irritation of meningitis.

B (subarachnoid hemorrhage) is incorrect. The headache of a subarachnoid hemorrhage occurs suddenly, with an intensity that is frequently described as "the worst headache of my life." The irritation of subarachnoid blood could cause stiff neck, but in the context of fever and listlessness, the stiff neck is more suggestive of meningeal infection.

C (tension headache) is incorrect. Tension headaches generally do worsen throughout the day, but only rarely are accompanied by other signs.

D (cluster headache) is incorrect. Cluster headaches occur suddenly, with maximum intensity reached within minutes rather than hours. Their duration is rarely more than 1 or 2 hours. Accompanying signs may include autonomic findings (tearing, runny nose, flushing) on the ipsilateral face, but fever and listlessness are not part of a cluster headache presentation.

27. **D** (tardive dyskinesia) is correct. Typical antipsychotics (e.g., haloperidol) are targeted to the mesolimbic system where they block D2 dopamine receptors. Unavoidably, they also block D2 receptors in the striatum. Chronic administration results in supersensitivity of dopamine D2 receptors in the striatum. The result is uncontrolled movements, including lip smacking and grimacing, termed *tardive dyskinesia*.

A (tremor), **B** (rigidity), and **C** (bradykinesia) are incorrect. Each represents a movement disorder that results from a loss of dopamine release into the striatum rather than a supersensitivity.

E (ballism) is incorrect. This uncontrolled limb flinging results from damage to the subthalamic nucleus of the basal ganglia, typically due to stroke.

28. **D** (axons terminating in the right cuneate gyrus) is correct. Losses in the left visual field result from damage in the right side of the brain. Damage above the calcarine sulcus, in the cuneate gyrus, in the primary visual cortex affects the lower visual field.

A (axons running in the optic radiation of the left temporal lobe) and **B** (axons running in the optic radiation of the right temporal lobe) are incorrect. Damage to axons of the optic radiation that run forward through the temporal lobe as Meyer loop will result in superior quadrant, not inferior quadrant, anopsia.

C (axons terminating in the left cuneate gyrus) is incorrect. Losses in the left visual field result from damage in the right side of the brain.

29. **A** (supratentorial tumor) is correct. Although most tumors do not initially present as headache, headache related to tumor is likely to be dull and not well localized. A headache that changes in quality, severity or location should always be investigated, as should any change in level of alertness associated with headache. A pupil that is newly dilated and unresponsive is a medical emergency that, coupled with other signs of intracranial mass, suggests compression of the ipsilateral oculomotor nerve secondary to temporal lobe (uncal) herniation.

B (cluster headache) is incorrect. Cluster headaches are severe with a stabbing (not a dull) quality. Individual headaches are brief, lasting minutes to 2 hours, although these headaches occur in groups (clusters) that may continue for weeks. They may cause tearing and redness in the ipsilateral eye, but the pupil will not become unreactive.

C (subarachnoid hemorrhage) is incorrect. Subarachnoid hemorrhage produces a severe headache ("worst headache of my life") with rapid onset, rather than a dull headache of several months' duration.

D (classic migraine) is incorrect. Migraines are throbbing, not dull. An individual headache may last hours to days, but not months. Migraine headaches commonly first occur in the second decade and only very rarely present first as late as the sixth decade. Photophobia is common, but a unilateral unreactive pupil is not part of a migraine presentation.

30. **E** (venous blood resulting from the rupture of bridging vessels) is correct. Blood that accumulates between the dura and arachnoid layers and forces open a subdural space most commonly arises from rupture of veins that carry venous blood from the brain to the sinuses. Rapid acceleration–deceleration events are sufficient to tear these veins.

A (arterial blood resulting from the rupture of the anterior cerebral artery) is incorrect. The cerebral arteries lie within the pial layer against the brain and are unlikely to rupture under the circumstances described. If a cerebral artery does rupture, the blood enters the subarachnoid space between the pia and the overlying arachnoid and mixes with the cerebrospinal fluid.

B (arterial blood resulting from the rupture of the middle meningeal artery) is incorrect. The middle meningeal artery is embedded within the dura and is most likely to rupture as a result of skull fracture. Blood from a meningeal artery will force its way between the dura and the skull, creating an epidural hematoma.

C (arterial blood resulting from the rupture of an aneurysm) is incorrect. Aneurysms that bleed outside the brain generally are located on cerebral arteries, especially those near the arterial circle (of Willis) on the anterior brainstem. Blood escaping from a cerebral artery enters the subarachnoid, not the subdural space.

D (venous blood resulting from the rupture of the superior sagittal sinus) is incorrect. The most common cause of rupture of the superior sagittal sinus is severe head trauma. The blood most commonly pools between the skull and dura as an epidural hematoma.

31. **A** (decreased homovanillic acid) is correct. This individual has Parkinson disease, a disorder resulting from a massive loss of dopaminergic neurons in the substantia nigra. Because HVA is the major metabolite of dopamine, CSF levels can be a useful marker for estimating the levels of turnover. HVA can also be measured in the urine.

B (decreased vanillylmandelic acid) is incorrect. VMA is a marker for norepinephrine and epinephrine, not dopamine. It can be measured in blood or urine. VMA levels are elevated with adrenal tumor (pheochromocytoma).

C (increased 3-methoxy-4-hydroxyphenylglycol) is incorrect. MHPG is a metabolite of norepinephrine, not dopamine. MHPG levels can be measured in both CSF and urine. MHPG levels are changed in a variety of mental disorders, including schizophrenia, anxiety, and depression.

D (increased 5-hydroxyindole acetic acid) is incorrect. 5-HIAA is a marker for serotonin, not dopamine. 5-HIAA levels are decreased in the CSF of individuals with idiopathic Parkinson disease.

32. **B** (right optic tract) is correct. Visual loss in the left visual field is caused by damage to the right visual pathway central to the optic chiasm. The expanding subdural hematoma on the right side with subsequent midline shift to the left began to compress the left cerebral peduncle, resulting in the right-sided weakness that sent him to the emergency department.

A (right optic nerve) and **C** (left optic nerve) are incorrect. Damage to an optic nerve will result in partial or complete blindness in that eye. Loss of part or all of a visual field requires loss of visual inputs originating from each eye.

D (left optic tract) is incorrect. Visual loss in the left visual field is caused by damage to the right visual pathway central to the optic chiasm.

E (optic chiasm) is incorrect. Damage to the central chiasm will yield bilateral loss of temporal visual fields, whereas damage to the lateral chiasm will yield a nasal visual field loss ipsilateral to the damage.

33. **D** (anterior spinal artery) is correct. Occlusion of the penetrating branches of the anterior spinal artery supplying the right medulla above the level of the pyramidal decussation results in this presentation of medial medullary syndrome. Paresis and eventual atrophy of right (ipsilateral) tongue is due to damage to the right hypoglossal nerve; acute flaccid paralysis of the left (contralateral) arm and leg is due to damage to the right medullary pyramid; and loss of touch, vibration, and proprioception from the left (contralateral) arm and leg is due to damage to the right medial lemniscus.

A (anterior cerebral artery) is incorrect. Occlusion of the ACA would affect the medial portion of the cerebral cortex and result in paresis or paralysis of contralateral leg and foot (not arm), paresthesia of contralateral leg and foot (not arm), and urinary incontinence.

B (posterior inferior cerebellar artery) is incorrect. Occlusion of the PICA would result in a lateral medullary syndrome. Tracts and nuclei damaged include spinothalamic (loss of pain and temperature sensation from the contralateral arm and leg) and spinal trigeminal tract and nucleus (ipsilateral face), descending autonomic pathways (ipsilateral Horner syndrome; miosis, ptosis, anhidrosis), vestibular nucleus (vertigo), and cerebellum (ipsilateral limb ataxia).

C (anterior inferior cerebellar artery) is incorrect. The labyrinthine artery is a major branch of the AICA, so occlusion would result in tinnitus or deafness on the side of the lesion.

E (posterior spinal artery) is incorrect. The paired PSAs rarely occlude because they receive collateral circulation from the radicular arteries. Although occlusion of the left PSA could result in some of the sensory and motor loss described, portions of the lateral funiculus receive blood from the ASA, so that complete arm and leg paralysis would be unlikely. Furthermore, occlusion of the left PSA would not cause weakness of the right side of the tongue.

34. **D** (epidural hematoma) is correct. This clinical presentation represents an epidural bleed from the right middle meningeal artery that has progressed to produce a space-occupying lesion shifting the right side of the brain across the midline and causing herniation of the medial temporal lobe through the tentorial notch (uncal herniation). The herniation results in the compression of the oculomotor nerve yielding a dilated, unresponsive pupil. The changes in consciousness and the dilated ("blown") pupil are hallmarks of this disorder.

A (subarachnoid hemorrhage) is incorrect. Subarachnoid hemorrhage is characterized by a severe headache ("worst headache of my life") with rapid onset due to the sudden increase in intracranial pressure, not the progressive changes in consciousness from lucid to semicomatose. It is unlikely to cause unilateral loss of pupil reactivity.

B (Horner syndrome) is incorrect. Horner syndrome (e.g., resulting from a neurovascular accident involving descending sympathetic pathways) would result in a constricted pupil, not a dilated pupil. The clinical triad of Horner syndrome includes miosis (constricted pupil), ptosis (drooping of the eyelid), and facial anhidrosis (loss of sweating), all affecting the ipsilateral side; there are no associated changes in the level of consciousness.

C (complex partial seizures) is incorrect. Confusion is immediate following complex partial seizures (CPS), not after a half-hour delay. CPS would not produce a unilateral dialated pupil.

35. **A** (right supratentorial brain) is correct. This is a stroke involving much of the territory supplied by the right middle cerebral artery. Only the lower face is involved because the upper face is controlled bilaterally by upper motor neuron in both the right and left cerebral cortex. The eyes cannot move to the left because of damage to the right frontal eye fields. Because this is an acute lesion, unbalanced activity from the left frontal eye fields continues to drive the eyes right. The flaccid paralysis is also consistent with the acute phase of the damage.

B (right midbrain) is incorrect. A stroke involving the right cerebral peduncle could cause the observed paralysis of face and arm and could damage the right oculomotor nerve. The result would be paralysis of the right eye (eye positioned "down and out"), paralysis of the right eyelid (severe ptosis or eyelid droop), and loss of parasympathetic innervation to the right eye (loss of pupil constriction and lens thickening). Movement of the left eye would be unaffected.

C (right pons) is incorrect. Damage involving portions of the right pontine base could cause the observed paralysis of the left arm. A sufficiently caudal lesion would also affect the right abducens nerve, causing paralysis of only the right eye on lateral gaze. If the damage extended to the posterior pons, it could involve the right abducens nucleus and right lateral gaze center, resulting in paralysis of right (not left) gaze. Damage extending to this region would likely affect the right facial motor nucleus and nerve, resulting in paralysis of the entire right face.

D (left spinal cord) is incorrect. Damage in the spinal cord cannot account for facial paralysis or gaze paralysis.

36. D (rapid transition from wakefulness to REM sleep) is correct. Sleep-onset REM is a hallmark of narcolepsy. Of the four major symptoms of narcolepsy, three (cataplexy, sleep paralysis, and hypnagogic hallucinations) are believed to represent the intrusion of REM sleep into the waking state. (The fourth symptom is excessive daytime sleepiness.)

A (abnormally long period of time spent initially in stage 1 sleep), B (a rapid transition from wakefulness to stage 2 sleep), and C (a direct transition from wakefulness to delta sleep) are incorrect. One feature of narcolepsy is the transition from wakefulness directly into REM sleep.

E (delay [90 minute] between sleep onset and the first episode of REM sleep) is incorrect. A 90-minute delay before first entering REM sleep is part of a normal sleep cycle. One feature of narcolepsy is the rapid transition to REM sleep, referred to as "sleep-onset REM."

37. C (overwhelming weakness when he is emotional) is correct. This case describes narcolepsy, the second most common cause of excessive daytime sleepiness (EDS). Cataplexy, sudden weakness or paralysis brought on by strong emotions, such as anger or uncontrollable laughter, is one of the hallmarks of narcolepsy. Other hallmarks include the hypnagogic hallucinations and the sleep paralysis that are described.

A (difficulty in falling asleep) is incorrect. On multiple sleep latency tests (MSLTs), narcolepsy is confirmed by unusually short sleep latency.

B (no REM sleep on an average night) is incorrect. The case describes narcolepsy, a hallmark of which is a rapid entrance into the first episode of REM sleep.

D (snoring) is incorrect. Snoring accompanies obstructive sleep apnea, the most common cause of EDS. This case describes three hallmarks of narcolepsy, the second most common cause of EDS.

E (frequent limb flailing during REM sleep) is incorrect. REM sleep is normally accompanied by paralysis of almost all voluntary muscles. A loss of this paralysis occurs in a disorder known as REM sleep behavior disorder. Individuals with this disorder may move and appear to act out dreams during sleep.

38. **C** (C) is correct. Damage to ventral posterior region of the right thalamus (VPL and VPM) would result in the acute loss of all somatic sensation from the left body and face. In a small percentage of individuals, thalamic pain (neuropathic pain) can occur weeks to months after damage to the thalamus. Conventional treatments (e.g., nonsteroidal anti-inflammatory drugs) are generally ineffective in managing neuropathic pain; antidepressants may be useful.

A and **D** (A and D) are incorrect. Damage to the caudate nuclei would not result in acute loss of sensation or the eventual return of thalamic pain. Degeneration of these nuclei is a later finding in Huntington disease, an autosomal dominant neurodegenerative disorder resulting from the expansion of the CAG trinucleotide repeat coding for huntingtin protein.

B and **E** (B and E) are incorrect. Damage to the posterior limb of the internal capsule would result in contralateral loss of sensation, without return of spontaneous pain, and in a dense contralateral hemiparesis or hemiparalysis

F (F) is incorrect. Damage to the left thalamus would result in acute loss of sensation and the potential for thalamic pain on the right side (not the left).

39. **A** (tachycardia) is correct. Atropine is a competitive antagonist for the muscarinic cholinergic receptor. It will block the action of parasympathetic postganglionic fibers at their target organs and can be used to relax smooth muscle (e.g., organophosphate poisoning antidote). Administration usually results in a slight increase in heart rate (excess dose can result in tachycardia). Atropine can also cause dry mouth and relaxation of the smooth muscle in the gastrointestinal tract and urinary tract.

B (weakness of respiratory muscles) is incorrect. Respiratory muscles, including the diaphragm and the intercostals, express nicotinic, not muscarinic receptors. Toxic overdoses of atropine can result in rapid respiration (not reduced respiration), flushing of the face, and central nervous system stimulation.

C (constricted pupils) is incorrect. Pupil constriction is mediated by the parasympathetic nervous system. Blocking the action of the parasympathetic fibers will allow pupil dilation.

D (transient Horner syndrome) is incorrect. Horner syndrome, consisting of eyelid droop (ptosis), pupil constriction (miosis), and decreased facial sweating (anhidrosis), is the result of loss of sympathetic nerve control of eye and face. Atropine, by antagonizing muscarinic ACh receptors, blocks parasympathetic, not sympathetic, control.

40. **C** (benign essential tremor) is correct. Benign essential tremor (ET) is a common movement disorder that can occur at any time during adult life. It typically affects the hands (usually symmetrically), head, and voice (diaphragm). It may initially appear as a transient nervousness (twitching) during periods of stress. ET is commonly relieved by alcohol intake, which helps to distinguish it from several other tremors. It usually presents as a postural tremor, seen in movements made against gravity. It may also occur as an action tremor, seen during voluntary movement. Although it does not affect life expectancy, it can affect the ability to perform many daily activities (e.g., eating, dressing, and writing). One type of essential tremor is known to be an inherited autosomal dominant disorder with almost complete penetrance by age 70 years. There may also be sporadic occurrence.

A (Parkinson disease) is incorrect. Other neurologic signs would be present, including bradykinesia, rigidity, and postural instability. The "pill-rolling" tremor in Parkinson disease is typically characterized by a frequency of 4 to 7 Hz and is present at rest, unlike most essential tremors. It is a pathologic tremor. As with other resting tremors, the intensity of the tremor in PD decreases with voluntary motor activity. ET may respond to β-adrenergic antagonists (e.g., propranolol), whereas the tremor of PD responds to L-dopa.

B (alcoholic cerebellar degeneration) is incorrect. Cerebellar degeneration due to alcohol localizes to the anterior cerebellar vermis. Major findings include loss of coordination affecting gait and propulsion. A wide-based (ataxic) gait is expected. The arms and face are generally spared. The described disorder, an essential tremor, is thought to involve the red nucleus, the inferior olivary nucleus, and the cerebellum, but it would not localize to the superior vermis.

D (dystonic tremor) is incorrect. This tremor, which is considered a "postural tremor," often affects the head, appears to be an attempt to overcome dystonia, and is worsened when the head is moved in the direction opposite the dystonic contraction. Other neurologic signs would be present, including twisting movements and abnormal postures (e.g., torticollis), that are thought to be related to the basal ganglia. Unlike essential tremor, dystonic tremor is not lessened by alcohol.

41. **A** (within a day, Schwann cells will begin to break down myelin of the axon distal to the lesion) is correct. This is an initial step of Wallerian degeneration, affecting the portion of the nerve distal to the injury. Schwann cells initially break down the myelin (forming myelin ovoids) and eventually engulf and remove fragmented axons.

B (axons distal to the lesion will degenerate owing to the loss of retrogradely transported trophic factors) is incorrect. Trophic factors needed to maintain the axon are moved by anterograde (not retrograde) transport.

C (axon regrowth will occur, dependent on the fast axonal transport of tubulin and actin) is incorrect. The growth of new axon is dependent on the slow component (2 mm/day) of axonal transport (formerly called "bulk flow") that is responsible for carrying intermediate filaments, actin, and tubulin to the newly growing nerve terminal.

D (microglia are recruited to the area to remove debris) is incorrect. Microglia are only found in the CNS. Macrophages and Schwann cells are responsible for phagocytosis in the periphery.

42. **D** (small infarct in the right pons) is correct. Loss of conjugate right eye movement could result from damage to the right lateral gaze center in the right paramedian pontine reticular formation in the posteromedial pons. The response to corneal touch should have included bilateral eye blink. Loss of right eye blink indicates possible damage to the right facial nerve or facial motor nucleus. The facial nerve wraps posteriorly around the abducens nucleus before exiting the anterolateral pons. A small infarct in the right posteromedial pons could affect both the right lateral gaze center and the right facial nerve.

A and **B** (Schwannoma in the left or right cerebellopontine angle) are incorrect. A schwannoma at the cerebellopontine angle is also known as an *acoustic neuroma*. It will first affect the vestibular, and then the auditory portion of CN VIII. The primary deficit associated with this slow-growing, benign tumor is hearing loss, although tinnitus, loss of balance, and nystagmus are relatively common. If the tumor expands to involve the facial nerve, paralysis of muscles of facial expression results, with loss of ipsilateral eye blink. Paralysis of eye movement should not occur.

C (small infarct in the left pons) is incorrect. This would affect the left lateral gaze center, preventing left conjugate gaze, and would affect the left facial nerve, preventing left eye blink.

spinal cord lesion has removed them from control by upper motor neurons.

43. **B** (his bladder empties reflexively when full, with urine retention) is correct. This case describes spinal cord damage. Loss of sensation below the umbilicus puts the damage just below the T10 spinal segment. Hyperreflexia and Babinski sign (rather than flaccid paralysis and muscle atrophy) in the legs requires that the spinal cord anterior horn is intact in the lumbar spinal cord. Therefore, this is a likely a low thoracic cord lesion. During the acute phase after injury (flaccid paralysis), the bladder is atonic, and catheterization is necessary. During the chronic phase after injury, reflexive emptying of the urinary bladder occurs because the parasympathetic fibers, emerging from sacral spinal cord, are intact. However, coordination of sphincter and detrusor muscles is lost, so bladder emptying may not be complete, and catheterization may still be important.

A (his bladder is atonic and does not empty reflexively) is incorrect. Atonic or flaccid neurogenic bladder, like flaccid paralysis, occurs acutely after spinal cord damage, but occurs chronically only if the nerves to the detrusor muscle are damaged, as would occur with a lesion of the sacral spinal cord or the cauda equina.

C (his bladder fills and empties completely and frequently, but without voluntary control) is incorrect. Full coordination of reflexive bladder filling and emptying occurs when the spinal cord is intact and communication exists between the sacral spinal cord and the pontine micturition center. Voluntary control in the adult arises from the frontal lobes.

D (control of the external urinary sphincter is intact) is incorrect. The external urinary sphincter is controlled by lower motor neurons with cell bodies at spinal levels S2–S4 whose axons travel in the pudendal nerve. Although these nerves are intact, the

44. **B** (sensory neuropathy of metabolic origin) is correct. A bilateral, symmetric neuropathy suggests a metabolic or systemic disorder rather than a focal lesion. A pattern of bilateral distal extremity involvement is more easily explained by a peripheral neuropathy than by CNS damage. There is damage to large, myelinated sensory fibers, because these carry both vibratory sensation and muscle spindle inputs necessary for deep tendon reflexes.

A (entrapment neuropathy) is incorrect. A bilaterally symmetric distal sensory loss is unlikely to result from two equivalent focal compressions.

C (radicular neuropathy affecting the anterior lumbar roots) is incorrect. This would not explain the sensory loss. In addition, the F response specifically tests conduction through anterior spinal roots.

D (damage to the posterior columns) is incorrect. Although a Romberg sign frequently results from damage to posterior columns, it actually indicates loss of proprioceptive input. Loss of peripheral sensory input could account for loss of proprioception and could produce a Romberg sign, but damage to the posterior columns could not account for the change in deep tendon reflexes.

45. **B** (hyperthermia) is correct. The anterior hypothalamic nuclei are important to heat dissipation. As body temperature rises, it acts through the autonomic nervous system to cause sweating and cutaneous vasodilation.

A (an increase in basal metabolism), **D** (cutaneous vasoconstriction), and **E** (uncontrolled shivering) are incorrect. These responses would be appropriate in a cold environment and would be triggered by the posterior hypothalamic nuclei, which are responsible for heat conservation.

C (cutaneous vasodilation) is incorrect. The anterior hypothalamic nuclei are responsible for triggering vasodilation in response to rising body temperature. Damage to this region interferes with thermoregulatory control and, specifically, with heat dissipation.

46. **B** (difficulty directing gaze while going down stairs) is correct. The only cranial nerve that exists from the posterior surface of the brainstem is the trochlear nerve, which exits just caudal to the inferior colliculus and innervates the superior oblique. This muscle acts to depress and intort the eye and is necessary to look down and in.

A (bitemporal hemianopsia ["tunnel vision"]) is incorrect. This would result from damage to the optic chiasm and is often related to pituitary tumor.

C (internuclear ophthalmoplegia) is incorrect. INO describes a paralysis of eye movement in which the adducting eye cannot move past midline on lateral gaze. It is due to damage to the medial longitudinal fasciculus, which runs through the posterior medial brainstem and connects the oculomotor, trochlear, abducens, and vestibular nuclei. INO may result from demyelination due to multiple sclerosis and can be unilateral or bilateral.

D (one or both eyes deviated down and out with eyelid droop) is incorrect. Paralysis of eye movement of this sort is due to damage to the oculomotor nerve, which exits anteriorly from the midbrain.

E (loss of corneal blink reflex) is incorrect. This reflex tests trigeminal and facial, both of which emerge from the anterolateral pons, not from the caudal posterior midbrain.

47. **D** (posterior column/medial lemniscal system) is correct. Loss of sensation coupled with loss of pupillary constriction to light but not to near focus (Argyll-Robertson pupil) is consistent with neurosyphilis (tertiary syphilis). The loss of sensation is due to an inflammatory reaction to infection by *Treponema pallidum,* which destroys posterior spinal roots and the posterior columns.

A (ventral posterolateral nuclei of the thalamus) is incorrect. Although damage to VPL of thalamus could account for the observed sensory loss, the additional information supplied by the observed Argyll-Robertson pupil (loss of pupillary constriction to light but not to near focus) is consistent with neurosyphilis, which damages the posterior spinal roots and columns.

B (dorsal reticular nuclei of the thalamus) is incorrect. Damage here would not account for either the sensory loss or the pupillary finding (Argyll-Robertson pupil).

C (cerebellum) is incorrect. The broad-based stance seen here is a result of loss of proprioceptive input, not cerebellar damage. The addition of the Argyll-Robertson pupil (loss of pupillary constriction to light but not to near focus) leads to a diagnosis of neurosyphilis with damage to posterior spinal roots and column.

E (posterior limb of the internal capsule) is incorrect. Damage to the IC could result in loss of sensation from the legs, but it would also likely produce paralysis of the legs, which is not reported. In addition, the Argyll-Robertson pupil (loss of pupillary constriction to light but not to near focus) leads to a diagnosis of neurosyphilis with damage to posterior spinal roots and column.

48. **C** (right cerebellar hemisphere) is correct. Hypotonia, dysmetria, decomposition of movement and pendular reflexes are all signs of cerebellar damage. Cerebellar control is exerted upon the ipsilateral body, so signs in the right body indicate right cerebellar damage. Falling to the right is consistent with right cerebellar damage, although under other circumstances, it can indicate vestibular damage without cerebellar involvement.

A (right ventrolateral nucleus of the thalamus) is incorrect. Damage to the right VLN of thalamus would affect the left body.

B (left frontal cortex) is incorrect. Damage to the left frontal cortex that affects movement will produce flaccid paralysis and areflexia if the damage is acute and severe, or will produce spastic paralysis and hyperreflexia if the damage is chronic.

D (left substantia nigra) is incorrect. Damage to the left SN will produce signs in the right body that are Parkinson-like and could include bradykinesia, rigidity, and resting tremor. Reflexes would not be affected.

E (right vestibular nucleus) is incorrect. The right vestibular nucleus does provide extensor tone to the right body, so damage to this nucleus could result in falling to the right. However, the other signs (hypotonia, dysmetria, decomposition of movement and pendular reflexes) cannot be explained by a vestibular lesion.

49. **B** (retinohypothalamic tract) is correct. The RHT carries light information from the retina to the suprachiasmatic nucleus of the hypothalamus, which is responsible for coordinating many aspects of the circadian cycle of physiologic activity.

A (supraoptic–hypophyseal tract) is incorrect. This tract supplies vasopressin from the supraoptic nucleus of the hypothalamus to the posterior pituitary.

C (tuberohypophyseal tract) is incorrect. This is one of three important dopamine pathways. It runs from the arcuate nucleus of the hypothalamus to the median eminence and

posterior pituitary. It serves to inhibit prolactin release and stimulate growth hormone release from the pituitary. The other two dopaminergic pathways are the nigrostriatal and the mesocortical/mesolimbic pathways.

D (retinogeniculate tract) is incorrect. This is the pathway from the retina to the lateral geniculate nucleus of the thalamus supports vision.

E (retinocollicular tract) is incorrect. This pathway from the retina to the superior colliculus supports reflexive eye movements in response to visual stimuli.

50. **A** (posterior and anterior roots) is correct. Muscle atrophy indicates that muscle innervation has been lost. Fasciculations, the visible twitches of individual motor units, occur during ongoing damage to the anterior horn or anterior roots. Loss of sensation is explained by posterior root damage.

B (posterior limb of the internal capsule) is incorrect. This would not account for fasciculations or for severe muscle wasting. It would be unlikely to account for such localized findings.

C (ipsilateral side of the spinal cord) is incorrect. To affect the arm, this lesion would be cervical. Such a lesion would cause upper motor neuron findings in the right leg, loss of fine touch, vibration, and proprioceptive sense in the right leg, and loss of pain and temperature in the left leg.

D (contralateral side of the spinal cord) is incorrect. This would not explain any findings, with the possible exception of a loss of pain and temperature.

E (ventrolateral medulla) is incorrect. This would not account for fasciculations, the severe muscle wasting, or the loss of fine touch, vibration, or proprioception. It would be unlikely to account for such localized findings.

questions

DIRECTIONS: Each numbered item or incomplete statement is followed by options arranged in alphabetical or logical order. Select the best answer to each question. Some options may be partially correct, but there is only **ONE BEST** answer.

1. A 29-year-old man is seen in the emergency department because of excruciating pain over his left cheek. The pain can be elicited by light touch on the cheek or changes in temperature. The pain is severe, has an acute onset, and lasts for only a few seconds. Which of the following is the most likely cause of this pain?

A. Nerve inflammation secondary to a bacterial infection such as Lyme disease

B. Nerve inflammation secondary to a viral infection such as herpes zoster

C. Nerve compression from an adjacent blood vessel

D. Hyperalgesia associated with temporal arteritis

2. A 57-year-old man is brought to the emergency department because of weakness in his right leg. Examination reveals flaccid paralysis and patellar reflex is absent on the right. Plantar reflex is normal. Sensory testing reveals sensitivity to pin-prick and vibration. Which of the following is the most likely site of damage given these findings?

A. Spinal cord hemisection at T12 on the right side

B. Posterior roots at L2, L3, and L4 on the right side

C. Anterior roots at L2, L3, and L4 on the right side

D. Lateral funiculus of spinal cord at midthoracic level on the right side

E. Medullary pyramids on the right side

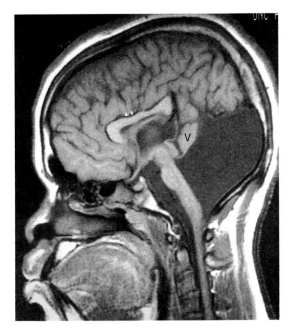

3. A 4-year boy is developmentally delayed and presents with extensive signs of CNS dysfunction, including hypotonia and ataxia. The accompanying MRI is obtained. Which of the following is most consistent with these findings?

A. Chiari malformation

B. Dandy-Walker malformation

C. Lissencephaly

D. Myelomeningocele

E. Syringomyelia

4. A 22-year-old woman presents with complex partial seizures. A CT scan reveals the presence of a tumor in the left temporal lobe. Visual field testing reveals a subtle visual field defect. Which of the following deficits is most likely to result from this tumor?
   A. Left inferior quadrant anopsia
   B. Right inferior quadrant anopsia
   C. Left superior quadrant anopsia
   D. Right superior quadrant anopsia

5. A 68-year-old woman is seen because of increasing forgetfulness. Her family expresses concern that she is frequently withdrawn and confused. She has become lost several times while returning from shopping. She does not always recognize her grandchildren and cannot remember that her daughter recently gave birth to twins. During the medical interview, she frequently searches for words in response to questions and scores an 18 on the mini-mental status exam, although she claims that she is just fine. Which of the following additional findings would you expect?
   A. Decreased acetylcholinesterase in the cerebral cortex
   B. Antibodies to nicotinic cholinergic receptors in the cerebral cortex
   C. Loss of cholinergic neurons in the basal forebrain
   D. Lewy bodies in the pars compacta of the substantia nigra
   E. Decreased levels of GABA in the striatum and substantia nigra

6. A 7-year-old girl experiences brief episodes, lasting less than 10 seconds, in which she is unresponsive. These occur without warning. Her eyes are open and, at times, her eyelids flutter. Following the spell, she is immediately aware of her surroundings and is not confused or disorientated. She has several hundred of these episodes every day and is diagnosed with a seizure disorder. Hyperventilation can induce her seizures, and an EEG recorded during one seizure reveals a 3-Hz spike-and-wave pattern that is found in all portions of both cerebral

hemispheres. Which of the following types of seizure is she most likely to be experiencing?
   A. Complex partial
   B. Pseudoseizure
   C. Tonic–clonic
   D. Absence
   E. Simple partial

7. A 72-year-old man is seen because he is having trouble remembering things and has increasing difficulty "finding words" in conversation. His wife reports that his memory problems and his ability to concentrate became noticeably worse about a year ago. She also reports he was always active, but now just sits and watches television. During the medical interview, he frequently searches for words in response to questions and scores a 17 on his mini-mental status exam. An MRI shows profound degeneration in the frontal lobe and the anterior temporal lobe. Which of the following is the most likely cause of his findings?
   A. Alzheimer disease
   B. Pick lobar atrophy
   C. Multiple system atrophy
   D. Progressive supranuclear palsy

8. A 22-year-old woman experiences severe cervical dystonia (torticollis). The spasms are worse when she is under excessive stress. Initially, she was able to relieve them by applying light pressure to her head opposite to the side to which she was turned. As this became less effective, she began receiving injections of botulinum toxin to relieve the dystonia. Which of the following is the most likely mechanism of action of the botulinum toxin treatment?
   A. Activate the same sensory pathway that the light touch activated, but at a central synapse
   B. Decrease the basal ganglia output responsible for the dystonia
   C. Inhibit cell bodies in the anterior horn of the cervical spinal cord
   D. Block release of acetylcholine at the neuromuscular junction
   E. Block acetylcholine receptors at the neuromuscular junction

9. A 16-year-old girl is seen because she is tired and losing weight. Examination reveals that she is jaundiced and has a ring of yellow-brown deposits around the cornea. Motor findings include reduced fine motor control, increased tone, unsteady gait, and coarse postural tremors. Which of the following is the most likely cause of her symptoms?
   A. Hepatolenticular degeneration
   B. Striatonigral degeneration
   C. Excessive deposition of iron in the globus pallidus
   D. Excessive deposition of inorganic lead in the cerebral cortex

10. A 44-year-old woman complains of daytime sleepiness and disrupted sleep. For several years, she has experienced leg discomfort that she describes as a deep aching and itching sensation. It is worse late at night and any time she is forced to sit motionless for an extended period of time. The uncomfortable sensations, although not painful, are only fully relieved by walking or deep knee bends. They make falling asleep difficult and sometimes cause her to wake from sleep and stretch her legs. Which of the following disorders is the most likely cause of her sleepiness?
   A. Restless leg syndrome
   B. Fibromyalgia
   C. Sleep apnea
   D. Narcolepsy
   E. REM sleep disorder

11. A 10-year-old boy is seen because of tics affecting the eye and face and constant throat clearing. His mother reports that the tics have been increasing in both frequency and intensity. She notes that he is having difficulty concentrating at school and that his teacher has recommended that he be placed in a class for the learning disabled. Examination confirms frequent motor tics around head and neck. When challenged, he can suppress the tics for about a minute, and then there is a burst of abnormal motor activity. Which of the following is the most likely cause of this disorder?

A. Decreased serotonergic activity in the cerebral cortex
B. Increased serotonergic activity in the cerebral cortex
C. Decreased dopaminergic activity in the striatum
D. Increased dopaminergic activity in the striatum
E. Decreased acetylcholinesterase activity in the basal forebrain

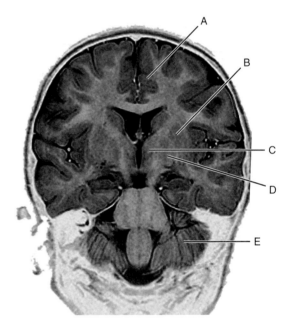

12. A 46-year-old woman presents with slight grimacing of the face, shrugging of the shoulders, and involuntary flinging of both the arms and legs. She has been treated for depression, which predates the uncontrolled movements. A mental status exam reveals some impairment of intellectual capacity. The history reveals that both her father and paternal grandmother had a similar disorder that became completely incapacitating before their deaths. Which brain region indicated in the accompanying normal MRI would be most likely to atrophy in this individual?

A. A
B. B
C. C
D. D
E. E

13. A 46-year-old man is seen because of painful cramping in his back and shoulder muscles. He reports that the spasms are particularly intense when he is stressed or overexerts. Examination reveals hypertonia and orthostatic tremor. When asked to walk, his gait looks stiff and rigid (e.g., tin soldier). Lab results indicate autoantibodies to glutamic acid decarboxylase. Which of the following is the most likely cause of these findings?
A. Huntington disease
B. Stiff-person syndrome
C. Parkinson disease
D. Progressive supranuclear palsy
E. Friedreich ataxia

14. A 28-year-old man was diagnosed 15 years earlier with a seizure disorder. Since that time, he has experienced between 2 and 25 seizures per week. Most of these episodes last less than 4 minutes and usually consist of very strong feelings of déjà vu (having previously experienced the current moment). Which of the following brain regions is most likely to be involved during these seizures?
A. Hypothalamus
B. Anterior calcarine sulcus
C. Orbitofrontal cortex
D. Precentral gyrus
E. Medial temporal lobe

15. A 28-year-old woman is seen because she is experiencing periods of double vision. The history reveals that she has had intermittent periods of numbness and tingling sensations that began in her feet and are slowly progressing up both legs. Examination reveals normal eye movement except when she gazes to the left (her left eye abducts normally, but her right eye does not adduct). MRI shows hyperintense periventricular lesions in the frontal and occipital lobes. Which of the following is most likely during periods when she is without symptoms?
A. Sprouting of small-diameter unmyelinated fibers that innervate muscles formerly innervated by larger myelinated fibers
B. Regrowth of myelin by Schwann cells
C. Depolarization in membrane potential due to decreased numbers of K^+ channels
D. Redistribution of Na^+ channels within demyelinated region of the axons

16. A 64-year-old man is brought to the physician by his wife because she is having difficulty understanding him. Examination reveals that his spontaneous speech has missing words and contains neologisms (nonwords). During normal conversation, he substitutes words that are phonetically similar, but with inappropriate meaning and context. He also has difficulty repeating words or phrases and reading aloud. His speech is fluent, and language comprehension is normal. Which of the following most likely describes his disorder?
A. Expressive aphasia
B. Transcortical sensory aphasia
C. Transcortical motor aphasia
D. Receptive aphasia
E. Conduction aphasia

17. A 37-year-old woman has a 4-month history of progressive weakness in her hands and arms. Examination reveals decreased ability to distinguish sharp from dull stimuli in both arms; vibration and position sensations are normal. Fasciculations can be seen in the upper left arm. Sensory and motor examination of the legs is unremarkable. Which of the following is the most likely cause of her findings?
A. Amyotrophic lateral sclerosis (motor neuron disease)
B. Acute inflammatory demyelinating polyradiculoneuropathy (Guillain-Barré disease)
C. Lambert-Eaton myasthenic syndrome
D. Syringomyelia

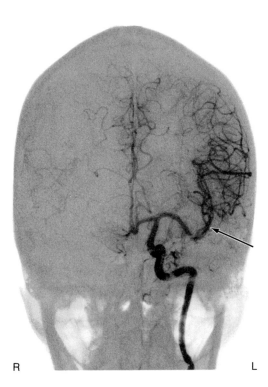

R   L

18. A 57-year-old man experiences a sudden occlusion of the artery indicated by the arrow in the accompanying normal angiogram. Which of the following signs is most likely to be present when he is seen 2 hours later in the emergency department?
A. Deviation of the tongue to the left upon protrusion
B. Fasciculations in the right tongue
C. Inability to wrinkle the right forehead
D. Flaccid paralysis of the right arm
E. Spastic paralysis of the right arm

19. A 75-year-old woman is unable to recognize objects placed in her right hand by feel, although she can recognize them with her left hand. Sensory testing for both arms and both legs is unremarkable. Muscle strength and tendon reflexes are normal. Which of the following regions is most likely damaged?
A. Left frontal cortex
B. Left parietal cortex
C. Left ventral posterior lateral thalamic nucleus

D. Left medial lemniscus
E. Right fasciculus cuneatus

20. A 5-year-old girl with a history of tonic, atonic, and tonic–clonic seizures is diagnosed with Lennox-Gastaut syndrome. Her seizures do not respond to medication and, by age 9 years, she experiences several seizures daily. A partial corpus callosotomy is performed, which is not fully successful in controlling her seizures. A second operation is performed to complete the callosotomy. This significantly reduces the number and intensity of her seizures. Which of the following is most likely to be affected by the callosotomy?
A. Generation of brain waves
B. Aspects of learning
C. Use of language
D. Maintenance of posture

21. A 61-year-old woman suffers a small hemorrhagic stroke involving the left medial geniculate nucleus of the thalamus. Which of the following is the most likely finding?
A. Right homonymous hemianopsia
B. Loss of sensation from right side of the face
C. Difficulty locating sounds on the right
D. Loss of vibration sensation from right side of the body

22. A 36-year-old man is seen because of repeated tripping and falling. The history reveals that he began to experience weakness in his left leg about 6 months ago and has recently begun to experience weakness in his right leg. He also reports twitching in his leg and arm muscles. Examination reveals weakness with hyperreflexia in leg and arm muscles. Fasciculations are observable in both thighs. Fasciculations and muscle atrophy are seen in the intrinsic hand muscles. There is no sensory involvement. Which of the following is the most likely cause of his symptoms?
A. Schwannoma
B. Amyotrophic lateral sclerosis
C. Myasthenia gravis
D. Lambert-Eaton myasthenic syndrome

23. A 73-year-old man has had increasing difficulty remembering names, dates, and tasks for 4 years. For the past 6 months, he has required some assistance with activities of daily living, such as dressing and bathing. He scores 18 on a mini-mental status exam. Neurologic exam reveals constructional apraxia. MRI reveals nonspecific, generalized atrophy of the cerebral hemispheres. Which of the following is most likely to be found in the brain of this individual?

A. Apolipoprotein E ε4
B. Abnormal huntingtin protein
C. Abnormal parkin protein
D. Abnormal prion protein

24. A 48-year-old woman is seen by her physician because she frequently wakes at night with a numb right hand. She reports a frequent "pins and needles" sensation her right hand when she is driving or working at the computer. Tapping her right wrist over the median nerve results in a tingling sensation over the second, third, and fourth digits. Compression of which of the following is the most likely cause of her symptoms?

A. Brachial plexus
B. Median nerve
C. Radial nerve
D. Ulnar nerve

25. A 63-year-old man undergoes surgery to remove a benign tumor in the spinal canal. As a result of the surgery, there is damage to fasciculus gracilis on the right side at T7–T10. Following recovery, he has a limited neurologic deficit due to this damage. Which of the following is most likely given these findings?

A. Dysmetria in the right arm
B. Dysmetria in the left arm
C. Decreased pain sensation from the right leg
D. Decreased pain sensation from the left leg
E. Decreased proprioceptive sensation from the right leg
F. Decreased proprioceptive sensation from the left leg

26. A 28-year-old woman is brought to the emergency department with fever and chills. She reports that foods have not tasted right and sounds have been uncomfortably loud in her left ear for about a day. Her temperature is 100.1°F and blood pressure is 142/90 mmHg. Corneal reflex testing reveals a weak response from the left eyelid and a normal response from the right. She has trouble holding the left eye closed against attempts to pry both eyes open. Which of the following is the most likely cause of her symptoms?

A. Acute trauma to the face damaging the ophthalmic division of the left trigeminal nerve
B. Inflammation of the left facial nerve from a viral infection
C. Acoustic neuroma pressing on the left facial and vestibulocochlear nerves
D. Hemorrhage into the left cavernous sinus damaging the oculomotor and trigeminal nerves

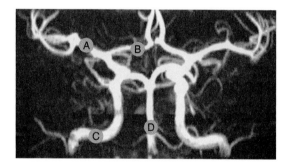

27. A 68-year-old woman is brought to the emergency department immobile and apparently unconscious. Careful examination reveals that she is conscious and able to look up and down. She has no other motor control. A limited sensory examination, in which she communicates through eye movements, suggests that sensory modalities are intact for arms and legs. Penetrating branches of which of the arteries indicated on the accompanying MRA (magnetic resonance angiogram) is most likely occluded?

A. A
B. B
C. C
D. D

A. L2 and L3
B. L3 and L4
C. L4 and L5
D. L5 and S1
E. S1 and S2

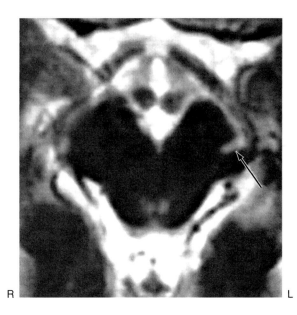

R   L

29. A 73-year-old man suffered a small stroke that resulted in weakness in his right lower leg. A series of MRIs were obtained several months later, one of which is presented here. Wallerian degeneration had produced an area of ischemic damage, as indicated by the arrow. Which of the following structures was most likely damaged by the stroke?

A. Right internal capsule, posterior limb
B. Left internal capsule, posterior limb
C. Right cerebral peduncle
D. Left cerebral peduncle
E. Right pontine base
F. Left pontine base
G. Right medullary pyramid
H. Left medullary pyramid

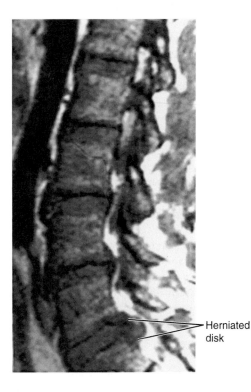

Herniated disk

28. A 48-year-old woman is brought to the emergency department with episodes of intense, stabbing pain that radiates down her left leg. She is suffering from a cold, and the pain is made worse when she coughs. Upon questioning, she adds that the outside (lateral aspect) of her left calf intermittently tingles and feels numb. Examination reveals that passively raising the leg 30 degrees from the supine position elicits excruciating pain. The accompanying MRI confirms that she has a herniated disk. It is most likely that this disk is compressing the nerve root exiting between which of the following pairs of vertebrae?

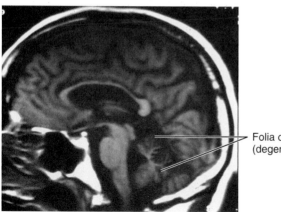

Folia of vermis (degenerated)

30. A 57-year-old man is brought to the emergency department after falling at home. He is observed to walk with a particularly wide-based gait and is very unstable, almost falling on several occasions. Attempts at a heel-to-shin maneuver reveal little coordination of the lower extremities. Finger-to-nose coordination tests are performed with little difficulty. The accompanying MRI shows degeneration of the vermis and anterior lobe of the cerebellum. Which of the following is most likely given these findings?

A. Friedreich ataxia
B. Progressive supranuclear palsy
C. Alcoholic cerebellar degeneration
D. Korsakoff psychosis
E. Tabes dorsalis

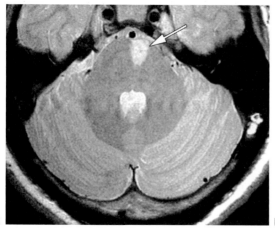

R   L

31. A 61-year-old man is brought to the emergency department with weakness of the right arm and leg. A Babinski sign is obtained on the right; the left planter reflex is normal. There is a tremor in his right arm on a finger-to-nose maneuver. There is paralysis of the left eye on left lateral gaze. The accompanying MRI, obtained 4 days after admission, shows an area of ischemic damage (arrow). A penetrating branch of which of the following vessels is most likely occluded in this individual?

A. Anterior inferior cerebellar artery
B. Anterior spinal artery
C. Basilar artery
D. Posterior cerebral artery
E. Posterior inferior cerebellar artery
F. Superior cerebellar artery

32. A 72-year-old man is treated with vincristine for Kaposi sarcoma. After several treatments, the patient begins to complain of numbness, tingling, and weakness in his lower legs and feet. Ankle reflexes are 1+ bilaterally. Patellar reflexes are 1+ on the right and 2+ on the left. Which of the following is the most likely explanation for the side effects of vincristine?

A. Compromise of the vascular supply to the extremities
B. Demyelination of the long tracts within the spinal cord
C. Disruption of the neuronal cytoskeleton
D. Disruption of slow anterograde transport

33. A 62-year-old man is brought to the emergency department with right arm weakness. He has a 10-year treatment history for high blood pressure, although he has had periods of noncompliance. Examination reveals weakness of the right hand with reduced tone in the arm. Triceps and biceps reflexes are graded 1+ on the right and 2+ on the left. The weakness remains unresolved 48 hours later. Vision, speech, and sensation from the face and body are all normal. Which of the following is the most likely cause of his symptoms?

A. Transient ischemic attack involving the left cerebral hemisphere

    B. Lacunar infarct in the posterior limb of the left internal capsule

    C. Cerebral infarct following occlusion of the left middle cerebral artery

    D. Brainstem infarction following occlusion of the posterior inferior cerebellar artery

34. A 13-month-old girl was brought to the emergency department with impaired consciousness and irregular breathing. A CT scan of her head revealed a subdural hematoma. Funduscopic exam showed retinal hemorrhages. A history reveals two previous trips to the emergency department, one of which was precipitated by an apparent fall down a flight of stairs, which resulted in severe bruising of the arms and the back of the head. Which of the following is the most likely cause of these findings?

    A. Fall from a high chair

    B. *Streptococcus pneumoniae* bacterial meningitis

    C. Herpes simplex virus type 1 encephalitis

    D. Shaken baby syndrome

    E. Infantile spasms

35. A 27-year-old man is seen in the emergency department after falling from a 16-ft extension ladder. He is treated and appears to recover completely. However, at his next physical, he is noted to have a minor head tilt to the left. A careful history and examination reveal that he tilts his head voluntarily in order to clear up some minor double vision. He reports that the double vision is worst when he attempts to look "down and in," as he must do when descending stairs. Damage to which of the following cranial nerves is most likely to be responsible for this double vision?

    A. Left oculomotor

    B. Right oculomotor

    C. Left trochlear

    D. Right trochlear

    E. Left abducens

    F. Right abducens

36. A 14-year-old boy has "drop attacks" (atonic seizures) that have not responded to drug therapy. On several occasions, he has fallen and sustained significant injury during a seizure. A complete callosotomy performed 6 months ago has significantly reduced the number and intensity of his seizures. Which of the following is most likely to be affected by the callosotomy?

    A. Ability to name verbally an object placed in the right hand

    B. Ability to name verbally an object placed in the left hand

    C. Ability to name verbally an object viewed with the right eye

    D. Ability to name verbally an object viewed with the left eye

37. An 88-year-old woman experiences a dizzy spell, falls, and is unable to rise, but summons help using a medical alert device. She is taken directly to the emergency department where she is found to be awake but very confused. Her level of consciousness and her ability to comprehend verbal instructions fluctuate over the next 18 hours. There are no focal sensory or motor findings. A family member is summoned who confirms that the woman has been previously healthy and lives alone without assistance. An emergent CT reveals some generalized brain atrophy. Which of the following is most likely given her symptoms?

    A. Alzheimer disease

    B. Huntington disease

    C. Multi-infarct dementia

    D. Systemic infection

38. An 87-year-old man is brought to the emergency department in a drowsy state. Examination reveals that he is obtunded with weakness in the left arm and leg. He has no obvious injuries. A CT scan reveals a mass over much of the right hemisphere consistent with hemorrhage. Family members report that he slipped on ice 3 weeks ago while getting in the car and bumped his head against the door frame. He had no signs of difficulty at that time and did not complain of headache. Which of the following is most likely given these findings?

A. Epidural hemorrhage
B. Subdural hemorrhage
C. Subarachnoid hemorrhage
D. Early signs of Alzheimer disease
E. Wernicke-Korsakoff syndrome

39. An 11-month-old girl with delayed development and mental retardation develops seizures and signs of brainstem dysfunction. A Dandy-Walker malformation is identified by MRI. A thorough history and interview is conducted with the mother. Maternal exposure to which of the following during pregnancy is considered a risk factor for Dandy-Walker malformation?
A. Alcohol
B. Folic acid
C. Lead
D. Mercury
E. Warfarin

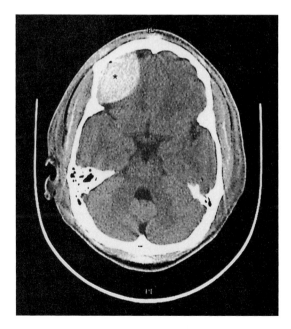

40. An unconscious 66-year-old man is brought to the emergency department after being struck in the head by a falling tree limb. He regains consciousness for several minutes and then loses consciousness again. An emergent CT taken upon his arrival (see image) reveals a skull fracture and a pool of blood (asterisk). Which of the following is the most likely source of the blood in the accompanying image?
A. Cerebral artery
B. Meningeal artery
C. Venous sinus
D. Bridging veins
E. Arteriovenous malformation

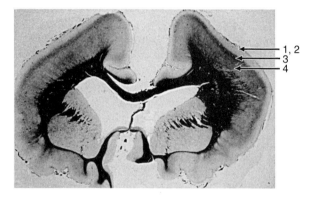

41. A 4-month-old girl is microcephalic and extremely developmentally delayed. She begins to suffer seizures that do not respond to medication. She dies at 13 months, an autopsy is performed, and brain sections are obtained. The accompanying myelin-stained section reveals four distinct layers within the region indicated. Which of the following developmental abnormalities is consistent with these findings?
A. Dandy-Walker syndrome
B. Holoprosencephaly
C. Lissencephaly
D. Megalencephaly
E. Polymicrogyria

42. A 29-year-old man is seen in the emergency department following a fall from a deck onto a concrete pavement. He reports that he had sudden weakness in his legs just before falling. Examination reveals weakness as well as diminished pain sensation in all four extremities. Proprioceptive sense is intact. Cranial nerve exam is normal. The patient is alert and oriented, but

the weakness progresses to flaccid paralysis of all four limbs. Deep tendon reflexes are absent, and a Babinski sign is present bilaterally. The history is positive for alcohol and cocaine use. Which of the following is the most likely cause of these findings?
A. Epidural hematoma
B. Infarct involving the anterior spinal artery at the level of the medulla
C. Infarct involving the anterior spinal artery at the level of the cervical spinal cord
D. Infarct involving a posterior spinal artery at the level of the cervical spinal cord
E. Acute inflammatory demyelinating disorder

43. A 39-year-old man is seen because of numbness and weakness in the hands and feet. Examination reveals bilateral internuclear ophthalmoplegia, hyperreflexia, and Babinski sign. A lumbar puncture shows elevated levels of myelin basic protein (MBP) in the CSF. MRI reveals periventricular plaques in the frontal and occipital horns of the lateral ventricles. Which of the following is the most likely cause of this disorder?
A. Amyotrophic lateral sclerosis
B. Poliomyelitis
C. Myasthenia gravis
D. Multiple sclerosis
E. Tabes dorsalis

44. A 78-year-old man seen for a routine physical exam is found to have gait instability, decreased speed of postural reflexes, and slowed reaction times. Vibration sensation is diminished. Six months later, he dies in an automobile accident. An autopsy reveals a loss of neurons, especially in the frontal and temporal lobes, the presence of neurofibrillary tangles, enlarged and calcified arachnoid granulations, and enlarged ventricles. Which of the following is most consistent with the history and autopsy findings?
A. Huntington disease
B. Korsakoff syndrome
C. Normal aging
D. Parkinson disease
E. Pick lobar atrophy

45. A 3-month-old boy is seen in the emergency department because of repeated episodes of vomiting. The mother reports that he has been irritable and has not been feeding. Examination reveals dilated scalp veins and disjoined sutures on palpation. There is hypertonia in both the upper and lower extremities. A CT scan confirms a diagnosis of hydrocephalus with expansion of the lateral and third ventricles. Which of the following is the most likely cause of this disorder?
A. Choroid plexus papilloma
B. Atresia of the arachnoid granulations
C. Obstruction of the cerebral aqueduct
D. Obstruction of the interventricular foramen
E. Atresia of the median and lateral apertures

46. A 62-year-old man suffers from chronic pain resulting from cancer to the head of the pancreas. He is legally using marijuana for relief of pain under a doctor's supervision. Which of the following is an endogenous ligand that acts upon the same CNS receptors as delta-9-tetrahydrocannabinol (THC), the active ingredient in marijuana?
A. Anandamide
B. Capsaicin
C. Enkephalin
D. Fatty acid amide hydroxylase

47. A 10-year-old girl is seen because of increasing episodes of apparent daydreaming in school. Although she had been an excellent student, her grades have declined over the last year. Her mother reports that she has frequent episodes of staring spells during which her eyes remain open, and her eyelids frequently flutter. Although each of these episodes lasts less than 10 seconds, she now has more than 500 of them per day. She is diagnosed with absence seizure disorder. Which of the following is the most likely additional finding?
A. Muscle twitches that begin in one hand, ascend through the arm, and eventually involve one side of her body
B. A 3-Hz spike-and-wave pattern in both cerebral hemispheres on EEG recording during a seizure

C. Muscle atonia causing her to fall and injure herself

D. Confusion and disorientation for up to half an hour after each seizure

48. A 45-year-old man is seen for an 8-week history of weakness in his arms and legs. Examination reveals a symmetric weakness in distal muscles of the arms and legs with hypotonia and hyporeflexia, with a lesser weakness of proximal musculature. Sensory testing reveals a mild paresthesia with a distal-to-proximal gradient. Electrodiagnostic testing shows segmental demyelination. A diagnosis of chronic inflammatory demyelinating polyradiculoneuro-pathy is made. Which of the following is most likely to occur as a result of a peripheral demye-linating disorder?

A. Sympathetic postganglionic fibers controlling heart rate and contractility are impaired.

B. Muscles of facial expression are weak or paralyzed.

C. Dull, burning pain sensation is lost, followed by a return of spontaneous, excruciating pain.

D. Vision is blurred.

49. A 57-year-old woman presents at the emergency department after awakening one morning with noticeable facial weakness. Her right nasolabial fold is somewhat flattened. She cannot maintain air in her right check against pressure, although her left is normal. Eye blink reflex is normal. When asked to raise her eyebrows and wrinkle her forehead, the movement is symmetric. Taste sensation is normal. Which of the following is the most likely site of the lesion responsible for the facial weakness?

A. Genu of left internal capsule

B. Genu of right internal capsule

C. Posterior limb of left internal capsule

D. Posterior limb of right internal capsule

E. Left facial nerve near the acoustic meatus

F. Right facial nerve near the acoustic meatus

G. Left facial nerve near the stylomastoid foramen

H. Right facial nerve near the stylomastoid foramen

50. An 8-year-old boy is seen in the emergency department because of dizziness and headaches and difficulty with walking, swallowing and speech, all of which occur only intermittently. A Dandy-Walker malformation is identified by MRI. Which of the following is the most likely finding shown on the MRI?

A. Smooth, agyric cerebral cortex

B. Syringomyelia, with the syrinx extending from C5 rostrally into the brainstem

C. Enlarged fourth ventricle and absent cerebellar vermis

D. Protrusion of the meningeal layers and underlying neural tissue in the lumbosacral region

E. Displacement of the cerebellar tonsils through the foramen magnum, extending over the cervical spinal cord

answers

1. **C** (nerve compression from an adjacent blood vessel) is correct. This case describes trigeminal neuralgia (tic douloureux), which typically presents with brief, intense, stabbing pain over one or more divisions of the trigeminal nerve. It is frequently caused by compression of the nerve by the anterior inferior cerebellar artery. The pain is usually limited to one side and can be triggered by cutaneous stimulation (e.g., touching the cheek, shaving, brushing teeth). Anticonvulsants (e.g., carbamazepine) and vascular microdecompression surgery are potential treatments.

A (nerve inflammation secondary to a bacterial infection, such as Lyme disease) is incorrect. A facial nerve paralysis (Bell palsy) is the most common cranial nerve finding associated with infection by the bacterium, *Borrelia burgdorferi*, that is responsible for Lyme disease.

B (nerve inflammation secondary to a viral infection such as herpes zoster) is incorrect. Herpes zoster (shingles), the reactivation of the chicken pox virus, can cause severe pain in the affected dermatome, but it is not brief, or elicited by touch. Characteristically, the skin of the infected dermatome will erupt with a vesicular rash during active expression. Postherpetic neuralgia may follow once the rash has resolved and may continue for a month or more.

D (hyperalgesia associated with temporal arteritis) is incorrect. The pain of temporal arteritis presents as tenderness over the temporal artery. It is more common in women, and risk increases with age, with most cases developing after age 50 years. Primary complaints are headache and visual loss.

2. **C** (anterior roots at L2, L3, and L4 on the right side) is correct. Axons of lower motor neurons travel through the anterior spinal roots. Damage to the axons results in LMN signs, including flaccid paralysis and areflexia. Over time, the denervated muscle will atrophy.

A (spinal cord hemisection at T12 on the right side) is incorrect. This represents an upper motor neuron lesion for the right leg. It would damage the axons of upper motor neurons as they descend through the lateral funiculus of the spinal cord en route to lower motor neuron targets in the lumbar anterior horn. Chronic UMN lesion signs include spastic paralysis and hyperreflexia. Acute signs include flaccid paralysis and areflexia. The plantar reflex would be abnormal, revealing up-going toes (Babinski). However, a spinal hemisection also disrupts vibration, proprioception, and fine touch from the ipsilateral body below the lesion and pain and temperature from the contralateral body below the lesion.

B (posterior roots at L2, L3, and L4 on the right side) is incorrect. Posterior roots carry sensory, not motor axons.

D (lateral funiculus of spinal cord at midthoracic level on the right side) is incorrect. This represents an upper motor neuron lesion for the right leg. Chronic UMN lesion signs include spastic paralysis and hyperreflexia. Acute signs include flaccid paralysis and areflexia. The plantar reflex would be abnormal, revealing up-going toes (Babinski).

E (medullary pyramids on the right side) is incorrect. This represents an upper motor neuron lesion that would affect the left leg.

3. **B** (Dandy-Walker malformation) is correct. Dandy-Walker malformations are a group of malformations resulting from disruptions in the development of the brainstem and cerebellum, probably related to the migration of the rhombic lip. The term is generally applied to malformations showing a triad of changes: (1) partial or complete agenesis of the cerebellar vermis, with anterior rotation; (2) dilation of the fourth ventricle; and (3) enlarged posterior fossa with superior displacement of the tentorium.

A (Chiari malformation) is incorrect. Chiari malformations are downward displacements of the cerebellum. Chiari type I refers to a developmental downward deviation of the cerebellar tonsils (as distinct from a pressure-gradient–induced tonsillar herniation). Chiari type II refers to an extrusion of the vermis of the cerebellum downward over the cervical spinal cord.

C (lissencephaly) is incorrect. This word, meaning "smooth brain" refers to a defect in neuronal migration that yields an agyric cerebral cortex in which the normal six neocortical layers have been reduced to four.

D (myelomeningocele) is incorrect. This developmental defect results when the caudal neural tube does not fully close during developmental days 26 to 28. It is recognized as a protrusion of the meningeal layers and underlying neural tissue in the lumbosacral region.

E (syringomyelia) is incorrect. Syringomyelia is a cystic cavitation of the central canal of the spinal cord. It is associated with Chiari type I malformations, in which case it is most likely

to occur in the midcervical region. Cystic enlargements in the lumbar region are less common, but do occur.

4. **D** (right superior quadrant anopsia) is correct. Right-sided visual field deficits reflect damage to the left side of the brain. The superior quadrant is carried in axons of Meyer loop that sweep forward through the temporal lobe and around the inferior horn of the lateral ventricle. These anopsias are sometimes referred to as "pie in the sky."

A (left inferior quadrant anopsia) and **C** (left superior quadrant anopsia) are incorrect. Damage in the left brain would cause a right-sided visual field defect.

B (right inferior quadrant anopsia) is incorrect. A tumor in the temporal lobe that also causes a visual field deficit would most likely compress axons of Meyer loop. These axons of the optic radiation swing anteriorly around the inferior horn of the lateral ventricle and carry input from the contralateral superior visual field of both eyes.

5. **C** (loss of cholinergic neurons in the basal forebrain) is correct. The case describes Alzheimer disease (AD), a progressive dementia characterized by memory loss and additional disturbances, including difficulty in acquiring new information, disorientation, difficulty with activities of daily living, apraxias, paranoia, and disrupted sleep cycle. AD is characterized by the loss of cholinergic neurons in the basal nucleus (of Meynert). Treatment options include the acetylcholinesterase inhibitors to increase the levels of acetylcholine in the brain.

A (decreased acetylcholinesterase in the cerebral cortex) is incorrect. Acetylcholinesterase is responsible for metabolizing acetylcholine in the synapse into choline and acetyl CoA. Current therapy for AD is centrally acting acetylcholinesterase inhibitors, although their benefit appears to be minimal, particularly as the disorder advances.

B (antibodies to nicotinic cholinergic receptors in the cerebral cortex) is incorrect. However, the case described, Alzheimer disease, is not linked to any type of nAChR antibody.

D (Lewy bodies in the pars compacta of the substantia nigra) is incorrect. Lewy bodies, which contain deposits of the protein α-synuclein, are found in the brains of both Parkinson and Alzheimer patients. Although they are primarily found in the substantia nigra of individuals with PD, they are widely distributed in patients with AD, such as the woman in this case.

E (decreased levels of GABA in the striatum and substantia nigra) is incorrect. The case describes Alzheimer disease. The neurotransmitter most closely associated with AD is ACh. GABA is an important neurotransmitter throughout the CNS. It is the major neurotransmitter used in communication within the basal ganglia. Atrophy of striatum in Huntington disease reflects loss of some of these GABAergic neurons. Dementia is a late finding in Huntington disease.

6. **D** (absence) is correct. Childhood absence epilepsy (petit mal) might be mistaken for inattention or for another type of seizure. It is not uncommon for a child with absence seizures to also have tonic–clonic seizures. However, the 3-Hz spike-and-wave pattern and the ability to induce through hyperventilation are not associated with other seizure types. The lack of postictal confusion is common with AE and uncommon with complex partial and tonic–clonic seizures.

A (complex partial) is incorrect. Complex partial seizures do involve alteration in consciousness. However, they do not produce the characteristic 3-Hz EEG finding bilaterally. The lack of postictal confusion is uncommon in complex partial seizure.

B (pseudoseizure) is incorrect. Pseudoseizure (nonepileptic seizure disorder) can have various presentations and can occur in individuals who also suffer from a seizure disorder. However, pseudoseizure has no organic cause and is not accompanied by changes in EEG pattern during or after the seizure episode.

C (tonic–clonic) is incorrect. This is a generalized seizure and is the most common type of seizure. It differs in several ways from the case described. Some warning before the seizure (prodromal symptoms) is common, as is postictal coma followed by confusion. The seizure itself may begin with bilateral muscle contractions that evolve into tonic contractions, with trunk flexion followed by body extension (tonic phase) that gives way to periods of alternating contraction and atonia (clonic phase). Tongue biting, incontinence, and injury related to falling are possible.

E (simple partial) is incorrect. This is a focal seizure that will not exhibit bilateral EEG changes. A simple seizure can produce sensory, motor, or psychic experience, but it does not cause alteration in consciousness.

7. **B** (Pick lobar atrophy) is correct. The case describes Pick disease, a progressive dementia characterized by memory loss and additional disturbances including speech that can be halting and dysarthric (progressive nonfluent aphasia), and marked difficulty naming objects (they can describe an object, but not name it). The pathognomonic feature is the profound degeneration in the frontal lobes and temporal poles. Histologic preparations would usually show Pick bodies (tangles of tau proteins) in affected brain cells. There are no known effective treatments for this progressive disorder.

A (Alzheimer disease) is incorrect. This is also a progressive dementia, but is characterized by lobar atrophy in most regions of the brain (particularly frontal, parietal, and temporal lobes), memory, difficulty in acquiring new information, disorientation, difficulty with activities of daily living, apraxias, paranoia, and disrupted sleep cycle. AD is characterized by the loss of cholinergic neurons in the basal nucleus (of Meynert).

C (multiple system atrophy) is incorrect. This group of Parkinson-like disorders is exemplified by olivopontocerebellar atrophy. Individuals usually have impaired motor abilities with depression. Actual dementia is rare.

D (progressive supranuclear palsy) is incorrect. This is also known as a Parkinson-plus syndrome. Individuals usually have the slowness of movement, rigidity, and cognitive impairment common in Parkinson disease, but do not have the tremor. The basal ganglia (diencephalon and midbrain) show the most profound loss of neurons and corresponding gliosis.

8. **D** (block release of acetylcholine at the neuromuscular junction) is correct. Botulinum toxin *(Clostridium botulinum)* is endocytosed by nerve terminals. It interferes with synaptic proteins required for vesicle docking and transmitter release, including VAMP (vesicle associated membrane protein, synaptobrevin), SNAP-25 (synaptosomal-associated protein, 25-KD), and syntaxin-1.

A (activate the same sensory pathway that the light touch activated, but at a central synapse) is incorrect. Sensory activation does seem to relieve some dystonias, for unknown reasons. Botulinum toxin does not act here, but at the neuromuscular junction.

B (decrease the basal ganglia output responsible for the dystonia) is incorrect. Botulinum toxin acts at the neuromuscular junction to relieve the muscle contraction of dystonia. There is, however, evidence that basal ganglia do play a role in some types of dystonia. For

instance, mutations in the *DYT1* gene, which codes for the protein torsion A, underlie early-onset torsion dystonia, a disorder related to basal ganglia dysfunction.

C (inhibit cell bodies in the anterior horn of the cervical spinal cord) is incorrect. Botulinum toxin acts on lower motor neurons, but at the neuromuscular junction, not at the soma, to relieve the muscle contraction of dystonia.

E (block acetylcholine receptors at the neuromuscular junction) is incorrect. Botulinum toxin acts presynaptically at the neuromuscular junction. Toxins like curare act postsynaptically to block ACh receptors on the motor end plate.

9. **A** (hepatolenticular degeneration) is correct. This case describes Wilson disease, an autosomal recessive disorder that results in increased deposits of copper in the brain (lenticular nuclei as well as other regions) and liver. Hallmarks of the disease include movement disorders (Parkinson-like symptoms), "wing-beating" tremor, and the yellow-brown ring around the cornea (Kayser-Fleischer ring). Treatment involves decreasing copper intake and increasing copper excretion (using copper-chelating agents).

B (striatonigral degeneration) is incorrect. Striatonigral degeneration is seen in Parkinson disease, which is characterized by tremor, rigidity, bradykinesia or akinesia, and postural instability (mnemonic: TRAP). Tremor in PD is "pill-rolling" instead of the postural (wing-beating) tremor seen in Wilson disease.

C (excessive disposition of iron in the globus pallidus) is incorrect. Excessive deposits of iron (not the excess copper deposition seen in Wilson disease) is a feature of a rare autosomal recessive disorder (Hallervorden-Spatz disease). Rigidity and abnormal tone are early clinical findings.

D (excessive deposition of inorganic lead in the cerebral cortex) is incorrect. Developing brain is a target for lead poisoning. Early signs of lead poisoning include changes in behavior, memory loss, and seizure. Tremor is not associated with this disorder.

10. **A** (restless leg syndrome) is correct. RLS is diagnosed by four criteria: discomfort or paresthesia in one or more extremities that produce a strong desire to move, symptoms that are exacerbated by inactivity and relieved by movement, symptoms that are worse at night, and motor restlessness. It may be a primary condition or secondary to another condition, such as end-stage renal failure. The cause of the primary condition is unknown. Some cases appear to have a genetic component. Treatments range from hot or cold compresses to various drug therapies.

B (fibromyalgia) is incorrect. This is a syndrome of chronic soft tissue pain with pain on pressure at specific points on the body. Some individuals do report paresthesias, and a subset of those diagnosed with FM may also be diagnosed with RLS.

C (sleep apnea) is incorrect. Sleep apnea is the cessation of breathing during sleep. Obstructive sleep apnea is the most common type and the most common cause of excessive daytime sleepiness. It is particularly common in thick-necked heavyset individuals and can be successfully treated in some by positive airway pressure supplied by a mask during sleep or by surgery (e.g., to remove tonsils, uvula, or soft palate tissue).

D (narcolepsy) is incorrect. Narcolepsy is the second most commonly diagnosed cause of excessive daytime sleepiness. It is a neurologic disorder that is believed to represent superimposition of aspects of REM sleep (e.g., paralysis, dreaming) on the waking state. There are aspects of the disorder that occur during the waking hours. These include loss of motor control (cataplexy) rather than constant movement.

E (REM sleep disorder) is incorrect. In this disorder, the paralysis of voluntary movement that accompanies REM sleep is lost, and the individual moves, even acting out dreams, during REM sleep.

11. **D** (Increased dopaminergic activity in the striatum) is correct. This case describes Tourette syndrome, a disorder that is initially characterized by simple motor tics (usually involving the face and head), simple vocal tics (e.g., hissing, snorting) and behavioral changes. Complex motor tics (compulsive movements) and vocal tics (e.g., shouting obscenities) can also occur. The disorder is thought to result from either supersensitivity of DA receptors in the striatum or hyperinnervation of DA terminals in the striatum. Neuroleptics are effective in treating the tics.

A (decreased serotonergic activity in the cerebral cortex) and **B** (increased serotonergic activity in the cerebral cortex) are incorrect. Serotonin, derived from the raphe nuclei in the pons, is thought to be involved in the regulation of arousal. It has no known effect on motor activity.

C (decreased dopaminergic activity in the striatum) is incorrect. Increased motor activity would result from increased (not decreased) dopamine activity in the striatum. DA receptor antagonists and DA-depleting drugs are used to treat Tourette syndrome.

E (decrease in acetylcholinesterase activity in the basal forebrain) is incorrect. Decreased acetylcholinesterase in basal forebrain is seen in Alzheimer disease, a progressive dementia that is characterized by memory loss, disorientation, and difficulty with daily living activities. AD is characterized by the loss of cholinergic neurons in the basal nucleus (of Meynert); motor function is either preserved or reduced.

12. **B** (B) is correct. The case describes Huntington disease, an autosomal dominant genetic disorder that causes early mood changes, including irritability and depression, followed by uncontrolled choreoathetotic movement, and eventually by dementia and death. The caudate nucleus and the putamen (B) of the basal ganglia atrophy as a part of this disease, which accounts for the uncontrolled limb movements.

A (A) is incorrect. This is within the motor region of cortex. Damage here would cause paresis or spastic paralysis of only the lower portion of the leg and foot.

C (C) is incorrect. This is the thalamus. Because sensory, cerebellar, and basal ganglia inputs all relay through the thalamus, damage to the thalamus can produce sensory and motor findings. However, the case described is Huntington disease, which produces atrophy of the striatum but not of the thalamus.

D (D) is incorrect. This is the globus pallidus of the basal ganglia. Huntington disease is a disease affecting the basal ganglia, but it does not cause atrophy of the GP.

E (E) is incorrect. This is the cerebellum. Damage to a cerebellar hemisphere would produce motor findings that would include loss of coordinated movement, decomposition of movement, and intention tremor. It would not produce involuntary flinging of the arms and legs.

13. **B** (stiff-person syndrome) is correct. Stiff-person syndrome is an autoimmune disorder that is related to the production of autoantibodies to glutamic acid decarboxylase, the enzyme responsible for the production of GABA. Decreasing the levels of GABA results in a disinhibition of the central nervous system and a corresponding increase in motor outflow, leading to muscle stiffness or spasms in the axial and proximal limb muscles.

A (Huntington disease) is incorrect. HD is an autosomal dominant genetic disorder that causes early mood changes, including irritability and depression, followed by uncontrolled choreoathetotic movement, and eventually by dementia and death.

C (Parkinson disease) is incorrect. PD is the result of degeneration of dopaminergic neurons (not GABAergic neurons) in the substantia nigra with subsequent loss of dopamine released into the caudate and putamen. The hallmark signs of PD are resting tremor, rigidity ("lead-pipe" or "cog-wheel"), and bradykinesia.

D (progressive supranuclear palsy) is incorrect. This is a Parkinson-plus syndrome that is characterized by slowness of movement, rigidity, and cognitive impairment (similar to Parkinson disease). Dopaminergic, cholinergic, and adrenergic transmitter systems (not GABA) are all affected in this disorder.

E (Friedreich ataxia) is incorrect. FA causes progressive limb and gait ataxia with loss of tendon reflexes rather than rigidity. Dysarthria and dysphagia are later symptoms. Most individuals are wheelchair bound by the third decade. The signs are due to loss of large myelinated axons, both sensory and motor, within the spinal cord and spinal roots. FA is an autosomal recessive disorder, resulting from a GAA trinucleotide repeat on chromosome 9. Although rare, it is the most common inherited ataxia.

14. **E** (medial temporal lobe) is correct. Seizures involving the hippocampus, parahippocampus, and amygdala of the temporal lobe may produce déjà vu. These may be classified as psychic simple partial seizures or, if consciousness is impaired, complex partial seizures.

A (hypothalamus) is incorrect. Hypothalamic activation could produce autonomic signs, but most autonomic seizures originate from the temporal lobe.

B (anterior calcarine sulcus) is incorrect. Seizures involving association visual cortex are likely to produce complex visual hallucinations.

C (orbitofrontal cortex) is incorrect. Seizures originating in orbitofrontal cortex may spread through the uncinate fasciculus to the piriform cortex of the temporal lobe. These may cause unpleasant olfactory hallucinations (e.g., burning rubber or sugar).

D (precentral gyrus) is incorrect. This is the primary motor strip. Seizure activity confined within this region will be a simple motor (Jacksonian march) seizure. These clonic contractions move across the body in a manner that reflects the passage of the uncontrolled electrical activity over the motor homunculus. The perioral region and great toe are common starting points for such seizures.

15. **D** (redistribution of Na+ channels within demyelinated region of the axons) is correct. The case describes CNS findings including the lesions apparent on MRI and the internuclear ophthalmoplegia (INO) on left lateral gaze. These are consistent with multiple sclerosis, a CNS demyelinating disorder. Within myelinated axons, voltage-gated Na+ channels are localized at the nodes of Ranvier. This localization is due to complex interactions between the axon and the myelinating oligodendrocyte. If the oligodendrocyte is removed by MS, and the localizing signal is removed, redistribution of these ion channels occurs, channels now appear in the internodal space, and the axon once again conducts action potentials down its full length.

A (sprouting of small-diameter unmyelinated fibers, which innervate muscles formerly innervated by larger myelinated fibers) is

incorrect. The case describes multiple sclerosis, a CNS demyelinating disorder. Nothing in it directly relates to muscle innervation. It is true that if a subpopulation of lower motor neurons is lost, leaving some muscle fibers denervated, lower motor neurons innervating adjacent muscle fibers may sprout new branches to innervate the denervated fibers. These, however, are additional large, myelinated branches.

B (regrowth of myelin by Schwann cells) is incorrect. The case describes multiple sclerosis, a CNS demyelinating disorder. Oligodendrocytes, not Schwann cells, provide CNS myelin.

C (depolarization in membrane potential due to decreased numbers of K+ channels) is incorrect. The case describes multiple sclerosis, a CNS demyelinating disorder. The major problem stems from the inability of demyelinated axons to conduct action potentials, not from an inability of portions of the membrane to reach threshold.

16. **E** (conduction aphasia) is correct. This describes conduction aphasia, which is characterized by difficulty with spontaneous speech (missing words and inserting nonwords) and the inability to repeat words or phrases. Speech is fluent, and comprehension is intact. Damage involves the arcuate fasciculus of the left hemisphere, which connects the receptive language (Wernicke) area with the expressive language (Broca) area and surrounding cortex.

A (expressive aphasia) is incorrect. Expressive (Broca) aphasia is characterized by a nonfluent aphasia word-finding difficulty, telegraphic speech, and few words produced. There is difficulty with repeating words/phrases and naming. Comprehension is good. Damage is in the left dorsolateral frontal lobe, in the region of the operculum.

B (transcortical sensory aphasia) is incorrect. Transcortical sensory aphasia is characterized by difficulty with comprehension and word meaning, whereas speech is relatively fluent. Repetition and naming are preserved. Damage generally involves the left parietal lobe in the region of the angular gyrus.

C (transcortical motor aphasia) is incorrect. Transcortical motor aphasia is similar to expressive aphasia (speech is nonfluent), except that repeating words and phrases is preserved. Damage is usually in the left medial frontal region.

D (receptive aphasia) is incorrect. Receptive (Wernicke) aphasia is characterized by difficulty with language comprehension. Speech is fluent, although there is difficulty with repeating words/phrases and word finding. Damage is in the posterior superior temporal lobe of the left hemisphere.

17. **D** (syringomyelia) is correct. In syringomyelia, a cyst or cavitation of the central canal of the spinal cord forms. It is more common at the cervical level as seen in this case, but lumbar cysts are possible. It can follow many types of injury, including those resulting from meningitis or from trauma. Many cases are associated with a congenital Chiari type I malformation, in which the inferior cerebellum becomes displaced downward. Because the cyst begins centrally, the axons of the anterior white commissure of the spinal cord are destroyed, resulting in segmental loss of pain and temperature. If the cavitation extends anterolaterally, it may destroy lower motor neurons, causing the observed weakness and fasciculations.

A (amyotrophic lateral sclerosis [motor neuron disease]) is incorrect. ALS does not present with sensory findings. It is diagnosed when both upper and lower motor neuron lesion signs appear in the same muscle mass. In the case described, there are no upper motor neuron findings.

B (acute inflammatory demyelinating polyradiculoneuropathy [Guillain-Barré

disease]) is incorrect. AIDP is an acute syndrome affecting peripheral nerves and causing severe weakness, sensory loss, and autonomic findings. It is acute, taking only hours to days to develop and reaching maximum weakness and paralysis by the second or third week. A time course extending into weeks is classified as chronic inflammatory demyelinating polyradiculoneuropathy. The most common course is weakness beginning in the legs and ascending.

C (Lambert-Eaton myasthenic syndrome) is incorrect. LEMS is an autoimmune disorder affecting presynaptic voltage-gated calcium channels in the nerve terminals of lower motor neurons. It presents with weakness, but not with fasciculations, because the cell body and proximal roots are not affected. There is no sensory component. About half of LEMS cases are associated with cancer, especially small cell lung cancer.

18. **D** (flaccid paralysis of the right arm) is correct. Occlusion of the left middle cerebral artery affects much of the lateral convexity of the left hemisphere, including the motor cortex related to the right arm. An acute upper motor neuron lesion will result in initial flaccid paralysis.

A (deviation of the tongue to the left upon protrusion) is incorrect. The tongue will deviate to the weak side upon protrusion. Stroke in the field of the left middle cerebral artery affects the right body, including right side of tongue. The tongue will protrude to the right.

B (fasciculations in the right tongue) is incorrect. Fasciculations are a result of activation of motor units. Pathologically, they can indicate damage to lower motor neurons or to proximal motor roots. An occlusion of a middle cerebral artery results in upper motor neuron damage.

C (inability to wrinkle the right forehead) is incorrect. The portion of the facial motor nucleus that innervates the right forehead is under bilateral cortical control. Damage to upper motor neurons in the left motor cortex for face will cause weakness or paralysis of the right lower face, but the right upper face will be spared because upper motor neurons communicating from the right motor cortex to the right facial motor nucleus are still intact.

E (spastic paralysis of the right arm) is incorrect. Occlusion of the left middle cerebral artery affects much of the lateral convexity of the left hemisphere, including the motor cortex related to the right arm. However, during the acute phase, an upper motor neuron lesion will result in initial flaccid paralysis, not spastic paralysis.

19. **B** (left parietal cortex) is correct. Discrete lesions of somatosensory cortex in the parietal lobe may cause astereognosis, the inability to recognize objects by feel, without loss of sensation. This will often be accompanied by some hemi-neglect or extinction of simultaneous stimulation, such that she may not report a touch to the right hand if it is accompanied by a simultaneous touch to the left hand.

A (left frontal cortex) is incorrect. The posterior frontal cortex is more important to motor than to sensory function. The prefrontal cortex is important to higher executive functions, such as inhibition of inappropriate behaviors.

C (left ventral posterior lateral thalamic nucleus) is incorrect. Damage to the VPL would be expected to cause reduction or loss of all somatic sensations from the contralateral arm and leg.

D (left medial lemniscus) is incorrect. Damage to this tract would result in reduction or loss of sensation from the contralateral arm and

leg. If the medial lemniscus is damaged within the rostral pons or midbrain, the contralateral face will also be affected. A lesion affecting the medial lemniscus in the more caudal pons could also affect the trigeminal nucleus on that side, resulting in loss of sensation from the ipsilateral face (all sensation) and contralateral body (fine touch, vibration, proprioception).

E (right fasciculus cuneatus) is incorrect. Fasciculus cuneatus carries fine touch, vibration, and proprioceptive sensation from the ipsilateral upper body (T6 and above). Damage to this tract would affect these sensations from the right hand.

20. **B** (aspects of learning) is correct. Although some tasks related to learning and memory may be relatively unaffected by callosotomy (e.g., verbal conjunction tests), others (e.g., paired associate tests) are impaired. Callosotomy may affect the storage of information as well as its later retrieval; both steps are necessary to successful learning.

A (generation of brain waves) is incorrect. Brain waves, as measured by EEG, reflect the underlying activity of neurons that lie between the two EEG leads. Each hemisphere continues to generate its own waves of activity, even in the absence of the corpus callosum, although the pattern of some waves will change, reflecting the loss of interhemispheric communication.

C (use of language) is incorrect. Complete callosotomy will produce a permanent sensory dissociation because visual, auditory, or tactile experiences presented to the nondominant hemisphere will not have access to the language-dominant (usually left) hemisphere. However, basic use of language can survive callosotomy.

D (maintenance of posture) is incorrect. Various forms of a loss of ability to maintain posture may follow damage to specific motor systems, but none are related to damage to the corpus callosum. Callosal apraxia, generally limited to the left hand, is an expected disorder of motor function following callosotomy.

21. **C** (difficulty locating sounds on the right) is correct. The medial geniculate nucleus is the relay nucleus of the thalamus projecting to primary auditory cortex (temporal lobe). Although the MGN receives auditory input from both ears, the predominant input is from the contralateral side, hence the loss of sound localization and not deafness.

A (right homonymous hemianopsia) is incorrect. Visual information to occipital cortex is relayed through the lateral geniculate (not the medial geniculate) nucleus. A contralateral homonymous hemianopsia can result from damage to either the optic tract (more likely) or the complete optic radiation (less likely).

B (loss of sensation from right side of the face) is incorrect. Sensation from the face is relayed through the ventral posteromedial (not the medial geniculate) nucleus of the thalamus. Damage to VPM can result in a loss of all sensation from the contralateral face.

D (loss of vibration sense from right side of the body) is incorrect. Vibration sensation from the body is carried by the posterior columns/medial lemniscal system. Information is relayed through the ventral postero-lateral (not the medial geniculate) nucleus of the thalamus to primary sensory cortex. Damage to VPL can result in loss of all sensation (pain, temperature, touch, vibration and position sense) from the contralateral body.

22. **B** (amyotrophic lateral sclerosis) is correct. Sporadic ALS is the most common acquired motor neuron disease, accounting for up to 80% of all such motor neuron diseases. It causes degeneration of both upper motor

neurons (e.g., pyramidal neurons of the cerebral cortex) and lower motor neurons (e.g., anterior horn neurons of spinal cord). Degeneration of the motor neuron cell bodies leads to loss of corticospinal tracts and anterior spinal roots. The afflicted individual presents with both upper motor neuron signs (hyperreflexia, spasticity, Babinski sign) and lower motor neuron signs (fasciculations, weakness, muscle atrophy).

A (Schwannoma) is incorrect. A schwannoma is a tumor of Schwann cells and, as such, involves only peripheral nerves. Commonly, schwannomas arise on the vestibular portion of CN VIII, although they can occur on other cranial and spinal nerve bundles. A schwannoma causes local compression and can be expected to produce local signs. These may be both sensory and motor, but will only involve lower motor neuron findings because only peripheral nerves are myelinated by Schwann cells.

C (myasthenia gravis) is incorrect. MG is an autoimmune disorder affecting nicotinic acetylcholine receptors at the neuromuscular junction. As expected of a postsynaptic disorder of the neuromuscular junction, it presents with weakness that increases with repeated activity. Ptosis and dysarthria are often early findings. Respiratory muscles can be affected; a myasthenic crisis will cause acute respiratory insufficiency and may require intubation. There will be no muscle atrophy and no upper motor neuron findings. The short-acting acetylcholinesterase inhibitor, edrophonium, rapidly reverses weakness of MG (edrophonium test), but other types of weakness also reverse to edrophonium. Electrodiagnostic testing using repetitive nerve stimulation will reveal a decrease in compound muscle action potential (CMAP).

D (Lambert-Eaton myasthenic syndrome) is incorrect. LEMS is an autoimmune disorder affecting voltage-gated calcium channels at the presynaptic terminal of the neuromuscular junction. It is rare and most commonly associated with small cell lung cancer. As expected of a presynaptic disorder of the neuromuscular junction, it presents with weakness that improves with repeated activity. This can be revealed by an increase in a hypoactive reflex following contraction of the tested muscle groups.

23. **A** (apolipoprotein E ε4) is correct. The individual has a history that is consistent with a diagnosis of Alzheimer disease. The APOE e4 allele is considered a risk factor for development of sporadic AD in a dose-dependent fashion, with two alleles conferring greater risk than a single allele. Conversely, APOE e3 is associated with a decreased risk for AD. However, presence of even two copies of the APOE e4 allele does not guarantee that an individual will develop AD, and sporadic AD also occurs in individuals without this allele.

B (abnormal huntingtin protein) is incorrect. Abnormal huntingtin protein is associated with Huntington disease. Early signs of HD include changes in personality, irritability, and depression. Motor signs, especially choreoathetotic movements, become apparent as the disease progresses. MRI will eventually reveal atrophy of the putamen and caudate nuclei, with concomitant enlargement of the lateral ventricles.

C (abnormal parkin protein) is incorrect. Normal parkin protein functions as a ubiquitin ligase, targeting specific proteins for degradation and removal from the cell. Mutation to the parkin gene, allowing ubiquitin-tagged proteins to accumulate and clump, is thought to be involved in the onset of certain forms of Parkinson disease. Cardinal features associated with PD include bradykinesia, rigidity, tremor (resting), and postural instability. Activities of daily living are affected in that they may

become slowed. PD is, on occasion, accompanied by dementia. However, subcortical dementias are not associated with apraxias.

D (abnormal prion protein) is incorrect. Prion diseases (transmissible spongiform encephalopathies) are a group of rare infectious diseases resulting when a normal prion protein (with alpha helix configuration) is induced to adopt an abnormal (β-pleated sheet) conformation. Several diseases have been described (e.g., Creutzfeldt-Jakob disease, fatal familial insomnia, Gerstmann-Sträussler-Scheinker syndrome, and kuru). The most common human prion disease, CJD, is still extremely rare, affecting as few as one person per million. Time course is generally very rapid, with the time from diagnosis to death less than 1 year in most cases. Myoclonus is observed in up to 90% of confirmed cases, and upper motor neuron signs are common. CJD also exhibits an identifiable periodic sharp wave complex on EEG.

24. **B** (median nerve) is correct. The nocturnal paresthesias are the most common finding with median nerve compression, better known as carpal tunnel syndrome (CTS). Tingling over the second, third, and fourth digits can frequently be elicited in CTS by tapping the region of the median nerve at the wrist (Tinel sign). Fourth-finger sensory innervation is split between the median and ulnar nerves, and presence of paresthesia only on the lateral aspect of the fourth finger can distinguish between CTS and malingering.

A (brachial plexus) is incorrect. Brachial plexus compression, which could be a component of thoracic outlet syndrome, compromises function of sensory and motor portions of both the medial and ulnar nerves.

C (radial nerve) is incorrect. Radial nerve compression is more likely to be acute than chronic. In addition, major findings are generally motor and include weakness on extension of the fingers and wrist. A compression of the superficial radial nerve may occur at the wrist (e.g., due to a tight wrist band or watch strap or to handcuffing), but the territory of this nerve is the dorsum of the hand, not the second through fourth digits.

D (ulnar nerve) is incorrect. Signs of ulnar compressive neuropathies may include paresthesia and weakness involving much of the hand, dorsally and ventrally, especially medially. Paresthesia will include the fifth digit and the medial aspect of the fourth finger (i.e., the regions not affected by carpal tunnel syndrome). Hand weakness is common. The ulnar nerve can be compressed within the condylar groove or in the cubital tunnel. These compressions may occur after lengthy periods of elbow flexion (i.e., during sleep) or leaning on the elbows.

25. **E** (decreased proprioceptive sensation from the right leg) is correct. Fasciculus gracilis, within the posterior columns, carries fine touch, proprioception, and vibration sensation from the ipsilateral lower body and leg (starting at about T6).

A (dysmetria in the right arm) and **B** (dysmetria in the left arm) are incorrect. Dysmetrias are errors in trajectory or end point in a movement and represent an inability to produce coordinated muscle activity to stop a movement. They result from cerebellar dysfunction. In addition, it is fasciculus cuneatus (not gracilis) that carries sensory input from the arms.

C (decreased pain sensation from the right leg) and **D** (decreased pain sensation from the left leg) are incorrect. Pain is transmitted primarily in the anterolateral spinal cord, whereas fasciculus gracilis and cuneatus of the posterior columns carry fine touch, vibration, and proprioceptive input.

F (decreased proprioceptive sensation from the left leg) is incorrect. Proprioception from the leg travels in the ipsilateral (not the contralateral) fasciculus gracilis.

26. **B** (inflammation of the left facial nerve from a viral infection) is correct. Damage (e.g., inflammation) to the facial nerve can result in loss of taste on the anterior two thirds of the tongue and a reduced stapedial reflex (inability to dampen loud noises). It can also compromise the corneal reflex because the lid muscles responsible for the blink response are supplied by the facial nerve. Facial nerve paralysis (Bell palsy) will also cause general weakness of the muscles of facial expression in the ipsilateral face. This could be revealed by an asymmetric smile, a flattened nasolabial fold, and inability to wrinkle the ipsilateral forehead.

A (acute trauma to the face damaging the ophthalmic division of the left trigeminal nerve) is incorrect. The ophthalmic division of the trigeminal nerve is responsible for sensation from upper face, including conjunctiva, cornea, forehead, eyelid, bridge of nose, dura, and vessels in the anterior brain. Damage to the ophthalmic division of the trigeminal nerve could account for a compromised corneal reflex, but the corneal reflex would be weak for both eyes when the left cornea is touched, whereas both eyes would show a normal blink in response to touch to the right cornea. This damage would not account for the loss of taste and the stapedial reflex (both related to the facial nerve).

C (acoustic neuroma pressing on the left facial and vestibulocochlear nerves) is incorrect. An acoustic neuroma (vestibular Schwannoma) could cause hearing loss (not increased sensitivity to sounds) and reduced control of facial muscles. These nerves can be damaged by a single small tumor because both nerves pass through the restricted space of the internal acoustic meatus.

D (hemorrhage into the left cavernous sinus damaging the oculomotor and trigeminal nerves) is incorrect. Damage to the oculomotor and trigeminal nerves would not affect taste or the stapedial reflex. Damage to the trigeminal nerve could compromise the corneal reflex because it carries sensation from the cornea (the facial carries the motor output to the eyelid muscles involved in the blink response). Damage to the oculomotor nerve would not interfere with closing the eye during eye blink, but would make raising the lid difficult. Eye position would be affected (eye "down and out") causing double vision (diplopia).

27. **D** (D) is correct. This is an example of "locked-in syndrome," in which the pontine base has been damaged, destroying all motor tracts to points caudal to this. Provided that the damage does not extend dorsally to include the medial lemniscus and spinothalamic tracts, all sensory modalities from the body remain intact. And provided that the damage does not extend dorsally and rostrally to involve the ascending reticular activating system, the lesion does not result in coma. Control of eye blink is variable, depending on whether the facial nerve and facial motor nucleus are involved. All control of vertical gaze, including the oculomotor nucleus and nerve and the vertical gaze center, resides within the midbrain and is spared. The blood supply to the pontine base is from penetrating branches of the basilar.

A (A) is incorrect. This is the middle cerebral artery (MCA). The portions of primary sensory and motor cortex representing the upper body are in the field of this artery, so occlusion could result in both sensory and motor loss, but only for the contralateral body. Lenticulostriate arteries supply the

internal capsule branch from the M1 segment of the MCA. Occlusion of these could result in a dense hemiplegia affecting only the contralateral body.

B (B) is incorrect. This is the anterior cerebral artery (ACA). The portions of primary sensory and motor cortex representing the lower body are in the field of this artery, so occlusion could result in both sensory and motor loss, but only for the contralateral body. On occasion, the A1 segment of one ACA is small caliber, and the remaining ACA may receive its primary blood supply from the contralateral ACA through the anterior communicating artery. In such cases, occlusion of the major A1 segment could eliminate blood supply to both ACAs distal to the occlusion, resulting in bilateral deficit. However, this deficit would be primarily to the lower body and would have both sensory and motor components.

C (C) is incorrect. This is the posterior cerebral artery (PCA). Proximally, branches of PCA supply much of ventral midbrain. Occlusion could damage the cerebral peduncle, resulting in a contralateral, not a bilateral, paralysis. Such damage would likely include the ipsilateral oculomotor nerve, resulting in paralysis of the ipsilateral eye, including "down and out" eye position, eyelid droop (ptosis) and pupil dilation (mydriasis) due to loss of parasympathetic fibers from the Edinger-Westphal nucleus.

28. **D** (L5 and S1) is correct. The L5 nerve root exits here and supplies the sensory innervation of the lateral calf and dorsal foot surface.

A (L2 and L3) is incorrect. The L2 nerve root supplies the dorsal aspect of the upper thigh and wraps around to include portions of the hip and lower back.

B (L3 and L4) is incorrect. The L3 nerve root supplies the dorsal and medial aspect of the leg around the knee.

C (L4 and L5) is incorrect. The L4 nerve root supplies the medial, not the lateral, aspect of the calf.

E (S1 and S2) is incorrect. The S1 nerve root supplies the plantar aspect of the foot, with a field that extends a short distant up the back of the leg. Damage to this root would disrupt the plantar reflex.

29. **B** (left internal capsule, posterior limb) is correct. The damage shown in the MRI is to the left cerebral peduncle of the midbrain. Wallerian degeneration is degeneration of the axon distal to the site of injury, which means that the injury is between this point and the motor neuron cell bodies. Corticospinal tract axons in the left cerebral peduncle originate in the left motor cortex and descend through the left internal capsule before passing through the left cerebral peduncle. They continue through the left pontine base and left medullary pyramid before crossing, descend in the right lateral spinal cord, and synapse on lower motor neurons cell bodies in the spinal cord. Damage to these axons at the level of the internal capsule, corona radiate, or motor cortex will cause the observed right leg weakness and the observed Wallerian degeneration of the distal axon as it passes through the cerebral peduncle.

A (right internal capsule, posterior limb), **C** (right cerebral peduncle), **E** (right pontine base), and **G** (right medullary pyramid) are all incorrect. Each of these would result in a left leg deficit, not a right leg deficit.

D (left cerebral peduncle), **F** (left pontine base), and **H** (left medullary pyramid) are incorrect. Although each of these could result in right leg weakness or paralysis, Wallerian degeneration implies degeneration of axons distal to the site of injury. Thus, the left cerebral peduncle is distal to the original injury site.

30. **C** (alcoholic cerebellar degeneration) is correct. The anterior lobe and vermis of the cerebellum are particularly vulnerable to damage from chronic alcohol abuse. Damage to this region of cerebellum causes severe gait ataxia while sparing the upper limbs.

A (Friedreich ataxia) is incorrect. This rare genetic disorder affects upper and lower limbs and causes both sensory and motor deficit. It is most commonly diagnosed in the second decade of life. Those with this form of ataxia are likely to become wheelchair bound by their 20s. Life expectancy is less than 40 years.

B (progressive supranuclear palsy) is incorrect. This idiopathic degenerative disorder is the most common of the Parkinson-plus syndromes. Patients commonly suffer from rigidity and severe postural instability.

D (Korsakoff psychosis) is incorrect. Although this does result from degeneration related to alcohol abuse, Korsakoff psychosis involves severe anterograde and retrograde memory loss, not gait disturbance. Amnestic confabulatory syndrome is a common finding accompanying this disorder.

E (tabes dorsalis) is incorrect. This degeneration of dorsal roots is seen in tertiary syphilis, occurring one to two decades after an initial (untreated) infection by *Treponema pallidum*. It produces instability due to sensory ataxia, not due to cerebellar damage. Romberg sign is a common early finding.

31. **C** (basilar artery) is correct. The MRI shows damage to the left pontine base. This infarction involved the corticospinal tracts before their decussation in the caudal medulla and is consistent with the right-sided weakness and a Babinski sign. The left abducens nerve also lies within the ischemic zone, accounting for the paralysis of the lateral rectus. In addition, communication from the left cerebral cortex to the right cerebellar hemisphere through pontine nuclei in the left pons is compromised, consistent with the intention tremor seen in the right arm.

A (anterior inferior cerebellar artery), **E** (posterior inferior cerebellar artery), and **F** (superior cerebellar artery) are incorrect. A Babinski sign indicates corticospinal tract damage. These axons do not run through the field of the AICA, PICA, or SCA. In addition, the MRI shows damage to the left pontine base. The artery that supplies this region is the basilar, which can be seen in the MRI on the anterior medial surface of the brainstem.

B (anterior spinal artery) and **D** (posterior cerebral artery) are incorrect. Although an infarct in either of these fields could result in the observed upper motor neuron signs (weakness, Babinski), the MRI shows damage to the left pontine base. In addition, the abducens involvement is consistent with a pontine infarction. The artery that supplies this region is the basilar, which can be seen in the MRI on the anterior medial surface of the brainstem.

32. **C** (disruption of the neuronal cytoskeleton) is correct. Vincristine disrupts microtubule assemblies and, in so doing, prevents spindle formation in dividing cancer cells, which is the presumed mechanism of action as an antineoplastic agent. The major dose-limiting side effect of vincristine is neurologic, commonly peripheral neuropathy. It is likely to produce these effects by disrupting axonal transport. Microtubules are a key component of the neuronal cytoskeleton necessary to fast anterograde and retrograde transport. They align along axons with their "+" ends directed away from the soma. Dynein translocates vesicles toward the "+" ends (fast anterograde), whereas kinesin moves vesicles toward the "−" end of these tubules.

A (compromise of the vascular supply to the extremities) is incorrect. The major effect of vincristine is to disrupt microtubule assemblies. A side effect of this action is to interfere with axonal transport.

B (demyelination of the long tracts within the spinal cord) is incorrect. Spinal cord damage involving motor pathways would constitute an upper motor neuron lesion and would present with increased, not decreased, reflexes. In addition, vincristine does not cross the blood–brain barrier and should not have access to the spinal long tracts.

D (disruption of slow anterograde transport) is incorrect. The major effect of vincristine is to disrupt microtubule assemblies. A side effect of this action is to interfere with axonal transport. However, it is fast anterograde and retrograde transport that rely on microtubules, not slow transport. In general, elements moved by slow transport are those too large to move through the microtubule-dynein assembly. Such elements would include the cytoskeletal elements required for repair and axon regrowth in the periphery, making the rate of slow transport the rate-limiting step in axon repair in the peripheral nervous system.

33. **B** (lacunar infarct in the posterior limb of the left internal capsule) is correct. Lacunar infarcts are frequently associated with chronic hypertensive vascular disease. The signs and symptoms can be precise (e.g., loss of sensation or weakness in the contralateral hand). Lacunar infarcts usually appear as slitlike hemorrhages because of the rupture of small penetrating arteries.

A (transient ischemic attack involving the left cerebral hemisphere) is incorrect. Transient ischemic attacks last less than 24 hours and commonly resolve within the first hour. Frequent causes include stenosis of carotid and vertebral arteries due to atherosclerosis. Transient blindness (e.g., patient reports a curtain is falling over their eyes) can be a symptom.

C (cerebral infarction following occlusion of the left middle cerebral artery) is incorrect. Occlusion of the middle cerebral typically results in a more encompassing set of signs and symptoms that may include weakness and loss of sensation in the contralateral face, hand, and arm; difficulties with speech (expressive and receptive aphasias); and Gerstmann syndrome (acalculia, agraphia, finger agnosia, right-left disorientation).

D (brainstem infarction following occlusion of the posterior inferior cerebellar artery) is incorrect. Occlusion of PICA results in lateral medullary (Wallenberg) syndrome that includes loss of pain and temperature sensation from the ipsilateral face and contralateral body, ipsilateral Horner syndrome, loss of gag reflex on the ipsilateral side, and dysarthria and dysphagia. Cerebellar involvement can result in vertigo, nausea, nystagmus, and limb ataxia.

34. **D** (shaken baby syndrome) is correct. SBS is best recognized by the combination of subdural hematoma and retinal hemorrhage. Infants are particularly susceptible to rupture of bridging veins leading to subdural hematoma. The smaller size of the brain relative to the skull means the subarachnoid space is large. In addition, because of limited development of muscles of the neck, coupled with a proportionally larger head relative to body size, shaking a young child causes greater head movement. Although retinal hemorrhage can be caused by delivery and by blunt trauma, when coupled with other injuries it is generally taken as a strong indication of shaking abuse. The extent of retinal hemorrhage correlates well with the extent of neurologic deficit.

A (fall from a high chair) is incorrect. Although it is possible that a fall could result in a subdural hematoma and retinal hemorrhage, such injuries, especially the retinal hemorrhage, are extremely rare under such circumstances. The combination of the subdural hematoma and the retinal hemorrhage, coupled with the history of previous injuries, very strongly suggests child abuse.

B (*Streptococcus pneumoniae* bacterial meningitis) is incorrect. *S. pneumoniae* is one of the most common causes of bacterial meningeal infection in this age group. However, meningitis most commonly presents with headache, fever, vomiting, and nuchal rigidity (stiff neck). The stiff neck may produce a Brudzinski or a Kernig sign. Seizures are possible, but evidence of a subdural hematoma tends to direct ones attention toward traumatic injury.

C (herpes simplex virus type 1 encephalitis) is incorrect. Viral encephalitis may produce seizure and petechial hemorrhages throughout the medial temporal and inferior frontal lobes. However, it would not cause a subdural hematoma; these are most commonly related to some type of trauma. Other signs that might accompany viral encephalitis would be those consistent with viral infection (e.g., fever, gastrointestinal and respiratory disturbance, general malaise and aching) followed by signs suggestive of CNS involvement (e.g., changes in level of consciousness, confusion, coma, changes in EEG pattern).

E (infantile spasms) is incorrect. Infantile spasms is a term that some use interchangeably with West syndrome. This syndrome consists of a triad of spasms, mental retardation, and a characteristic hypoarrhythmic interictal EEG pattern, two of which are required for diagnosis. West syndrome accounts for a quarter of the epilepsy syndromes seen in the first year of life. However, it would not account for the subdural hematoma or the retinal hemorrhage.

35. **D** (right trochlear) is correct. Trochlear nerve damage results in double vision, in particular when looking "down and in." A characteristic of this double vision is that the individual can align the eyes and reduce or eliminate the double vision by tilting the head toward the "good" eye, thus overcoming the loss of ability to rotate the eye down and in.

A (left oculomotor) and **B** (right oculomotor) are incorrect. Significant damage to an oculomotor nerve results in deviation of the affected eye "down and out," with significant eyelid droop and pupil dilation.

C (left trochlear) is incorrect. Double vision due to damage to this nerve could be overcome by tilting the head to the right.

E (left abducens) and **F** (right abducens) are incorrect. The abducens nerves are long and the most frequently damaged cranial nerves. Damage to an abducens results in double vision on attempted lateral gaze.

36. **B** (ability to name verbally an object placed in the left hand) is correct. Tactile representation from the left hand is first presented to the right somatosensory cortex. Identification of an object by tactile manipulation (stereognosis) requires additional involvement of the right somatosensory association cortex, all of which can occur without hemispheric transfer. However, in order to verbally name an identified object, information must be passed from the right to the left hemisphere, and this is prevented by complete callosotomy.

A (ability to name verbally an object placed in the right hand) is incorrect. Tactile representation from the right hand is presented to the left primary and then association somatosensory cortices. Once identified, information is presented to language-related areas in the left hemisphere in order to verbally name the identified object. Because all this processing occurs in the left hemisphere, it is unaffected by complete callosotomy.

C (ability to name verbally an object viewed with the right eye) and **D** (ability to name verbally an object viewed with the left eye) are incorrect. Information presented to the right visual field of either eye will be processed in the left visual cortex. From there, this information can be passed forward to association cortex and eventually to language-related areas of the left hemisphere. However, an object viewed only in the left visual field, which will be processed in right visual cortex, cannot be named verbally.

37. **D** (systemic infection) is correct. An acutely fluctuating level of consciousness is a delirium. Infection presents very differently in elderly and younger patients. Delirium and falls are two of the most common manifestations of infection in the elderly. In contrast, fever may be reduced or absent. Some brain atrophy, as revealed by CT, is considered normal in very elderly people.

A (Alzheimer disease) is incorrect. The rapid onset is not consistent with AD, which is a progressive degenerative disorder in which an individual may show difficulties with memory and with learning new tasks months or years before requiring assistance with activities of daily living.

B (Huntington disease) is incorrect. The rapid onset is not consistent with HD, which is a progressive degenerative disorder. Early signs of Huntington disease include changes in personality, irritability, and depression. Motor signs, especially choreoathetotic movements, become apparent as the disease progresses. MRI will eventually reveal atrophy of the putamen and caudate nuclei, with concomitant enlargement of the lateral ventricles, rather than generalized atrophy of the cerebral cortex.

C (multi-infarct dementia) is incorrect. A rapid onset of symptoms is consistent with MID. However, in MID, there is a step-wise progression and, frequently, focal sensory or motor deficit. In addition, the fluctuating level of consciousness and responsiveness described are more consistent with delirium than dementia. Only those signs remaining after the delirium has been resolved can be considered in a diagnosis of a vascular dementia.

38. **B** (subdural hemorrhage) is correct. This case describes a likely chronic subdural hemorrhage. Subdural hematomas occur as a result of tearing of bridging veins that span the distance between the brain and the venous sinuses. Any rapid acceleration–deceleration event may cause the brain to move relative to the skull, tearing these veins. In elderly or alcoholic patients, brain atrophy increases the distance that bridging veins must extend. A very minor event that goes unnoticed may be sufficient to tear some of these veins. It may take several weeks for signs and symptoms to develop.

A (epidural hemorrhage) is incorrect. Epidural hematomas are rapidly developing events. They are most commonly associated with tearing of the middle meningeal artery due to impact to, and fracture of, the temporal skull.

C (subarachnoid hemorrhage) is incorrect. Subarachnoid hemorrhage most commonly results from rupture of an aneurysm on the vertebral-basilar arteries or arterial circle (of Willis). It presents with sudden, excruciating headache ("the worst headache of my life"). SAH is more common in adults younger than 60 years of age.

D (early signs of Alzheimer disease) is incorrect. Obtundation that develops over hours to days is not consistent with early AD. AD presents first with difficulties with memory and with learning new tasks. It is not associated with focal signs such as unilateral weakness.

E (Wernicke-Korsakoff syndrome) is incorrect. WKS is associated with chronic alcohol abuse. Motor signs reflect cerebellar damage and include gait ataxia. Other signs include anterograde and retrograde memory loss, but not rapidly developing obtundation.

39. **E** (warfarin) is correct. The causes of Dandy-Walker malformations are unknown. Some likely have a genetic component. Others are sporadic. Risk factors for sporadic DW include exposure to the anticoagulant, warfarin, and retinoic acid.

A (alcohol) is incorrect. Consumption of alcohol during pregnancy can result in fetal alcohol syndrome. FAS is diagnosed on the basis of slowed prenatal or postnatal growth, facial malformations (e.g., small palpebral fissures, flattened or shorted nose), and CNS dysfunction, which may include mental retardation, microcephaly, and behavioral problems such as attention deficit hyperactivity disorder.

B (folic acid) is incorrect. Lack of folic acid availability in the maternal diet during pregnancy is believed to be a major risk factor for birth defects, but not Dandy-Walker syndrome.

C (lead) is incorrect. Lead exposure during pregnancy can lead to spontaneous abortion and, in term infants, to neurologic impairment including subnormal cognitive and memory function. It is also correlated with minor congenital malformations and low birth weight, but not with Dandy-Walker syndrome.

D (mercury) is incorrect. Like lead exposure, mercury exposure during pregnancy can result in spontaneous abortion or physical and mental retardation in the infant.

40. **B** (meningeal artery) is correct. The meningeal arteries are embedded in the dura and are most likely to rupture as a result of a skull fracture. Blood forces its way between the dura and the skull, creating a lens-shaped epidural hematoma that is bounded by the skull and the dura. The individual experienced a lucid interval (the period of consciousness between the initial and the second period of loss of consciousness). It is estimated that less than one third of epidural hematomas are accompanied by a lucid interval; subdural hematomas may have a similar presentation.

A (cerebral artery) is incorrect. Cerebral arteries on the surface of the brain bleed into the subarachnoid space (commonly due to rupture of aneurysm) or into the parenchyma of the brain.

C (venous sinus) is incorrect. Severe head trauma can cause a venous sinus to rupture resulting in an epidural hematoma. Venous sinus rupture is more common in posterior regions (parieto-occipital and posterior fossa). However, rupture of the superior sagittal sinus would be expected to extend to the midline, and venous ruptures are less common than arterial bleeds in causing the classic lens-shaped epidural hematoma.

D (bridging veins) is incorrect. Tearing of bridging veins is generally due to severe head trauma that causes rapid acceleration–deceleration. The result is a subdural hematoma with a generally crescent shape because it is bounded medially by the arachnoid membrane rather than the dura.

E (arteriovenous malformation) is incorrect. AVMs are a tangle of abnormal vessels where arteries connect directly to veins without intervening capillaries. They do not generally bleed as a result of a blow to the head. When one does bleed, it can be expected to bleed into the subarachnoid space or into the parenchyma of the brain, depending on the location of the AVM. About 90% of AVMs are found in cerebral hemispheres and are not associated with surface bleeds.

41. **C** (lissencephaly) is correct. Lissencephaly, meaning "smooth brain," refers to a defect in neuronal migration that yields an agyric cerebral cortex in which the normal six neocortical layers have been reduced to four, as seen in this coronal section.

A (Dandy-Walker syndrome) is incorrect. Dandy-Walker malformations are primarily recognized by an enlarged fourth ventricle with a partial or fully absent cerebellar vermis and a vermal region that is anteriorly rotated. The tentorium is deflected upward, reflecting the enlarged posterior fossa.

B (holoprosencephaly) is incorrect. During the fifth and sixth weeks of development, following closure of the neural tube, the prosencephalon divides into two hemispheres. A midline developmental defect at this time causes abnormal separation of the neural tube without development of two hemispheres, called *holoprosencephaly.*

D (megalencephaly) is incorrect. This is a defect resulting in abnormally large gray- and white-matter regions (the word means "large brain"). It has many causes, some genetic, some metabolic, and some unknown. The abnormally large brain causes an abnormally large head. Although some individuals have few neurologic signs, many will have delayed development, motor control problems, and seizures, depending on the cause of the defect. Hemimegalencephaly is generally associated with intractable seizures and has a poor prognosis.

E (polymicrogyria) is incorrect. This neuronal migration defect probably occurs in the second trimester and results in numerous small gyri and abnormalities in cortical layer 1 in some areas, with normal six-layer cortex in adjacent regions.

42. **C** (infarct involving the anterior spinal artery at the level of the cervical spinal cord) is correct. Cocaine use is associated with increased risk for stroke. In this case, the rapidly developing flaccid paralysis of all four extremities could be explained by infarct involving the pyramids or the cervical spinal cord. However, loss of pain sensation in the presence of proprioceptive sense is more consistent with a spinal cord lesion that has spared the posterior columns. The paralysis will evolve and reflexes will become hyperactive over time.

A (epidural hematoma) is incorrect. An epidural hematoma might result from the fall. It could compromise sensory and motor function of the ipsilateral cortex, affecting the contralateral body. With sufficient expansion, it could cause a midline shift with compression of the contralateral cerebral peduncle against the tentorial notch, causing ipsilateral paralysis. However, these findings would be expected to involve the face and body, they would not spare proprioception, and the patient would not continue to be alert and responsive.

B (infarct involving the anterior spinal artery at the level of the medulla) is incorrect. Such an infarct might involve the medullary pyramids bilaterally, producing the observed paralysis. It would also involve the medial lemniscus, resulting in loss of proprioception, while sparing the spinothalamic tract and pain sensation.

D (infarct involving a posterior spinal artery at the level of the cervical spinal cord) is incorrect. This would predominantly cause loss of vibration and proprioceptive sense.

E (acute inflammatory demyelinating polyneuropathy) is incorrect. AIDP, or Guillain-Barré syndrome, develops over days, not minutes to hours. Sensory abnormalities are common and may include paresthesias and numbness. But, because this is a demyelinating disorder, it should affect proprioception at least as much as pain sensation.

43. **D** (multiple sclerosis) is correct. MS is an inflammatory disease affecting CNS myelin and axons. Diagnosis requires evidence of lesions disseminated in space and time. The numbness, INO, and upper motor neuron lesion signs can all be caused by MS. Elevated CSF MBP is common in MS. Demonstration of multiple lesions on MRI is important to diagnosis.

A (amyotrophic lateral sclerosis) is incorrect. Sporadic ALS, the most common acquired motor neuron disease, causes degeneration of both upper and lower motor neurons. Degeneration of motor neuron cell bodies leads to loss of corticospinal tracts and anterior spinal roots. Signs include hyperreflexia, spasticity, and Babinski sign (upper motor neuron) and fasciculations, weakness, and muscle atrophy (lower motor neuron signs).

B (poliomyelitis) is incorrect. Polio causes degeneration of motor neurons in the anterior horn of the spinal cord and in the brainstem. Most individuals (90%–95%) exposed to this enterovirus remain asymptomatic. A small percentage (~1%) can develop either nonparalytic or paralytic poliomyelitis. With nonparalytic poliomyelitis, the individual may have recurring episodes of headache, fever, and vomiting. There can be pain in neck, trunk, arm, and leg muscles and stiffness in the neck. With paralytic poliomyelitis, muscles weakness is followed by flaccid paralysis and muscle atrophy. The individual has difficulty swallowing and breathing. Because this is a lower motor neuron disorder, reflexes are reduced instead of exaggerated.

C (myasthenia gravis) is incorrect. MG is an autoimmune disorder affecting nicotinic acetylcholine receptors at the neuromuscular junction. It presents with weakness that increases with repeated activity, ptosis, and dysarthria. Respiratory muscles can be affected. There will be no muscle atrophy or upper motor neuron findings. The acetylcholinesterase inhibitor, edrophonium, rapidly reverses weakness of MG (edrophonium test).

E (tabes dorsalis) is incorrect. Tabes dorsalis results from spirochete damage to the dorsal (sensory) roots. Individuals will typically experience impaired joint position sense, ataxia, and reduced or absent deep tendon reflexes. They lose their balance when their eyes are closed but are able to compensate the loss of balance if the eyes are open (Romberg sign). Pain sensation is reduced or lost, which can result in Charcot joints. So called "lightning pains" are characteristic of the disorder.

44. **C** (normal aging) is correct. The brain undergoes changes in gross appearance as well as cellular and molecular composition during the aging process. There is a progressive loss of neurons from the seventh decade on, with significant loss of small neurons of layers II and IV in the frontal and superior temporal regions. Neurofibrillary tangles, senile plaques, and calcified arachnoid granulations can all be seen in normal aged brain. Neurologic findings can include a decrease in the rate and strength of motor activity as well as a slowed reaction time. Vibration sensation diminishes. There appears to be a decline in cognitive function and memory, although not all elderly individuals exhibit such changes. However, many aspects of mental decline once viewed as part of normal aging are now believed to reflect underlying pathologies.

A (Huntington disease) is incorrect. HD results from a genetic defect in the short arm of chromosome 4. The pathology is characterized by a severely atrophied neostriatum with loss of both projecting neurons and local interneurons. Typically, the frontal cortex shows a reduction is size and volume. Symptoms begin to appear between the ages of 30 and 50 years. Initially there is disinterest and apathy, followed by a movement disorder that often begins with fidgeting. As the disease progresses, the abnormal movements increase in frequency, affecting speech, swallowing, and walking.

B (Korsakoff syndrome) is incorrect. Korsakoff syndrome (amnestic confabulatory syndrome) results from degeneration in a number of regions, including the thalamus and mammillary bodies. It is commonly seen in chronic alcoholism. Signs and symptoms include a loss of recent memory (retrograde amnesia) with a tendency to confusion and fabrication, a loss of spontaneity and initiative, and difficulty establishing new memories (anterograde amnesia). It is frequently part of a combined Wernicke-Korsakoff syndrome, which includes cerebellar ataxia related to degeneration of the anterior vermis of the cerebellum.

D (Parkinson disease) is incorrect. PD is a neurodegenerative disease that is characterized by the loss (usually >70%) of dopaminergic neurons in the substantia nigra (pars compact). Diagnosis depends on the presence of three of the following: rigidity, bradykinesia, postural instability, and tremor at rest. PD can have an insidious onset with a slight tremor or stiffness in the hand that is followed by more pronounced symptoms, like a slowing of movement. The characteristic "pill-rolling" tremor is at rest and continual.

E (Pick lobar atrophy) is incorrect. This is a rare, progressive dementia characterized by personality changes and language disorders. Postural reflexes and reaction time are not affected. The brain shows atrophy of the frontal and temporal lobes. Microscopic examination reveals a loss of neurons, with many remaining neurons containing Pick bodies (cytoplasmic, round, filamentous inclusions that are only weakly basophilic).

45. **C** (obstruction of the cerebral aqueduct) is correct. Cerebrospinal fluid produced by choroid plexus on the floor of the lateral ventricles and roof of the third ventricle circulates through the paired lateral ventricles and third ventricle before exiting through the cerebral aqueduct to the fourth ventricle. Occlusion of the cerebral aqueduct prevents CSF from exiting the third ventricle. In general, the ventricle immediately upstream enlarges first.

A (choroid plexus papilloma) is incorrect. A choroid plexus papilloma, which produces excess cerebrospinal fluid, could result in fluid buildup and expansion of all ventricles (lateral, third, and fourth). However, it should be noted that a papilloma may grow to a size sufficient to obstruct CSF flow, in which case the resulting hydrocephalus would be primarily upstream of the obstruction.

B (atresia of the arachnoid granulations) is incorrect. Atresia, or absence, of arachnoid granulations would result in fluid buildup and expansion of all ventricles (lateral, third, and fourth).

D (obstruction of the interventricular foramen) is incorrect. Occlusion of an interventricular foramen prevents CSF produced from the choroid plexus on the floor of the lateral ventricle from flowing into the third ventricle. This results in dilation of the affected lateral ventricle.

E (atresia of the median and lateral apertures) is incorrect. Failure of opening of the median and lateral apertures (foramina of Magendie and Luschka) would block the flow of CSF from the fourth ventricle to the subarachnoid space. This results in a hydrocephalus with expansion of the fourth ventricle and is believed to be one factor related to Dandy-Walker malformation.

46. **A** (anandamide) is correct. Marijuana affects the nervous system through several cannabinoid receptor subtypes. These are found in numerous areas of the CNS and PNS. Some of these receptors have been demonstrated to reduce neurotransmission within pain transmission pathways.

B (capsaicin) is incorrect. Capsaicin is an exogenous substance found in hot chili peppers. It binds to the vanilloid receptor. The ability of capsaicin to relieve pain derives from several of its actions. Capsaicin exposure can induce receptor desensitization, block voltage-gated calcium channels, and decrease substance P, a peptide transmitter important in pain transmission in the spinal cord.

C (enkephalin) is incorrect. Enkephalinergic interneurons in the spinal cord dorsal horn inhibit transmission between primary nociceptive afferents and pain transmission neurons. These interneurons can be activated from brainstem centers as part of an intrinsic analgesia system. It is likely that cannabinoid receptor activation is a component of this intrinsic analgesia system, but enkephalin is a transmitter of the opioid, not the cannabinoid, system.

D (fatty acid amide hydroxylase) is incorrect. FAAH is the endogenous enzyme that is responsible for degradation of the endogenous cannabinoid receptor ligand, anandamide.

47. **B** (a 3-Hz spike-and-wave pattern in both cerebral hemispheres on EEG recording during a seizure) is correct. Absence seizures are associated with 3-Hz spike-and-slow-wave complexes. Absence seizures in children are typically brief (lasting 3 to 10 seconds) and can be repeated hundreds of times per day. This is in contrast to other seizure types that can last for minutes and may occur a couple of times a day. Absence seizures are frequently idiopathic, but also occur in symptomatic epilepsies.

A (muscle twitches that begin in one hand, ascend through the arm, and eventually involve one side of her body) is incorrect. This describes a simple partial motor seizure known as a *jacksonian march*. The seizure results from abnormal electrical activity that begins within the motor cortex and spreads along the motor strip. These so-called jacksonian epilepsies or epileptic marches cannot be stopped once started. Like all simple partial seizures, they do not affect state of consciousness.

C (muscle atonia causing her to fall and injure herself) is incorrect. By definition, the individual experiencing an absence seizure simply stops moving for a few seconds and then resumes normal activities without realizing that they have experienced a seizure. The seizure is brief enough that the individual does not fall. A seizure that produces muscle atonia, causing the individual to fall, is known as a "drop attack" and has a much poorer prognosis than an absence seizure.

D (confusion and disorientation for up to half an hour following each seizure) is incorrect. Recovery from an absence seizure is immediate. In contrast, complex partial seizures, which cause disruptions in consciousness during the seizure event, may be followed by an extended postdromal phase. Careful examination and EEG may be necessary to distinguish some types of complex partial seizure from absence. However, the distinction is important because treatments for the two seizure types differ. Tonic–clonic seizures similarly cause confusion in the postictal period, but are unlikely to be mistaken for absence seizures.

48. **B** (muscles of facial expression are weak or paralyzed) is correct. The muscles of facial expression are innervated by CN VII, the facial nerve. This is a peripheral nerve and is subject to PNS demyelinating disorders. Although chronic inflammatory demyelinating polyradiculoneuropathy and the more common closely related disorder, acute inflammatory demyelinating polyradiculoneuropathy (a Guillain-Barré variant), normally begin in the legs and ascend, cranial nerve involvement can be seen in both.

A (sympathetic postganglionic fibers controlling heart rate and contractility are impaired) is incorrect. Postganglionic autonomic fibers are unmyelinated.

C (dull, burning pain sensation is lost, followed by a return of spontaneous, excruciating pain) is incorrect. Dull burning pain is carried primarily by unmyelinated C fibers. Loss of pain sensation followed by return of spontaneous pain is a feature of thalamic pain syndrome, which results from localized thalamic infarct.

D (vision is blurred) is incorrect. Blurred vision accompanies optic neuritis and may be an indication of an ongoing demyelination process such as multiple sclerosis. However, the optic nerve consists of CNS axons, not PNS axons. It is demyelinated by central, not peripheral, demyelinating disorder.

49. **A** (genu of left internal capsule) is correct. Weakness affecting the lower face but sparing the upper face is a sign of an upper motor neuron lesion. Corticobulbar axons destined for the portion of the right facial motor nucleus that innervates the right lower face travel through the genu of the left internal capsule.

B (genu of right internal capsule) is incorrect. Weakness affecting the lower face but sparing the upper face is a sign of an upper motor neuron lesion. However, the right lower face, like the right body, is controlled by upper motor neurons that originate from the left motor cortex. Their axons course through the left, not the right, internal capsule.

C (posterior limb of left internal capsule) and **D** (posterior limb of right internal capsule) are incorrect. The face and head region are represented in the genu of the internal capsule. The arm and leg are represented in the posterior limb.

E (left facial nerve at the internal acoustic meatus) and **G** (left facial nerve at the stylomastoid foramen) are incorrect. The left facial nerve innervates muscle of facial expression in the left face.

F (right facial nerve at the internal acoustic meatus) is incorrect. The right facial nerve innervates muscle of facial expression in the right face. However, damage at the acoustic meatus will affect the complete facial nerve. Because the right facial nerve innervates the right portion of frontalis, the right forehead will not wrinkle. The right facial nerve also innervates the right orbicularis oculi, so the right eye will not close fully. The right facial nerve carries taste sensation from the front of the right side of the tongue, so taste sensation, if carefully tested, will be abnormal. Furthermore, CN VIII, the vestibulocochlear, also travels through the internal acoustic meatus. Thus, vertigo, tinnitus, and loss of hearing are likely to be found.

H (right facial nerve near the stylomastoid foramen) is incorrect. The right facial nerve innervates muscle of facial expression in the right face. Damage at the stylomastoid foramen will spare the portion of the facial nerve that carries taste sensation and will not affect CN VIII. However, it will affect the complete facial nerve. Thus, right frontalis and right orbicularis oculi will be weak or paralyzed, as discussed in F.

50. **C** (enlarged fourth ventricle and absent cerebellar vermis) is correct. Dandy-Walker malformations are a group of malformations reflecting disruptions in the development of the brainstem and cerebellum, probably related to the migration of the rhombic lip. The term is generally applied to malformations showing a triad of changes: (1) partial or complete agenesis of the cerebellar vermis, with anterior rotation; (2) dilation of the fourth ventricle; and (3) enlarged posterior fossa with superior displacement of the tentorium. Most cases are diagnosed within the first year, but less severe cases may not be recognized until childhood or, occasionally, adulthood.

A (smooth, agyric cerebral cortex) is incorrect. The term for such a malformation is a lissencephaly (meaning "smooth brain" from the Greek, *lissos,* meaning smooth, and *encephalos,* meaning brain). Most infants born with this malformation will have extremely limited development, will be unable to sit or feed themselves, and will not live to adulthood.

B (syringomyelia, with the syrinx extending from C5 rostrally into the brainstem) is incorrect. Syringomyelia is a cystic cavitation of the central canal of the spinal cord. It is particularly associated with Chiari type I malformations, in which the cerebellar tonsils are displaced downward and overlie the cervical spinal cord. Primary findings with cervical syringomyelia include loss of pain and temperature sensation in a capelike distribution.

D (protrusion of the meningeal layers and underlying neural tissue in the lumbosacral region) is incorrect. This is referred to as a myelomeningocele. It represents a disruption to neural tube closure and is the most severe form of spina bifida. Minimally, such a developmental abnormality may affect control of the lower limbs and bladder.

E (displacement of the cerebellar tonsils through the foramen magnum, extending over the cervical spinal cord) is incorrect. This is a Chiari type I malformation. Signs and symptoms range widely, but frequently do not appear until the second decade of life or later. They may include neck pain and torticollis, brainstem and cerebellar findings, and findings that would be associated with a syringomyelia, which is frequently associated with a Chiari type I malformation (see answer B discussion).

Index

Note: Page numbers followed by f indicate figures; those followed by t indicate tables.